Biology and Pathology of Trophoblast

This is the first dedicated, in-depth account of trophoblast: the tissue derived from the fertilised egg that nourishes and protects the developing fetus. The cells of the trophoblast have many unique qualities, and exhibit great variability across different species. It has a fascinating role in the development of the placenta and as a regulator during early growth of the embryo. These aspects are all fully covered as well as studies on why it is not rejected by the mother as 'foreign' tissue. Disorders of trophoblast during development also manifest themselves in several clinical conditions during pregnancy, including gestational trophoblastic disease and pre-eclampsia. From stem cells through to epigenetics, implantation and X-chromosome inactivation, there is still a lot to be learned about trophoblast: this volume provides an up-to-date summary of the state of current knowledge and offers some glimpses as to future development on the scientific and clinical front.

Biology and Pathology of
Trophoblast

Edited by

Ashley Moffett

Charlie Loke

Anne McLaren

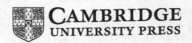

CAMBRIDGE
UNIVERSITY PRESS

CAMBRIDGE UNIVERSITY PRESS
Cambridge, New York, Melbourne, Madrid, Cape Town,
Singapore, São Paulo, Delhi, Tokyo, Mexico City

Cambridge University Press
The Edinburgh Building, Cambridge CB2 8RU, UK

Published in the United States of America by Cambridge University Press, New York

www.cambridge.org
Information on this title: www.cambridge.org/9781107403154

First published 2006
First paperback edition 2011

A catalogue record for this publication is available from the British Library

ISBN 978-0-521-85165-7 Hardback
ISBN 978-1-107-40315-4 Paperback

Additional resources for this publication at www.cambridge.org/9781107403154

Contents

Contributors

Neil Brockdorff
MRC Clinical Sciences Centre, ICSM,
Hammersmith Hospital, DuCane Road,
London W12 0NN, UK

Graham Burton
University of Cambridge, Department of
Anatomy, Downing Street, Cambridge CB2
3DY, UK

James Cross
University of Calgary, Department of
Biochemistry and Molecular Biology, Faculty
of Medicine, HSC Room 2279, 3330 Hospital
Drive NW, Calgary, Alberta T2N 4N1,
Canada

S. K. Dey
Division of Reproductive and Developmental
Biology, Vanderbilt University Medical
Center, Nashville, TN 37232-2678, USA

S. E. Erhardt
LBNL, 1 Cyclotron Road, MS 84-171,
Berkeley CA 94720, USA

Rosemary Fisher
Imperial College London, Faculty of
Medicine, Department of Cancer Medicine,
Charing Cross Hospital, Fulham Palace Road,
London W6 8RF, UK

Susan Fisher
UCSF, Biomedical Sciences Program, Box
0512, San Francisco, CA 94143-0512, USA

Russell Foulk
The Nevada Center for Reproductive
Medicine, 6630 S. McCarran Blvd, Reno, NV
89509, USA

Olga Genbacev
Department of Cell and Tissue Biology,
University of California San Francisco, 513
Parnassus Avenue, San Francisco, CA
94143-0512, USA

Petra Hajkova
Wellcome Trust/Cancer Research UK, Gurdon
Institute of Cancer and Developmental
Biology, Tennis Court Road, Cambridge CB2
1QR, UK

Eric Jauniaux
Academic Department of Obstetrics and
Gynaecology, Royal Free and University
College London, UK

Barry Keverne
University of Cambridge, Department of
Zoology, Downing Street, Cambridge CB2
3EJ, UK

Tilo Kunath
Institute for Stem Cell Research, University
of Edinburgh, Roger Land Building, King's
Buildings, West Mains Road, Edinburgh
EH9 3JQ, UK

E. A. Linton
Department of Obstetrics & Gynaecology,
Nuffield Department, John Radcliffe Hospital,
Oxford, OX3 9DU, UK

Y. W. Loke
Kings College, University of Cambridge,
Cambridge CB2 1ST, UK

Anne McLaren
(*Chair*) Wellcome Trust Cancer Research UK
Gurdon Institute of Cancer and
Developmental Biology, Tennis Court Road,
Cambridge CB2 1QR, UK

Ashley Moffett
Research Group in Human Reproductive
Immunobiology, Department of Pathology,
University of Cambridge, Tennis Court Road,
Cambridge CB2 1QP, UK

Akraporn Prakobphol
Department of Cell and Tissue Biology,
University of California San Francisco,
513 Parnassus Avenue, San Francisco,
CA 94143-0512

Chris Redman
Department of Obstetrics & Gynaecology,
Nuffield Department, John Radcliffe
Hospital, Oxford, OX3 9DU, UK

I. L. Sargent
Department of Obstetrics & Gynaecology,
Nuffield Department, John Radcliffe Hospital,
Oxford, OX3 9DU, UK

N. J. Sebire
Department of Histopathology,
Charing Cross Hospital, Fulham Palace Road,
London W6 8RF, UK

Azim Surani
Wellcome Trust/Cancer Research UK Gurdon
Institute of Cancer and Developmental
Biology, Tennis Court Road, Cambridge
CB2 1QR, UK

Susanne Tranguch
Division of Reproductive and Developmental
Biology, Vanderbilt University Medical
Center, Nashville, TN 37232-2678,
USA

Participants

Peter Braude
10th floor, North Wing, St Thomas' Hospital, Lambeth Palace Road, London SE1 7EH, UK

Neil Brockdorff
MRC Clinical Sciences Centre, ICSM, Hammersmith Hospital, DuCane Road, London W12 0NN, UK

Graham Burton
University of Cambridge, Department of Anatomy, Downing Street, Cambridge CB2 3DY, UK

James Cross
University of Calgary, Department of Biochemistry and Molecular Biology, Faculty of Medicine, HSC Room 2279, 3330 Hospital Drive NW, Calgary, Alberta T2N 4N1, Canada

S. K. Dey
Division of Reproductive and Developmental Biology, Vanderbilt University Medical Center, Nashville, TN 37232-2678, USA

Danielle Evain-Brion
Inserm U427, Faculty des Sciences Pharmaceutiques et Biologiques, Universite Rene-Descartes, Paris V, 4 Avenue de l'Observatoire, 75006 Paris, France

Anne Ferguson-Smith
University of Cambridge, Department of Anatomy, Downing Street, Cambridge CB2 3DY, UK

Rosemary Fisher
Imperial College London, Faculty of Medicine, Department of Cancer Medicine, Charing Cross Hospital, Fulham Palace Road, London W6 8RF, UK

Susan Fisher
UCSF, Biomedical Sciences Program, Box 0512, San Francisco, CA 94143-0512, USA

Abby Fowden
University of Cambridge, Downing Street, Cambridge, CB2 3EG, UK

Petra Hajkova
Wellcome Trust/Cancer Research UK Gurdon Institute of Cancer and Developmental Biology, Tennis Court Road, Cambridge CB2 1QR, UK

Myriam Hemberger
The Babraham Institute, Babraham Hall, Babraham, Cambridge CB2 4AT, UK

P. Jacobs
Department of Human Genetics, Salisbury District Hospital, Salisbury, Wilts SP2 8BJ, UK

Barry Keverne
University of Cambridge, Department of
Zoology, Downing Street, Cambridge CB2
3EJ, UK

Tilo Kunath
Institute for Stem Cell Research, University of
Edinburgh, Roger Land Building, King's
Buildings, West Mains Road, Edinburgh EH9
3JQ, UK

Andrew Lever
Level 5, Addenbrooke's Hospital, Hills Road,
Cambridge, CB2 2QQ, UK

Y. W. Loke
Kings College, University of Cambridge,
Cambridge CB2 1ST, UK

Anne McLaren
(*Chair*) Wellcome Trust Cancer Research
UK Gurdon Institute of Cancer and
Developmental Biology, Tennis Court
Road, Cambridge CB2 1QR, UK

Ashley Moffett
Research Group in Human Reproductive
Immunobiology, Department of Pathology,
University of Cambridge, Tennis Court Road,
Cambridge CB2 1QP, UK

Robert Pijnenborg
Universitaire Ziekenhuizen Leuven,
Obstetrics-Gynaecology, UZ Gasthuisberg,
Herestraat 49, B3000 Leuven, Belgium

Chris Redman
Department of Obstetrics & Gynaecology,
Nuffield Department, John Radcliffe Hospital,
Oxford OX3 9DU, UK

Wolf Reik
The Babraham Institute, Babraham,
Cambridge CB2 4AT, UK

Marilyn Renfree
Department of Zoology, University of
Melbourne, Victoria, Australia

Andrew Sharkey
Department of Pathology, University of
Cambridge, Tennis Court Road, Cambridge
CB2 1QP, UK

Colin Sibley
The Medical School, University of Manchester,
St Mary's Hospital, Manchester M13 0JH,
UK

Azim Surani
Wellcome Trust/Cancer Research UK Gurdon
Institute of Cancer and Developmental
Biology, Tennis Court Road, Cambridge CB2
1QR, UK

John Trowsdale
Department of Pathology, University of
Cambridge, Tennis Court Road, Cambridge
CB2 1QP, UK

Preface

Y. W. (Charlie) Loke

A major step in the evolution of eutherian mammals was the formation of the trophoblast, a specialised layer of cells derived early in embryogenesis. From this separate compartment, trophoblast is able to organise its own programme of development within a well-defined time span that is independent of the embryo, thereby enabling it to fulfil unique functions during ontogeny. While trophoblast contributes to the formation of the placenta in all eutherians, the manner by which it does so varies significantly among species (Carter 2001). It is important to recognise the pattern and extent of these variations if dialogue between investigators using human and those using animal material is to be meaningful. The trophoblast cell itself occurs in different forms ranging from uninuclear to multinuclear varieties, the latter appearing either as large giant cells or as a syncytium. Some of the giant cells are polytenic whilst others are polyploid but it is not known why these occur in different locations and time points of gestation in different species.

Trophoblast cells have remarkable growth and invasive properties in vivo, so much so that they resemble neoplastic cells, yet the in vitro culture and propagation of human trophoblast cells have still not met with much success. The recent realisation that some 'trophoblast' cell lines presently available are not what they seem to be has raised questions about how these cells should be characterised (King et al. 2000). Murine trophoblast stem cells have been identified, but in humans they have been elusive and the search continues.

Targeted mutation studies in mice have identified many genes involved in trophoblast development, some of which are specific to trophoblast, such as *Mash2*, a member of the basic helix-loop-helix gene family, while others also have roles in other cell lineages. It is becoming increasingly clear that different phases of trophoblast development are controlled by different regulatory genes (Rossant & Cross 2001). Interestingly, *Mash2* and the human equivalent *HASH2* show imprinting. Indeed, a significant number of imprinted genes so far identified are expressed in trophoblast (John & Surani 2000). The pattern of imprinting in trophoblast can differ from that in somatic tissues. An example of this is the selective inactivation of the paternal X chromosome in trophoblast, while this process is random in somatic tissues. In marsupials, the paternal X chromosome is inactivated in all tissues so it appears that, with the evolution of eutherians, this selective process is retained only in extraembryonic tissues. Transcription and translation of endogenous retroviral genes have also been frequently observed in trophoblast (Taruscio & Mantovani 1998). What role these extraneous gene sequences might play in trophoblast development is not clear but the ability of one such retroviral protein (syncytin) to cause cell fusion and syncytialisation raises the intriguing possibility that they could contribute to trophoblast differentiation.

The term 'trophoblast' (Greek for nutrition) was introduced by Hubrecht (1889), who viewed it as a layer that serves to nourish the embryo. While this histiotrophic role is indeed important, there are many others, still poorly understood, that are equally critical for development. In spite of its physical separation early in ontogeny, trophoblast remains an important source of signalling molecules involved in embryonic patterning. Trophoblast also has influence on the mother. Its products regulate both the prenatal behaviour of the female (increased feeding, inhibition of sexual behaviour) and the production of milk by the mammary glands; it also primes the female's brain to ensure a prompt onset of maternal behaviour and milk let-down postnatally (Keverne 2001). Hence, its position at the interface between the fetus and its mother makes trophoblast a vital link in the pathway for maternal communication, with influence directed simultaneously at two genetically distinct individuals. The placenta separates the fetus and mother, so trophoblast must also hold the key to the immunological paradox of pregnancy, an enigma which has remained unexplained ever since the elucidation half a century ago, that transplant rejection is caused by genetic differences of polymorphic major histocompatability complex (MHC) molecules between graft and recipient. In humans, trophoblast expresses a unique combination of MHC molecules and receptors for these paternally derived MHC molecules are expressed by a distinctive population of uterine leukocytes (natural killer cells) (Loke & King 2001). This provides a molecular mechanism for maternal recognition of the allogeneic trophoblast. In addition, the physiological transport of important molecules, such as antibodies, from mother to fetus is a selective receptor-mediated process by trophoblast. Thus, it is not surprising that trophoblast should have a range of functions far more varied than other tissues of the developing embryo.

The study of trophoblast, therefore, transcends disciplinary boundaries. Investigators interested in one aspect of trophoblast would greatly benefit from knowledge gained from research in areas other than their own. This became apparent recently when several of us at King's College, Cambridge discovered that although we have an overlapping interest in trophoblast, we are ignorant about the work being done by the others and would like to learn more from each other. For this reason, we have gathered together scientists and clinicians from diverse disciplines to share their expertise in an intimate workshop environment characteristic of a Novartis Foundation Symposium. The presented papers and discussions are now published by Cambridge University Press and should serve as a valuable, comprehensive source of information for the future.

REFERENCES

Carter, A. M. (2001). Evolution of the placenta and fetal membranes seen in the light of molecular phylogenetics. *Placenta*, **22**, 800–7.

Hubrecht, A. A. W. (1889). Studies in mammalian embryology. 1. The placentation of *Erinaceus europaeus*, with remarks on the phylogeny of the placenta. *Q. J. Microsc. Sci.* **30**, 284–404.

John, R. M. & Surani, M. A. (2000). Genomic imprinting, mammalian evolution, and the mystery of egg-laying mammals. *Cell*, **10**, 585–8.

Keverne, E. B. (2001). Genomic imprinting and the maternal brain. *Prog. Brain Res.*, **133**, 279–87.

King, A., Thomas, L. & Bischof, P. (2000). Cell culture models of trophoblast. II. Trophoblast cell lines. *Placenta*, **21**, S113–19.

Loke, Y. W. & King, A. (2001). HLA class I molecules in implantation. *Fetal Maternal Med. Rev.*, **12**, 299–314.

Rossant, J. & Cross, J. C. (2001). Placental development: lessons from mouse mutants. *Nat. Rev. Genet.*, **2**, 538–48.

Taruscio, D. & Mantovani, A. (1998). Human endogenous retroviral sequences: possible roles in reproductive physiopathology. *Biol. Reprod.*, **59**, 713–24.

Chair's introduction

Anne McLaren

The origin of this meeting was a rather good dinner in King's College Cambridge, at which Charlie Loke, Ashley Moffett, Barry Keverne, Azim Surani and myself got together, and it occurred to us that the trophoblast as a tissue was shamefully neglected. Since the definition of the word 'trophoblast' clearly means 'original feeding tissue' it is perhaps appropriate that the meeting had its origins in a good dinner!

Because I have spent a lot of time looking at sections of mouse implantation, seeing the giant mouse trophoblast cells, I have always found trophoblast rather scary. These cells are huge: they are so big they can be seen with the naked eye. In sections they seem to engulf the uterine epithelium and then they engulf the stromal cells. They are very aggressive cells, but they do a remarkable job. Those primary trophoblast cells are directly responsible for the very explosive growth that occurs in mouse implantation during gastrulation. It has been estimated that from the inner cell mass of the 3-day blastocyst (i.e. 3–4 days *post coitum* (dpc)) up to the 7-day embryo there is a more than 500-fold increase in tissue volume. This is all due to the yolk sac placenta, which does a remarkable job in nourishing and supporting this explosive growth. At 8 days the allantois is growing: it hasn't quite reached the chorion, so we don't have a chorioallantoic placenta, but it is the chorioallantoic placenta which is in a way more remarkable because this supports the entire human fetal growth up to full term – in most cases, fortunately, rather successfully. Animals of course eat their placentas and derive considerable nutritional benefit from doing so. This is rare in humans, but I believe recipes have been published.

The chorioallantoic placenta has certainly been a source of wonder in many parts of the world for centuries. I have read in Maureen Young's book (Young 2001) that the Balinese, for example, wash the placenta in perfumed water after birth, wrap it in a cloth and then bury it on the threshold of the family home in a carefully

Biology and Pathology of Trophoblast, eds. Ashley Moffett, Charlie Loke and Anne McLaren.
Published by Cambridge University Press © Cambridge University Press 2005.

prepared coconut. Think of that next time you see a placenta! The Japanese used to bury it in a cedar wood placental pot. If it was from a boy then it had Indian ink and a writing brush with it; from a girl it would have a needle and thread. The Egyptians were also very keen on the placenta. It was considered to be the seat of the eternal soul and after a pharaoh died his placenta was preserved in a jar.

In our first talk, Jay Cross is going to tell us how the various trophoblast cell lineages contribute to this seat of the eternal soul – the placenta.

REFERENCE

Young, M. (2001). *What is Baby Expecting? How We Are Fed to Grow Before We Are Born.* Toft, Cambridgeshire: Maureen Young.

Trophoblast cell fate specification

James Cross

University of Calgary, Canada

The trophoblast cell lineage is the first cell type to be specified during mammalian development – as the trophectoderm layer in the blastocyst – and is fated to form the epithelial cell compartment of the placenta (Cross *et al.* 1994, Rossant 1995). Trophoblast cells can be derived from blastocysts, at least in mice, that show properties expected of trophoblast stem (TS) cells in that they can differentiate into a range of differentiated trophoblast cell subtypes both in vitro and in vivo (Tanaka *et al.* 1998, Hughes *et al.* 2004). The trophoblast cell lineage is relatively simple in mice, in that TS cells differentiate into only four major differentiated cell types: trophoblast giant cells, spongiotrophoblast, glycogen trophoblast cells and syncytiotrophoblast (Cross *et al.* 2003) (Fig 1.1). Considerable progress has been made in the last few years in defining the molecular mechanisms that regulate the maintenance of the stem cell fate as well as the formation of the alternative differentiated cell types. This review focuses on the key transcription factors that specify trophoblast cell fates and the emerging evidence as to how signalling pathways interact with these transcription factors ultimately to regulate alternative cell fate decisions.

Trophoblast stem cells

Trophoblast stem cell lines can be derived from mice by culturing blastocysts or dissected extraembryonic ectoderm (chorionic trophoblast) in the presence of fibroblast growth factor (FGF)4 and feeder-cell conditioned medium (Tanaka *et al.* 1998). The identification of FGF4 as a critical factor was based on the findings that mutations in both the *Fgf4* gene, which is expressed by embryonic ectoderm (Feldman *et al.* 1995, Goldin & Papaioannou 2003), or the FGF receptor gene *Fgfr2*, which is expressed in trophectoderm (Arman *et al.* 1998), result in early post-implantation lethality due to a failure in trophoblast proliferation. The homeobox transcription factor genes *Cdx2* (Chawengsaksophak *et al.* 1997) and *Eomes* (Russ *et al.* 2000) are

Biology and Pathology of Trophoblast, eds. Ashley Moffett, Charlie Loke and Anne McLaren.
Published by Cambridge University Press © Cambridge University Press 2005.

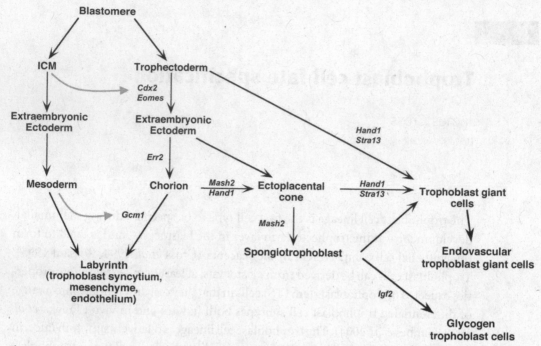

Figure 1.1   Outline of murine trophoblast cell lineage and regulatory genes. ICM, inner cell mass.

activated by FGF signalling and are clearly somehow required in turn for maintenance of TS cell fate, as mutations in either gene result in early post-implantation
lethality similar to the *Fgf4* and *Fgfr2* mutants. Removal of FGF4 from cultured
TS cells results in rapid down-regulation of *Cdx2* and *Eomes* expression and the
cells stop dividing soon thereafter (Tanaka *et al.* 1998), and the vast majority of
cells differentiate into trophoblast giant cells (Hughes *et al.* 2004). This implies that
differentiation of trophoblast giant cells does not require specific external cues. The
Err2 (Luo *et al.* 1997, Tremblay *et al.* 2001) and *AP*γ (Auman *et al.* 2002) transcription factor genes are also required for maintenance of the trophoblast stem cell fate,
but are only required at a slightly later stage.

Trophoblast giant cells

Trophoblast giant cells are large polyploid cells that mediate implantation and
invasion of the conceptus into the uterus. They also produce several growth factors
and hormones that promote both local and systemic physiological adaptations in
the mother that are necessary for embryonic growth and survival (Linzer & Fisher
1999, Cross *et al.* 2002). Primary trophoblast giant cells arise directly from the mural
trophectoderm at the blastocyst stage (Cross *et al.* 1994, Cross 2000). These cells

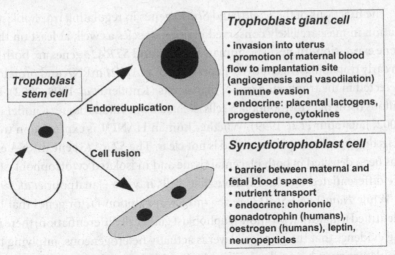

Trophoblast stem cell

Endoreduplication

Cell fusion

Trophoblast giant cell

- invasion into uterus
- promotion of maternal blood flow to implantation site (angiogenesis and vasodilation)
- immune evasion
- endocrine: placental lactogens, progesterone, cytokines

Syncytiotrophoblast cell

- barrier between maternal and fetal blood spaces
- nutrient transport
- endocrine: chorionic gonadotrophin (humans), oestrogen (humans), leptin, neuropeptides

Figure 1.2   Comparison of trophoblast giant cells and syncytiotrophoblast cells.

exit the mitotic cell cycle and stop dividing, but continue to go through rounds of DNA replication without intervening mitoses (endoreduplication) to become polyploid (MacAuley *et al.* 1998, Nakayama *et al.* 1998) (Fig 1.2). While there are only ~50 mural trophectoderm/primary giant cells in the peri-implantation blastocyst, the number of trophoblast giant cells increases to over 400 over the next few days through the process of secondary giant cell differentiation in which cells of the ectoplacental cone (precursor to the spongiotrophoblast layer) differentiate into giant cells (Cross *et al.* 1994, Cross 2000).

The differentiation of trophoblast giant cells is promoted by two basic helix-loop-helix (bHLH) transcription factor genes, *Hand1* and *Stra13*. Expression of *Hand1* mRNA is low or undetectable in TS cells but is induced as they differentiate into giant cells (Cross *et al.* 1995, Scott *et al.* 2000, Hughes *et al.* 2004). Ectopic expression of *Hand1* in growing TS cells is sufficient to promote their differentiation into giant cells, even if the cells are maintained in FGF4 (Hughes *et al.* 2004). By contrast, while *Hand1*-deficient embryos are able to implant, they arrest their development within a few days and both primary and secondary giant cell differentiation is blocked (Riley *et al.* 1998, Scott *et al.* 2000). The *Stra13* gene is a retinoic acid-inducible bHLH transcription factor gene that is also induced during giant cell differentiation (Hughes *et al.* 2004). Both retinoic acid treatment (Yan *et al.* 2001) and ectopic expression of *Stra13* (Hughes *et al.* 2004) in TS cells promote rapid arrest of cell proliferation and giant cell differentiation. While bHLH factors form dimers in general in order to bind DNA, the Hand1 and Stra13 proteins do not appear to interact directly (Hughes *et al.* 2004).

The functions of the *Hand1* and *Stra13* genes in regulating trophoblast differentiation in mice are likely conserved in other species as well, at least on the basis of gene expression studies. The human *HAND1* and *STRA13* genes are both expressed in early trophoblast derivatives. Expression of *HAND1* mRNA and protein has been detected in the trophectoderm of blastocysts (Knofler *et al.* 1998, 2002), but not in villous tissue or cytotrophoblast cells isolated from villous tissue (Knofler *et al.* 1998, 2002, Janatpour *et al.* 1999). Whether human HAND1 is expressed in trophoblast cells that invade the placental bed is not clear. The *STRA13* gene mRNA expression has been detected in both placental tissue and in isolated cytotrophoblast cells that are differentiated into 'extravillous-like' cells in vitro (Janatpour *et al.* 1999).

While *Hand1* and *Stra13* are the only transcription factor genes that have been identified to date that promote trophoblast giant cell differentiation, there is mounting evidence that the giant cell layer is actually heterogeneous, implying that other regulators must be involved. First, the Stra13 protein is detectable in only a small subset of the Hand1-positive giant cells (Hughes *et al.* 2004). Second, several giant-cell restricted genes such as *Mrj* (Hunter *et al.* 1999), *Ctps7* (Hemberger *et al.* 2000) and *Mps1* (Hemberger *et al.* 2000) show non-uniform expression within the giant cell layer in vivo. Finally, some giant-cell specific genes such as *Pl1* and *Pl2* are temporally regulated, such that *Pl1* expression is restricted to giant cells within the first few days after implantation, whereas *Pl2* expression begins only after embryonic day 9 (Yamaguchi *et al.* 1994).

Endovascular trophoblast giant cells

After implantation, a subtype of trophoblast giant cell invades into the spiral arteries that bring maternal blood to the implantation site, thereby promoting the transition from endothelial-lined arteries to the haemochorial blood spaces typical of rodent and primate placentas (Adamson *et al.* 2002). Although these endovascular trophoblast cells are not as large as primary giant cells surrounding the implantation site, nor do they express genes like *Pl1*, they do have enlarged nuclei compared with other uterine bed cells and they also express the *Plf* gene, a gene that in the placenta is otherwise specifically expressed in trophoblast giant cells. The factors that mediate the differentiation of endovascular trophoblast giant cells are unknown.

Spongiotrophoblast

The spongiotrophoblast layer forms the middle layer of the placenta between the outermost giant cells and the innermost labyrinth layer. The function of the spongiotrophoblast layer is unknown, although it probably has a structural role and also produces several layer-specific secreted factors. For example, spongiotrophoblast cells express anti-angiogenic factors that may prevent the growth of maternal blood vessels into the fetal placenta, including soluble Flt1 (a vascular endothelial growth factor (VEGF) antagonist) and Prp (an antagonist of Plf) (Cross *et al.* 2002).

The formation and/or maintenance of the spongiotrophoblast layer is dependent on the *Mash2* bHLH transcription factor gene. The *Mash2* gene mRNA is expressed in the ectoplacental cone and later the spongiotrophoblast layer in mice, and expression is normally down-regulated in trophoblast giant cells (Guillemot *et al.* 1994, Scott *et al.* 2000). In *Mash2* mutants, the spongiotrophoblast layer is lost by embryonic day 10 and more trophoblast giant cells are formed (Guillemot *et al.* 1994, Tanaka *et al.* 1997). The latter finding implies that spongiotrophoblast cells can differentiate into giant cells and that Mash2 regulates this step. Consistent with this, ectopic expression of Mash2 in Rcho-1 cells, which are derived from a rat trophoblast tumour (choriocarcinoma), blocks giant cell differentiation (Cross *et al.* 1995, Kraut *et al.* 1998, Scott *et al.* 2000). The ability of Mash2 to suppress trophoblast giant cell differentiation may be mediated in part by its ability to suppress Hand1-induced differentiation (Scott *et al.* 2000, Hughes *et al.* 2004). Interestingly, however, Mash2 overexpression cannot block Stra13-induced differentiation (Hughes *et al.* 2004). Given these functions of Mash2, the *Mash2* mutant phenotype could be explained by premature differentiation of spongiotrophoblast to trophoblast giant cells. In addition, though, recent evidence suggests that Mash2 may also directly promote proliferation of trophoblast cells (Hughes *et al.* 2004).

The actions of Mash2 may be modified by two other (non-bHLH) transcriptional regulators, I-mfa and Sna. The I-mfa protein inhibits the ability of some bHLH proteins including Mash2 to bind DNA. Consistent with an essential function in suppressing Mash2 function, I-mfa-deficient mice show a defect in the differentiation of trophoblast giant cells (Kraut *et al.*, 1998), albeit not as severe as Hand1 mutants. The zinc-finger transcription factor Sna has a consensus DNA recognition sequence similar to Mash2, and like Mash2 can block trophoblast giant cell differentiation (Nakayama *et al.*, 1998).

Glycogen trophoblast cells

Glycogen trophoblast cells appear only late in gestation, first within the spongiotrophoblast layer. After embryonic day 12, the glycogen trophoblast cells then invade into the uterus in a diffuse interstitial pattern that is quite distinct from the endovascular trophoblast giant cells (Adamson *et al.* 2002). Indeed, the glycogen cells appear to invade everywhere except for within or even close to the spiral arteries. The distinctive feature of glycogen cells is their accumulation of glycogen-rich granules, but its function is unknown. The developmental origin of these cells is not entirely clear, though their appearance first within the spongiotrophoblast layer and their expression of spongiotrophoblast-specific genes (e.g. *Tpbpa*) implies that glycogen trophoblast cells are a specialised subtype of spongiotrophoblast cell (Adamson *et al.* 2002). The only molecular insight that we have into the regulation of their development is that the number of glycogen trophoblast cells is reduced in *Igf2* mutants, implying a potential role for Igf2 in promoting either their differentiation or glycogen storage (Lopez *et al.* 1996).

Syncytiotrophoblast and chorionic villi

Syncytiotrophoblast cells form the major nutrient transport surfaces within the labyrinth layer of the rodent placenta and covering the chorionic villi in the primate placenta. Whereas trophoblast giant cells are mononuclear (occasionally binucleate) polyploid cells that arise as a result of endoreduplication, syncytiotrophoblast cells arise from the fusion of cells that have left the cell cycle (Cross 2000) (Fig 1.2). As a result, syncytiotrophoblast cells contain multiple diploid nuclei. In rodents, syncytiotrophoblast cell formation is first detected at the time that villous morphogenesis begins and indeed the two processes are dependent on a single transcription factor gene, *Gcm1* (Anson-Cartwright *et al.* 2000). Expression of *Gcm1* mRNA appears in small clusters of cells within the chorion layer that is otherwise comprised of cells with trophoblast stem cell potential (Basyuk *et al.* 1999, Anson-Cartwright *et al.* 2000). Ectopic expression of the *Gcm1* gene in TS cells is sufficient to force them out of the cell cycle, and to block their ability to differentiate into trophoblast giant cells but instead poise them to initiate morphogenesis and fuse into a syncytium (Hughes *et al.* 2004). In humans, GCM1 directly activates the transcription of the *Syncytin* gene (Yu *et al.* 2002), a gene encoding a cell surface, fusogenic protein (Mi *et al.* 2000). In *Gcm1* mutant mice, the chorioallantoic interface fails to initiate morphogenesis and syncytiotrophoblast cells fail to form (Anson-Cartwright *et al.* 2000).

The restricted and clustered pattern of *Gcm1/GCM1* expression in the developing villi of the mouse (Anson-Cartwright *et al.* 2000) and human (Baczyk *et al.* 2004) placenta implies very tight control over its expression. In mice, at least, the pattern appears within the chorion layer cell autonomously, but maintenance of the expression is dependent on attachment of the allantois to the chorion at embryonic day 8.5 (Hunter *et al.* 1999, Stecca *et al.* 2002). Indeed, syncytiotrophoblast differentiation does not normally begin until after the allantois makes contact. Likewise, TS cells do not normally develop into syncytiotrophoblast very efficiently in vitro (Hughes *et al.* 2004). However, addition of an allantois to an explanted chorion or to monolayers of TS cultured cells promotes Gcm1 expression (J. Cross, unpublished observation). The signal(s) from the allantois that regulates Gcm1 expression is unknown but is likely to be cell surface associated.

Conclusions

The molecular and genetic studies of the last few years have identified several critical regulators of placental development such that we now know of key regulators for most of the major cell differentiation steps in the trophoblast cell lineage. The identification of these factors will allow the more complete regulatory network to be described as upstream and downstream genes are identified. However, even as it stands now several important general principles of trophoblast development have emerged. First, the formation of distinct trophoblast cell subtypes appears to be specified by distinct molecular mechanisms. This implies that the spectrum of placental changes observed in human diseases like pre-eclampsia and intrauterine growth restriction, in which both villous and extravillous trophoblast defects have been described (Pijnenborg *et al.* 1981, Cross 1996, Pijnenborg 1996), cannot be explained by a single, direct molecular mechanism. Second, paracrine interactions regulate the development of the trophoblast lineage, at least in part, by modifying the expression if not the activity of key transcriptional regulators (e.g. FGF4 expression by embryonic ectoderm promoting TS cell proliferation/maintenance through Cdx2 and Eomes; allantoic factor promoting Gcm1 expression). Third, the ability of the Hand1, Stra13 and Gcm1 transcription factors to promote differentiation of TS cells, and even override the ability of FGF4 to maintain their stem cell character, implies that normally suppressing their expression and function within the stem cell compartment is critical for maintenance of the TS cell phenotype.

ACKNOWLEDGEMENTS

This work was supported by operating grants from the Canadian Institutes of Health Research (CIHR). Dr Cross is an Investigator of the CIHR and a Senior Scholar of the Alberta Heritage Foundation for Medical Research.

REFERENCES

Adamson, S.L., Lu, Y., Whiteley, K.J. *et al.* (2002). Interactions between trophoblast cells and the maternal and fetal circulation in the mouse placenta. *Dev. Biol.,* **250**, 358–73.

Anson-Cartwright, L., Dawson, K., Holmyard, D. *et al.* (2000). The glial cells missing-1 protein is essential for branching morphogenesis in the chorioallantoic placenta. *Nat. Genet.,* **25**, 311–14.

Arman, E., Haffner-Krausz, R., Chen, Y., Heath, J.K. & Lonai, P. (1998). Targeted disruption of fibroblast growth factor (FGF) receptor 2 suggests a role for FGF signaling in pregastrulation mammalian development. *Proc. Natl. Acad. Sci. U.S.A.,* **95**, 5082–7.

Auman, H.J., Nottoli, T., Lakiza, O. *et al.* (2002). Transcription factor AP-2gamma is essential in the extra-embryonic lineages for early postimplantation development. *Development,* **129**, 2733–47.

Baczyk, D., Satkunaratnam, A., Nait-Oumesmar, B. *et al.* (2004). Complex patterns of GCM1 mRNA and protein in villous and extravillous trophoblast cells of the human placenta. *Placenta*, **25**, 553–9.

Basyuk, E., Cross, J.C., Corbin, J. *et al.* (1999). The murine *Gcm1* gene is expressed in a subset of placental trophoblast cells. *Dev. Dyn.*, **214**, 303–11.

Chawengsaksophak, K., James, R., Hammond, V.E., Kontgen, F. & Beck, F. (1997). Homeosis and intestinal tumors in Cdx2 mutant mice. *Nature*, **386**, 84–7.

Cross, J.C. (1996). Trophoblast function in normal and preeclamptic pregnancy. *Fetal Maternal Med. Rev.*, **8**, 57–66.

  (2000). Genetic insights into trophoblast differentiation and placental morphogenesis. *Semin. Cell. Dev. Biol.*, **11**, 105–13.

Cross, J.C., Werb, Z. & Fisher, S.J. (1994). Implantation and the placenta: key pieces of the development puzzle. *Science*, **266**, 1508–18.

Cross, J.C., Flannery, M.L., Blanar, M.A. *et al.* (1995). Hxt encodes a basic helix-loop-helix transcription factor that regulates trophoblast cell development. *Development*, **121**, 2513–23.

Cross, J.C., Hemberger, M., Lu, Y. *et al.* (2002). Trophoblast functions, angiogenesis and remodeling of the maternal vasculature in the placenta. *Mol. Cell. Endocrinol.*, **187**, 207–12.

Cross, J.C., Baczyk, D., Dobric, N. *et al.* (2003). Genes, development and evolution of the placenta. *Placenta*, **24**, 123–30.

Feldman, B., Poueymirou, W., Papaioannou, V.E., DeChaira, T.M. & Goldfarb, M. (1995). Requirement of FGF-4 for postimplantation mouse development. *Science*, **267**, 246–9.

Goldin, S.N. & Papaioannou, V.E. (2003). Paracrine action of FGF4 during periimplantation development maintains trophectoderm and primitive endoderm. *Genesis*, **36**, 40–7.

Guillemot, F., Nagy, A., Auerbach, A., Rossant, J. & Joyner, A.L. (1994). Essential role of Mash-2 in extra-embryonic development. *Nature*, **371**, 333–6.

Hemberger, M., Himmelbauer, H., Ruschmann, J., Zeitz, C. & Fundele, R. (2000). cDNA subtraction cloning reveals novel genes whose temporal and spatial expression indicates association with trophoblast invasion. *Dev. Biol.*, **222**, 158–69.

Hughes, M., Dobric, N., Scott, I. *et al.* (2004). The Hand1, Stra13 and Gcm1 transcription factors override FGF signaling to promote terminal differentiation of trophoblast stem cells. *Dev. Biol.*, **271**, 27–38.

Hunter, P.J., Swanson, B.J., Haendel, M.A., Lyons, G.E. & Cross, J.C. (1999). *Mrj* encodes a DnaJ-related co-chaperone that is essential for murine placental development. *Development*, **126**, 1247–58.

Janatpour, M.J., Utset, M.F., Cross, J.C. *et al.* (1999). A repertoire of differentially expressed transcription factors that offers insight into mechanisms of human cytotrophoblast differentiation. *Dev. Genet.*, **25**, 146–57.

Knofler, M., Meinhardt, G., Vasicek, R., Husslein, P. & Egarter, C. (1998). Molecular cloning of the human *Hand1* gene/cDNA and its tissue-restricted expression in cytotrophoblastic cells and heart. *Gene*, **224**, 77–86.

Knofler, M., Meinhardt, G., Bauer, S. *et al.* (2002). Human Hand1 basic helix-loop-helix (bHLH) protein: extra-embryonic expression pattern, interaction partners and identification of its transcriptional repressor domains. *Biochem. J.*, **361**, 641–51.

Kraut, N., Snider, L., Chen, C., Tapscott, S.J. & Groudine, M. (1998). Requirement of the mouse I-mfa gene for placental development and skeletal patterning. *EMBO J.*, **17**, 6276–88.

Linzer, D.I. & Fisher, S.J. (1999). The placenta and the prolactin family of hormones: regulation of the physiology of pregnancy. *Mol. Endocrinol.*, **13**, 837–40.

Lopez, M.F., Dikkes, P., Zurakowski, D. & Villa-Komaroff, L. (1996). Insulin-like growth factor II affects the appearance and glycogen content of glycogen cells in the murine placenta. *Endocrinology*, **137**, 2100–8.

Luo, J., Sladek, R. & Bader, J-A. (1997). Placental abnormalities in mouse embryos lacking the orphan nuclear receptor ERR-b. *Nature*, **388**, 778–82.

MacAuley, A., Cross, J.C. & Werb, Z. (1998). Reprogramming the cell cycle for endoreduplication in rodent trophoblast cells. *Mol. Biol. Cell*, **9**, 795–807.

Mi, S., Lee, X., Li, X. *et al.* (2000). Syncytin is a captive retroviral envelope protein involved in human placental morphogenesis. *Nature*, **403**, 785–9.

Nakayama, H., Scott, I.C. & Cross, J.C. (1998). The transition to endoreduplication in trophoblast giant cells is regulated by the mSNA zinc-finger transcription factor. *Dev. Biol.*, **199**, 150–63.

Pijnenborg, R. (1996). The placental bed. *Hypertens. Pregnancy*, **15**, 7–23.

Pijnenborg, R., Robertson, W.B., Brosens, I. & Dixon, G. (1981). Review article: trophoblast invasion and the establishment of haemochorial placentation in man and laboratory animals. *Placenta*, **2**, 71–91.

Riley, P., Anson-Cartwright, L. & Cross, J.C. (1998). The Hand1 bHLH transcription factor is essential for placentation and cardiac morphogenesis. *Nat. Genet.*, **18**, 271–5.

Rossant, J. (1995). Development of the extra-embryonic lineages. *Semin. Dev. Biol.*, **6**, 237–47.

Russ, A.P., Wattler, S., Colledge, W.H. *et al.* (2000). Eomesodermin is required for mouse trophoblast development and mesoderm formation. *Nature*, **404**, 95–9.

Scott, I.C., Anson-Cartwright, L., Riley, P., Reda, D. & Cross, J.C. (2000). The Hand1 basic helix-loop-helix transcription factor regulates trophoblast giant cell differentiation via multiple mechanisms. *Mol. Cell. Biol.*, **20**, 530–41.

Stecca, B., Nait-Oumesmar, B., Kelley, K.A. *et al.* (2002). Gcm1 expression defines three stages of chorio-allantoic interaction during placental development. *Mech. Dev.*, **115**, 27–34.

Tanaka, M., Gertsenstein, M., Rossant, J. & Nagy, A. (1997). *Mash2* acts cell autonomously in mouse spongiotrophoblast development. *Dev. Biol.*, **190**, 55–65.

Tanaka, S., Kunath, T., Hadjantonakis, A.K., Nagy, A. & Rossant, J. (1998). Promotion of trophoblast stem cell proliferation by FGF4. *Science*, **282**, 2072–5.

Tremblay, G.B., Kunath, T., Bergeron, D. *et al.* (2001). Diethylstilbestrol regulates trophoblast stem cell differentiation as a ligand of orphan nuclear receptor ERR beta. *Genes Dev.*, **15**, 833–8.

Yamaguchi, M., Ogren, L., Endo, H., Soares, M.J. & Talamantes, F. (1994). Co-localization of placental lactogen-I, placental lactogen-II, and proliferin in the mouse placenta at midpregnancy. *Biol. Reprod.*, **51**, 1188–92.

Yan, J., Tanaka, S. & Oda, M. (2001). Retinoic acid promotes differentiation of trophoblast stem cells to a giant cell fate. *Dev. Biol.*, **235**, 422–32.

Yu, C., Shen, K., Lin, M. *et al.* (2002). GCMa regulates the syncytin-mediated trophoblastic fusion. *J. Biol. Chem.*, **277**, 50062–8.

DISCUSSION

McLaren For obvious reasons, most of what you said was about mouse trophoblast. I know that the implantation process and placentas vary a lot among different species: what about the actual trophoblast cell lineages? One probably doesn't know anything about the molecular basis, but what about the cell lineages themselves?

Cross Actually, we now know quite a bit about the molecular basis, at least in terms of comparing mouse to human. There are human homologues of *Gcm1*, *Hand1*, *Mash2* and *Stra13*. A few papers have been published documenting the expression of *GCM1* mRNA, and there will be a paper coming out soon showing that in human placenta *GCM1* is localised to small clusters of cells within the villous cytotrophoblast layer underlying the syncytium. If you catch a cell at the right phase you can see a *GCM1*-expressing cell as part of the villous cytotrophoblast compartment that is in the process of fusing to the overlying syncytium. The *HAND1* gene is expressed at the early blastocyst stage but its expression has been undetectable to date at later stages, unless reverse transcriptase (RT)-PCR is used. Expression of *MASH2* seems to be restricted to column cytotrophoblast cells that anchor the villi to the decidua. In this way, it is sort of analogous to the expression in mouse spongiotrophoblast that anchors the labyrinth to the decidual tissue. Expression of *STRA13* has been looked at in Susan Fisher's lab. If one cultures first trimester cytotrophoblast cells, its expression rises during the differentiation time course. This is consistent with expression in giant cells coming on as differentiation occurs. If you were asking a molecular biologist to compare the mouse and human placenta given that information, they could put comparable cell types together. Limited studies have been done in other species. The *Hand1* gene was initially cloned from a sheep blastocyst library. It is expressed in the cells analogous to giant cells in the sheep placenta. Francesca Stewart also detected expression in the chorionic girdle of equine conceptuses.

S. Fisher One of the things that we have seen in the human system is modulation of the expression of the partners – the IDs. I was curious: Jay Cross, have you seen any differential association of bHLH factors with any of the Ids?

Cross No, but we haven't put much effort into this. Just within the HLH transcription factor family we have looked at the expression and activities of a lot more than what I have described. In particular, E proteins are very dynamically expressed, and at least three of the Id proteins are dynamically expressed also.

McLaren Robert Pijnenborg, I know you have experience of a lot of different species. Would you like to comment on this question?

Pijnenborg   Yes, I have two questions. The first concerns morphology: why do you call the vascular trophoblastic cells in the mouse 'giant' cells? In my opinion, there is quite a difference in size and shape between the real giant cells and the vascular cells. Is there any evidence that they undergo endoreduplication of their DNA?

Cross   We haven't formally isolated the cells and shown that they endoreduplicate. But I agree that the endovascular cells are localised both within the vessel as well as around it. Although they are not as large as the primary giant cells, they are certainly much larger than the decidual cells or the endothelial cells that are adjacent. If we could isolate them and quantitate their DNA content, I would be very surprised if we couldn't show endoreduplication. The most compelling bit of information is that those cells express a subset of trophoblast giant cell-specific markers, and they don't express markers typical of spongiotrophoblast or other subtypes. We are trying to do formal cell lineage tracing experiments in the mouse using Cre-mediated recombination for activation of a marker gene to show formally that they originate in the normal giant cell compartment.

Pijnenborg   For historical and other reasons, a lot of the molecular biology is concentrated on the mouse. I am a trophoblast invasion person. In the mouse trophoblast invasion is restricted compared with the rat, for example. In the mouse this invasion is restricted to the mesometrial decidua, while in the rat it is much deeper, going into the overlying mesometrial triangle. Can the molecular biologists work on rats too? To my mind, for people interested in the mechanisms of trophoblast invasion the mouse looks more like a rhesus monkey or a pre-eclamptic woman. What happens in the rat is much more like a normal human pregnancy.

Cross   I am not going to make any apologies for having worked on the mouse. It has served us very well on the molecular side. What I can say is that there are mouse mutant lines that show much deeper patterns of invasion. One of these is the work of Anne Croy using natural killer (NK) cell-deficient mice. In this case, trophoblast invasion is much deeper.

Pijnenborg   Could it be that it is more the maternal environment which may be directly influencing the depth of invasion, rather than the molecular programming?

Cross   I think it will turn out to be a combination of factors. There has to be a molecular programme to make these invasive cells different from their cell type of origin. Not all giant cells show this endovascular pattern of invasion; not all spongiotrophoblast cells invade into the uterus.

McLaren   Aren't there some species, such as hamster, where the endovascular-invading trophoblast cells get way beyond the spiral arteries and out into the vascular system?

Pijnenborg   That is true. Also, they get deeper into the uterine vasculature. There are two different pathways of invasion in the hamster. Besides the invasion from the chorioallantoic placenta, as occurs in rats and mice, there is also migration starting from the primary giant cells that form the mural trophoblast layer overlying the inverted yolk sac. And from there, these giant cells migrate into the radial arteries and circumferential arteries, moving high into the mesometrial arteries. It is quite fascinating (Pijnenborg *et al.* 1974).

Ferguson-Smith   Jay Cross, do you think that all trophoblast giant cells are created equal and respond differently to their environment? Or are there different subpopulations of trophoblast giant cells?

Cross   I can't really answer that, but what I can say is that the more markers that we look at which are expressed in giant cells, the more diversity we see. Many of the genes that Myriam Hemberger has cloned light up different subpopulations of the giant cells. There may be some connection with whether the cells are associated with maternal blood space or not.

Ferguson-Smith   Have you found any consistent patterns?

Cross   No. Until we can isolate and separate cells we can't answer that.

Hemberger   Even if we were able to microdissect the invading cells and compare them with other cells in the giant cell layer, we wouldn't know whether a potential difference was observed because they were different giant cell subpopulations per se or because they were responding to the uterus. We would need to knock out the genes that we suspect make those cells more invasive and see whether that population is then gone or not.

Evain-Brion   In your culture system in which you differentiated trophoblast stem cells into giant cells or syncytia, you showed a slide with a syncytium with two nuclei. Have you seen syncytia with more nuclei?

Cross   Typically we see two, occasionally three, but never many more nuclei. The number of cells that become syncytiotrophoblasts in culture is very few. If we add allantoic tissue on top of a monolayer of trophoblast stem cells we get much more extensive syncytiotrophoblast differentiation, and morphogenesis in places of contact. Normally, syncytiotrophoblast doesn't form in vivo until after the allantois makes contact. That is why we initially did that experiment. We hope to be able to work out what the allantois is producing that gives the more robust response.

REFERENCE

Pijnenborg, R., Robertson, W.B. & Brosens, I. (1974). The arterial migration of trophoblast in the uterus of the golden hamster, *Mesocricetus auratus. J. Reprod. Fertil.*, **40**, 269–80.

2

Stem cells: pluripotency and extraembryonic differentiation in the mouse

Tilo Kunath

Institute for Stem Cell Research, University of Edinburgh

Abstract. Two distinct classes of stem cell lines can be derived from the mouse blastocyst: embryonic stem (ES) cells and trophoblast stem (TS) cells. Embryonic stem cells can differentiate into all embryonic lineages and extraembryonic mesoderm in chimeras, but are strictly excluded from the trophoblast lineage and rarely contribute to extraembryonic endoderm. In contrast, TS cells have the capacity to populate all trophoblast lineages, but are unable to make embryonic tissues or extraembryonic mesoderm and endoderm. A novel class of blastocyst-derived lines representative of the primitive endoderm lineage have been derived and characterised. Extraembryonic endoderm (XEN) cell lines contribute to derivatives of the primitive endoderm in vivo, but not to epiblast or trophoblast tissues. The signals required to maintain XEN cells in culture are not well characterised. However, the signals and critical transcription factors required for maintenance of ES and TS cell cultures have been partially determined. Embryonic stem cells require signalling through at least two pathways. The first is activated by leukaemia inhibitory factor (LIF) and transduced through the cell-surface receptor, gp130, and the intracellular protein, signal transducer and activator of transcription 3 (STAT3). The second pathway leads to activation of Smad proteins, which may be mediated by several factors, including bone morphogenetic proteins (BMPs). In contrast, TS cells require signalling from fibroblast growth factors (FGFs) and activation of mitogen-activated protein kinases (MAPKs). Trophoblast stem cells exhibit sustained activated MAPK activity that is FGF-dependent in vivo and they require transcription factors from diverse families such as eomesodermin (Eomes), Cdx2 and Errβ. Trophoblast stem cells also require the HMG-box domain protein, Sox2, a transcription factor also essential for ES cells. Two critical transcription factors required for ES cell pluripotency are Oct4 and Nanog. An important role of Oct4 is to suppress trophoblast differentiation, as the inner cell mass of $Oct4^{-/-}$ embryos differentiates into trophectoderm and $Oct4$ knock-down ES cells differentiate into

Biology and Pathology of Trophoblast, eds. Ashley Moffett, Charlie Loke and Anne McLaren.
Published by Cambridge University Press © Cambridge University Press 2005.

trophoblast giant cells and can also be transformed into TS cells in the presence of FGF4. Embryonic stem cells mutant for another pluripotency factor, Nanog, differentiate into an entirely different extraembryonic lineage, primitive endoderm. $Nanog^{-/-}$ ES cells are similar to the XEN cell lines described above. These observations led to a model which proposes that a major role of key pluripotency factors in ES cells is to actively suppress differentiation into extraembryonic lineages. Down-regulation of Oct4 and Nanog may also be necessary for differentiation of distinct extraembryonic lineages in vivo.

Pluripotency of embryonic stem cells

Embryonic stem cells are an excellent model system to study pluripotency and multi-lineage differentiation (Rathjen & Rathjen 2001, Smith 2001, Wassarman & Keller 2003). Since their derivation in 1981 (Evans & Kaufman 1981, Martin 1981), several mechanisms required for ES cell self-renewal have been revealed. The first major finding was the identification of LIF as the soluble factor secreted by feeder cells required for ES cell maintenance (Smith *et al.* 1988). Signalling via LIF or related cytokines promotes ES cell self-renewal by activation of the gp130 receptor (Yoshida *et al.* 1994) and the downstream effector, STAT3 (Niwa *et al.* 1998, Matsuda *et al.* 1999). Engagement of the gp130 receptor also activates the Ras–MAPK pathway, which acts to promote differentiation of ES cells (Burdon *et al.* 1999). Thus inhibition of this arm of the LIF signal actually enhances self-renewal and improves the efficiency of ES-cell-line derivations (Burdon *et al.* 1999, Buehr & Smith 2003). A second major pathway important for ES cell self-renewal has recently been described. Bone morphogenetic protein/Smad signalling in collaboration with LIF can maintain ES cells in serum-free conditions (Ying *et al.* 2003). Critical downstream target genes of the BMP/Smad signal were determined to be the *Id* genes. Overexpression of Id1 abrogated the need for exogenous BMP in serum-free LIF medium (Ying *et al.* 2003).

Several transcription factors are required for ES cell self-renewal. Two of the best characterised are the POU domain protein, Oct4, and the homeodomain protein, Nanog (Nichols *et al.* 1998, Chambers *et al.* 2003, Mitsui *et al.* 2003). The Oct4 protein is specifically expressed in undifferentiated cells of the early embryo and cells of the germline (Palmieri *et al.* 1994). In agreement with the in vivo expression pattern, the only cell lines that express Oct4 are ES cells, embryonal germ cells and embryonal carcinoma cells cultured in non-differentiating conditions (Palmieri *et al.* 1994, Pesce *et al.* 1998). Thus, *Oct4* expression is tightly correlated with cells in a pluripotent state and mutant analysis showed it was critical for the maintenance of this state. The *Oct4*-null mutant blastocysts do not produce a pluripotent inner cell mass (ICM) and they are unable to produce ES cell lines. The ICM is

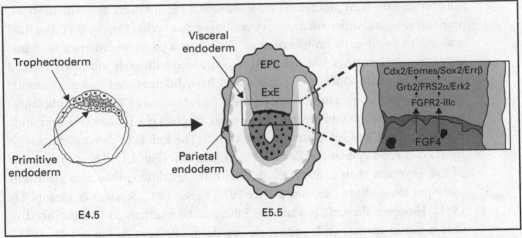

Figure 2.1   Early mouse lineages and model of trophoblast stem cell maintenance in vivo. The late blastocyst is composed of three distinct lineages; inner cell mass (ICM) in dark grey, primitive endoderm in light grey and trophectoderm (TE) in mid grey. After implantation, the polar TE gives rise to the extraembryonic ectoderm (ExE) adjacent to the ICM-derived epiblast (central dark grey area) and the ectoplacental cone (EPC). The interface between the epiblast and ExE is a region rich in inter-lineage signalling. Of relevance here is the FGF signal from the epiblast to ExE. Fibroblast growth factor 4 produced by the epiblast signals to the adjacent ExE resulting in an activation of Erk1/2. The model proposed here states that FGFR2-IIIc is the functional receptor in vivo and additional signalling molecules include Grb2, FRS2 and Erk2 (not Erk1). Some of the critical transcription factors required for trophoblast stem cell maintenance, such as Cdx2, Eomes, Sox2 and Errβ, may be directly or indirectly downstream of FGF signalling.

morphologically present at the blastocyst stage, but the cells have differentiated into trophoblast (Nichols *et al.* 1998). Acute down-regulation of this gene in ES cells also resulted in differentiation to trophoblast (Niwa *et al.* 2000), a cell type that ES cells do not normally produce in culture or in chimeras. Disruption of the *Nanog* locus in ES cells also resulted in a loss of pluripotency, but the cells differentiated into an entirely different lineage, extraembryonic endoderm (Mitsui *et al.* 2003). The mechanisms by which Oct4 and Nanog prevent ES cell differentiation into extraembryonic lineages will be explored further below. First, two classes of blastocyst-derived lines representative of distinct extraembryonic lineages will be described.

Trophoblast stem cells

The trophoblast lineage is first evident at the blastocyst stage as a sphere of epithelial-like cells known as trophectoderm (TE). At its formation, TE is a single-cell layer and it contains the ICM and a fluid-filled cavity, the blastocoel (Fig. 2.1). The polar

TE overlying the ICM proliferates while the mural TE, not in contact with the ICM, stops dividing and differentiates into trophoblast giant cells (Copp 1978). The ICM was shown to promote proliferation of TE cells in a paracrine manner by transplantation experiments. Isolated ICMs reconstituted with early mural TE induced proliferation of trophoblast cells that would have differentiated into post-mitotic giant cells during unperturbed development (Gardner *et al.* 1973). After implantation of the blastocyst into the uterus, the polar TE gives rise to the extraembryonic ectoderm (ExE) and ectoplacental cone (EPC). The ExE is in direct contact with the ICM-derived epiblast, while the EPC is distal to it (Fig. 2.1). The mitotic index of ExE is greater than that of EPC, but both tissues differentiate into giant cells when put into culture (Rossant & Ofer 1977, Ilgren 1981, Rossant & Tamura-Lis 1981). However, the ExE, but not the EPC, can be maintained in a proliferative state if put in contact with embryonic ectoderm (Rossant & Tamura-Lis 1981), supporting the model that the ICM, and later the epiblast, produces a local signal that promotes trophoblast proliferation. This model also predicted that the early trophoblast progenitor pool or stem cell population would be located in the ExE closest to the epiblast.

Expression and genetic ablation studies implicated FGF4 as the embryo-derived ligand necessary to promote proliferation of early trophoblast tissue. The reciprocal expression of FGF receptor 2 (*Fgfr2*) in the TE and ExE, and *Fgf4* in the ICM and epiblast, fits with the proposed paracrine signal required for trophoblast maintenance (Niswander & Martin 1992, Ciruna & Rossant 1999, Haffner-Krausz *et al.* 1999). Targeted disruption of *Fgf4* and *Fgfr2* further implicated FGF signalling in initial trophoblast expansion. Embryos mutant for *Fgf4* formed blastocysts and implanted, but did not develop further (Feldman *et al.* 1995). The polar TE did not expand into ExE suggesting FGF4 is required for this to occur. *Fgf4* mutant ES cells could be derived, suggesting that FGF4 is not required for maintenance of pluripotency (Wilder *et al.* 1997). Two different *Fgfr2* mutations resulted in embryonic lethality due to trophoblast defects, but at drastically different stages. One mutation caused lethality just after implantation, similar to $Fgf4^{-/-}$ embryos (Arman *et al.* 1998), while the other *Fgfr2* mutation resulted in failure of placental labyrinth development and lethality at embryonic day 10.5 (E10.5) (Xu *et al.* 1998). The differences between these two mutations have been discussed elsewhere (Kunath *et al.* 2001, 2004). The *Fgfr2* gene is alternatively spliced and two of its major isoforms, IIIb and IIIc, have different ligand specificity. The IIIc receptor has a high affinity for FGF4 and 9, while the IIIb isoform preferentially binds FGF3 and 7 (Ornitz *et al.* 1996). The *Fgfr2 IIIb* isoform-specific knockout embryos do not have trophoblast defects, but die at birth with limb and lung abnormalities (De Moerlooze *et al.* 2000). This phenotype resembles *Fgfr2* mutant pups that have had their placental defect rescued in chimeras (Arman *et al.* 1999). These mutant phenotypes, in addition to the biochemical data, strongly implicate FGFR2 IIIc as the receptor in trophoblast cells receiving the epiblast-derived FGF4 signal (Fig. 2.1).

In agreement with the in vivo observations, the derivation and maintenance of TS cell lines from blastocysts or ExE is critically dependent on FGF signalling (Tanaka *et al.* 1998). Although we consider FGF4 to be the ligand promoting early trophoblast expansion in vivo, cultured TS cells can also be maintained in FGF1 or FGF2. Trophoblast stem cells also require mouse embryonic fibroblasts (MEFs) or a critical concentration of MEF-conditioned medium to be maintained. Removal of the MEFs, FGF ligand, or its cofactor heparin results in differentiation to several trophoblast subtypes, including trophoblast giant cells (Tanaka *et al.* 1998). When cultured in stem cell conditions, TS cells express markers of ExE such as *Cdx2*, *Eomes*, *Errβ* and *Fgfr2*. Upon differentiation, expression of EPC markers, such as *Mash2* and *4311* (*Tpbp*), and the giant-cell marker, *Placental lactogen 1*, are observed (Tanaka *et al.* 1998).

The developmental potential of TS cells was investigated in chimeras. Trophoblast stem cells derived from enhanced green fluorescent protein (EGFP) transgenic embryos (Hadjantonakis *et al.* 1998) were injected into wild-type blastocysts or aggregated with morulae and the resulting chimeras were analysed from E6.5 to term. In all the chimeras obtained, the EGFP-TS cells were exclusively found in trophoblast tissue (Tanaka *et al.* 1998, Kunath *et al.* 2001). Contributions were observed to the ExE, EPC and giant cells of early conceptuses, and to the chorionic ectoderm, spongiotrophoblast and labyrinthine trophoblast at later stages, including term placentas. The EGFP-TS cells were never found in the embryo proper or extraembryonic membranes, such as the definitive yolk sac and amnion. Thus TS cells have the same developmental restrictions as nascent trophectoderm.

Since TS cell lines can be derived from both preimplantation and post-implantation embryos, it is useful to ask when and where this cell type resides in vivo. Extraembryonic tissues with TS cell competence were investigated throughout early development (Uy *et al.* 2002). Trophoblast stem cell lines can be derived from all regions of the ExE, but not from the EPC or embryo proper. Formation of the chorionic ectoderm and loss of direct contact with the epiblast did not make this tissue refractory to TS-cell-line derivations. In fact, TS cells could be obtained from chorionic ectoderm up to the 10-somite-pair stage (~E8.0), but not later (Uy *et al.* 2002). The source of FGF ligand at later stages is unknown, but it may be supplied by the extraembryonic mesoderm or endoderm.

The atlas of activated Erk1/2 during mouse development supported the embryological studies. At early stages (E5.5–E6.5), activated diphosphorylated MAPK (dpMAPK) was observed in the EPC and the region of the ExE closest to the epiblast (Corson *et al.* 2003). Erk1/2 activity in the ExE, but not the EPC, could be abolished during embryo culture with an FGFR-specific inhibitor (SU5402). The chorionic ectoderm was also positive for dpMAPK in agreement with its competence to produce TS cells (Uy *et al.* 2002). The phenotype of *Erk2* mutant embryos implicated this MAPK as the enzyme necessary for early trophoblast expansion. *Erk2* mutant embryos failed to form ExE and died shortly after implantation (Saba-El-Leil *et al.* 2003). A second report of the *Erk2*$^{-/-}$ phenotype claimed defects in mesoderm formation, but this is almost certainly a secondary defect due to failure of trophoblast development (Yao *et al.* 2003), since it shows that Erk activity is restricted to the ExE. The former study also showed that *Erk2* was cell-autonomously required in the trophoblast in chimeric studies (Saba-El-Leil *et al.* 2003). *Erk1* mutant animals are viable and fertile, suggesting that this MAPK is not essential for early trophoblast development (Pages *et al.* 1999). The FRS2α adaptor protein may also be important for TS cell maintenance as *FRS2α*$^{-/-}$ embryos die during early development and FRS2α is required for FGF signalling (Hadari *et al.* 2001). The expression domain of *Fgfr2* extended beyond the region of Erk activity, suggesting that ExE distal to the epiblast could respond to FGF signals in culture, but was not doing so in vivo. This was confirmed by the derivation of TS cell lines from the dpMAPK-negative region of ExE closest to the EPC (Uy *et al.* 2002). In contrast to *Fgfr2* expression, several other genes displayed more restricted ExE expression that closely coincided with dpMAPK staining. They include *Cdx2*, *Eomes*, *Sox2* and *Bmp4* (Beck *et al.* 1995, Ciruna & Rossant 1999, Coucouvanis & Martin 1999, Avilion *et al.* 2003). Some of these may be direct downstream targets of the FGF/Erk signal.

Sox2 was shown to be essential for TS cell line derivation (Avilion *et al.* 2003), and the early lethality of *Eomes* and *Cdx2* mutant embryos suggest that they may also be essential for TS cells (Chawengsaksophak *et al.* 1997, Russ *et al.* 2000). A recent study has demonstrated that *Cdx2* and *Eomes* are indeed required to make TS cells, and that *Cdx2* in the most upstream transcription factor in the specification of trophectoderm. By comparing *Cdx2* and *Eomes* homozygous mutant embryos, they demonstrated that *Cdx2*$^{-/-}$ blastocysts exhibit a more severe defect in trophectoderm development (Strumpf *et al.* 2005). The orphan nuclear receptor, Errβ, is also essential for early trophoblast development and the maintenance of TS cells (Luo *et al.* 1997, Tremblay *et al.* 2001). Rsk4 has been identified as a receptor tyrosine kinase inhibitor and is expressed in the ExE in a complementary pattern to the region of active MAPK (Myers *et al.* 2004). It may serve to restrict the extent to which FGF4 can signal in vivo. Mutations in the gene encoding the adaptor molecule, Grb2, also point to an essential role for MAPK signalling in trophoblast development (Cheng *et al.* 1998, Saxton *et al.* 2001). The current model of early TS cell maintenance places FGF4 and the FGFR/MAPK signalling pathway in a central position. The direct regulation of critical trophoblast-specific transcription factors by FGF signalling has not been demonstrated yet, but evidence from other species suggests that *Cdx2* and *Eomes* may be direct target genes (Griffin *et al.* 1998, Isaacs *et al.* 1998, Pownall *et al.* 1998).

Extraembryonic endoderm (XEN) cell lines

The implanting blastocyst consists of three cell types; trophectoderm, primitive ectoderm and primitive endoderm. Embryonic stem cells and TS cells are representative of primitive ectoderm and trophectoderm, respectively. Blastocyst-derived cell lines representative of extraembryonic endoderm have been reported (Fowler *et al.* 1990) and they have recently been extensively characterised (Kunath *et al.* 2005). Although the original cell lines were considered entirely parietal endoderm (PE), re-examination revealed them to exhibit some characteristics of visceral endoderm (VE) and have thus been named extraembryonic endoderm (XEN) cell lines to reflect this (Kunath *et al.* 2005). These cell lines can be derived from blastocysts in a number of ways. Isolated ICMs cultured on gelatin in the presence of LIF will often result in round, highly refractile cells migrating away from the outgrowth. These cells may be passaged and permanent cell lines derived. The outgrowth need not be disaggregated, as this may lead to the derivation of ES cell lines. A similar procedure can be followed for intact blastocyst outgrowths, but the efficiency is reduced. The original report of these cell lines showed that they express large amounts of extracellular matrix proteins associated with Reichert's membrane, such as laminin and type IV collagen (Fowler *et al.* 1990). Expression analysis by reverse transcriptase (RT)-PCR and Affymetrix profiling of XEN cells also showed high expression of PE matrix genes and other markers of this cell type, such as *Snail, thrombomodulin, tissue-type plasminogen activator* and *Platelet-derived growth factor receptor* α (PDGFRα) (Kunath *et al.* 2005). However, moderate to low expression of the VE markers, *Foxa2, Hex* and *Ihh* were also detected in all cultures, while α-*fetoprotein* (AFP) could be induced in some culture conditions (Kunath *et al.* 2005). Genes that are characteristic of the entire extraembryonic endoderm lineage, such as *Gata4, Gata6, Sox17, Sox7* and *Disabled*, were also highly expressed in XEN cells.

To examine their developmental potential, EGFP/LacZ XEN cells were injected into wild-type blastocysts to generate chimeras. Of the 50 chimeras examined, 49 had contributions to the parietal endoderm, and one exhibited a coherent clone in the visceral endoderm. Enhanced green fluorescent protein/LacZ cells were never observed in the embryo proper or trophoblast lineages (Kunath *et al.* 2005). Thus, XEN cells can contribute to PE, and rarely VE, in chimeras. The blastocyst-injection assay may not be the best method to test the full potential of this cell type, since injection of freshly isolated primitive endoderm or nascent VE cells into blastocysts

Table 2.1 Markers for ES, TS and XEN cell lines

Gene	ES cells	TS cells	XEN cells
Oct4	+	−	−
Nanog	+	−	−
Rex1	+	−	−
Fgf4	+	−	−
Sox2	+	+	−
Stat3	+	−	+
Cdx2	−	+	−
Eomes	−	+	−
Errβ	+	+	−
Gata4	−	−	+
Gata6	−	−	+
Sox7	−	−	+
Sox17	−	−	+
Disabled 2	−	−	+
Snail	−	−	+

also resulted in a strong bias towards PE (Gardner 1982). Although the donor cells in these experiments have the potential to make VE, this was not reflected in the chimera studies. The blastocoel environment and contact with trophectoderm may promote PE differentiation (Verheijen *et al.* 1999).

The morphology and gene expression profile of XEN cells is very distinct from ES and TS cells (Plate 1 and Table 2.1). Although they are all derived from mouse blastocysts, they are representative of different early embryonic lineages and contribute to non-overlapping tissues in chimeras (Plate 1).

TS cells and XEN cells derived from ES cells

Embryonic stem cell, TS cell and XEN cell lines can all be derived from the same stage mouse embryo, and are representative of the primitive ectoderm, trophectoderm and primitive endoderm lineages, respectively. In vivo, these lineages are restricted at E4.5 and cross-lineage contributions do not occur after this developmental time point. However, ES cells appear to be more plastic than primitive ectoderm. Particular genetic ablations of pluripotency factors or up-regulation of critical lineage-specific transcription factors can drive differentiation of ES cells into TS cell or XEN cell lines.

Analysis of $Oct4^{-/-}$ embryos suggested that this transcription factor was a repressor of the trophoblast lineage (Nichols *et al.* 1998). Isolated $Oct4^{-/-}$ ICMs expressed the trophoblast markers *Mash2* and *H19*, and the ICM outgrowths produced TS-cell-like colonies that could be expanded with FGF4 (Nichols *et al.* 1998). Since $Oct4^{-/-}$ ES cell lines could not be derived, a repressible transgenic Oct4 system was established (Niwa *et al.* 2000). An ES cell line (ZHBTc4) was derived that was null for both endogenous alleles of *Oct4* and was maintained by an *Oct4* transgene that could be repressed upon tetracycline (Tet) treatment. This ES cell line could self-renew in the presence of LIF, but Tet-mediated down-regulation of *Oct4* resulted in trophoblast differentiation and expression of the trophoblast markers, *Hand1*, *Cdx2* and *H19* (Niwa *et al.* 2000). Furthermore, if FGF4 was added to the Tet-treated cultures, the ES cells were transformed to TS cell lines that could be maintained for more than ten passages and could differentiate to EPC and trophoblast giant cells upon removal of FGF4 (Niwa *et al.* 2000). Two additional studies using RNA interference for *Oct4* confirmed that ES cells differentiate into trophoblast cells upon *Oct4* knock-down (Velkey & O'Shea 2003, Hay *et al.* 2004). An alternative way to transform ES cells to TS cells is to overexpress the caudal-related gene, *Cdx2* (Niwa 2003). This transcription factor was ectopically expressed in *Oct4*-deficient embryos and ES cells and may be directly repressed by Oct4. Whether other TS cell-specific transcription factors, such as Eomes and Errβ can transform ES cells to TS cells remains to be determined. Since Sox2 is essential for both ES cells and TS cells (Avilion *et al.* 2003), it is unlikely to be sufficient for ES cell to TS cell transformation, but may play a more general role in the maintenance of a stem cell state.

The homozygous knockout of *Nanog* in ES cells produced viable cell lines that could be passaged, but their morphology was unlike ES cells. $Nanog^{-/-}$ cells did not grow as tight epithelial colonies. They proliferated as dispersed cells and were large, round or stellate and highly refractile (Mitsui *et al.* 2003). Northern and RT-PCR analysis revealed they expressed markers of the extraembryonic endoderm, such as *Gata6*, *Hnf4α*, *Disabled 2 (Dab2)* and *AFP*, but not *Cdx2* like *Oct4*-deficient ES cells (Mitsui *et al.* 2003). The marker analysis and cell morphology strongly suggested that $Nanog^{-/-}$ cells were similar to the embryo-derived XEN cell lines. Overexpression of several endoderm-specific transcription factors in ES cells identified GATA4 and GATA6 as potent inducers of extraembryonic endoderm. Overexpression of *Hnf1α*, *Hnf4α*, *Pdx1* and other genes was unable to elicit this differentiation event (Fujikura *et al.* 2002). The cell morphology of the GATA4 and GATA6 overexpressing cell lines resembled $Nanog^{-/-}$ ES cells and XEN cell lines. The expression of extraembryonic endoderm markers, such as *Dab2*, *Hnf3β*, *Hnf4α* and, in some culture conditions, *AFP*, were induced and pluripotent markers, such as *Oct4* and

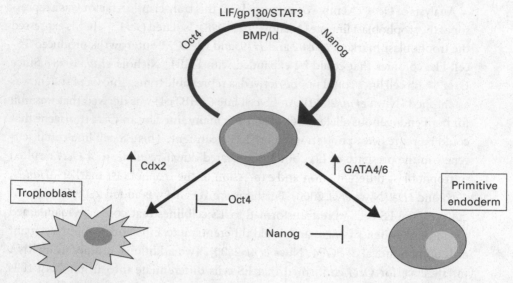

Figure 2.2   Inhibitory model of pluripotency. Embryonic stem cell self-renewal (central cell) requires several signalling pathways and critical transcription factors. LIF/gp130/STAT3 and BMP/Id signalling maintains ES cells in a pluripotent state. Oct4 and Nanog are also essential for ES cells, but their mechanisms of action are not well understood. This model postulates that an important mode of action for Oct4 and Nanog is to actively suppress trophoblast and primitive endoderm lineages, respectively. Deletion of either in ES cells leads to differentiation to these extraembryonic lineages in culture. Identical differentiation events from ES cells could be attained by overexpression of lineage-promoting transcription factors, Cdx2 (for trophoblast) and GATA4 or GATA6 (for primitive endoderm). Although speculative at present, the mechanism of action of Oct4 and Nanog may be to actively repress Cdx2 and GATA4/6, respectively.

Rex1, were repressed (Fujikura *et al.* 2002). Although *Nanog* was not cloned at the time, this gene is likely also repressed in GATA4/6-overexpressing ES cells.

Is it possible to revert ES-cell-derived TS cell or XEN cell lines back to ES cells? Or blastocyst-derived TS or XEN cell lines into ES cells? This could be attempted by returning Oct4 or Nanog (or both) to TS cells or XEN cells, respectively. It is encouraging to note that *Oct4* can be reactivated in TS cells more efficiently than in NIH/3T3 cells when treated with the histone deacetylase inhibitor, trichostatin A or the DNA methylation inhibitor, 5′-aza-2′-deoxycytidine (Hattori *et al.* 2004). As more of the molecular requirements for pluripotency are uncovered, the closer we will get to experimentally inducing this state in differentiated cells. Trophoblast stem cells and XEN cells are a good place to start, since they can be derived from ES cells in one step and they can be derived from direct sister lineages of the cell type (ICM) that gives rise to ES cells.

Inhibitory model of pluripotency

What are the molecular determinants of ES cell pluripotency? Although it is not possible to answer this question at the moment, we are in a position to construct a working model. Since Oct4 was discovered, it was considered a pluripotency factor and efforts were made to identify genes that it positively regulates (Saijoh *et al.* 1996, Du *et al.* 2001). It now appears that Oct4 may be mediating a significant proportion of its effects by transcriptional repression, not activation. Oct4 has been shown to repress some trophoblast genes (Liu & Roberts 1996, Liu *et al.* 1997, Ezashi *et al.* 2001), and analysis of *Oct4*-deficient embryos and ES cells suggested that it directly or indirectly represses a critical trophoblast determinant, *Cdx2*. Similarly, the *Nanog* mutant analysis suggested that it may be a repressor of a master regulator for the extraembryonic endoderm lineage, *Gata6* (Mitsui *et al.* 2003). Therefore, an important mechanism of action for two critical pluripotent transcription factors is to actively inhibit differentiation into extraembryonic lineages by repressing master regulatory genes (Fig. 2.2). A further example of an inhibitory mechanism to maintain ES cell pluripotency is BMP/Smad signalling and repression of neural commitment (Ying *et al.* 2003). This is mediated by antagonising the MAPK pathway and by up-regulation of Id proteins, inhibitors of basic helix-loop-helix transcription factors (Ying *et al.* 2003, Qi *et al.* 2004). Thus a common theme emerging from these mechanistic studies is that ES cells maintain their pluripotent status by actively and simultaneously inhibiting key differentiation determinants. This is accomplished, in part, by expression of Oct4 and Nanog, repressors of two distinct extraembryonic lineages, trophoblast and primitive endoderm, respectively.

REFERENCES

Arman, E., Haffner-Krausz, R., Chen, Y., Heath, J.K. & Lonai, P. (1998). Targeted disruption of fibroblast growth factor (FGF) receptor 2 suggests a role for FGF signaling in pregastrulation mammalian development. *Proc. Natl. Acad. Sci. U.S.A.*, **95**, 5082–7.

Arman, E., Haffner-Krausz, R., Gorivodsky, M. & Lonai, P. (1999). Fgfr2 is required for limb outgrowth and lung-branching morphogenesis. *Proc. Natl. Acad. Sci. U.S.A.*, **96**, 11895–9.

Avilion, A.A., Nicolis, S.K., Pevny, L.H. *et al.* (2003). Multipotent cell lineages in early mouse development depend on SOX2 function. *Genes Dev.*, **17**, 126–40.

Beck, F., Erler, T., Russell, A. & James, R. (1995). Expression of Cdx-2 in the mouse embryo and placenta: possible role in patterning of the extra-embryonic membranes. *Dev. Dyn.*, **204**, 219–27.

Buehr, M. & Smith, A. (2003). Genesis of embryonic stem cells. *Philos. Trans. R. Soc. Lond. B Biol. Sci.*, **358**, 1397–402; discussion 1402.

Burdon, T., Stracey, C., Chambers, I., Nichols, J. & Smith, A. (1999). Suppression of SHP-2 and ERK signaling promotes self-renewal of mouse embryonic stem cells. *Dev. Biol.*, **210**, 30–43.

Chambers, I., Colby, D., Robertson, M. *et al.* (2003). Functional expression cloning of Nanog, a pluripotency sustaining factor in embryonic stem cells. *Cell*, **113**, 643–55.

Chawengsaksophak, K., James, R., Hammond, V. E., Kontgen, F. & Beck, F. (1997). Homeosis and intestinal tumors in Cdx2 mutant mice. *Nature*, **386**, 84–7.

Cheng, A. M., Saxton, T. M., Sakai, R. *et al.* (1998). Mammalian Grb2 regulates multiple steps in embryonic development and malignant transformation. *Cell*, **95**, 793–803.

Ciruna, B. G. & Rossant, J. (1999). Expression of the T-box gene Eomesodermin during early mouse development. *Mech. Dev.*, **81**, 199–203.

Copp, A. J. (1978). Interaction between inner cell mass and trophectoderm of the mouse blastocyst. I. A study of cellular proliferation. *J. Embryol. Exp. Morphol.*, **48**, 109–25.

Corson, L. B., Yamanaka, Y., Lai, K. M. & Rossant, J. (2003). Spatial and temporal patterns of ERK signaling during mouse embryogenesis. *Development*, **130**, 4527–37.

Coucouvanis, E. & Martin, G. R. (1999). BMP signaling plays a role in visceral endoderm differentiation and cavitation in the early mouse embryo. *Development*, **126**, 535–46.

De Moerlooze, L., Spencer-Dene, B., Revest, J. *et al.* (2000). An important role for the IIIb isoform of fibroblast growth factor receptor 2 (FGFR2) in mesenchymal-epithelial signaling during mouse organogenesis. *Development*, **127**, 483–92.

Du, Z., Cong, H. & Yao, Z. (2001). Identification of putative downstream genes of Oct-4 by suppression-subtractive hybridisation. *Biochem. Biophys. Res. Commun.*, **282**, 701–6.

Evans, M. J. & Kaufman, M. H. (1981). Establishment in culture of pluripotential cells from mouse embryos. *Nature*, **292**, 154–6.

Ezashi, T., Ghosh, D. & Roberts, R. M. (2001). Repression of Ets-2-induced transactivation of the tau interferon promoter by Oct-4. *Mol. Cell. Biol.*, **21**, 7883–91.

Feldman, B., Poueymirou, W., Papaioannou, V. E., DeChiara, T. M. & Goldfarb, M. (1995). Requirement of FGF-4 for postimplantation mouse development. *Science*, **267**, 246–9.

Fowler, K. J., Mitrangas, K. & Dziadek, M. (1990). *In vitro* production of Reichert's membrane by mouse embryo-derived parietal endoderm cell lines. *Exp. Cell Res.*, **191**, 194–203.

Fujikura, J., Yamato, E., Yonemura, S. *et al.* (2002). Differentiation of embryonic stem cells is induced by GATA factors. *Genes Dev.*, **16**, 784–9.

Gardner, R. L. (1982). Investigation of cell lineage and differentiation in the extra-embryonic endoderm of the mouse embryo. *J. Embryol. Exp. Morphol.*, **68**, 175–98.

Gardner, R. L., Papaioannou, V. E. & Barton, S. C. (1973). Origin of the ectoplacental cone and secondary giant cells in mouse blastocysts reconstituted from isolated trophoblast and inner cell mass. *J. Embryol. Exp. Morphol.*, **30**, 561–72.

Griffin, K. J., Amacher, S. L., Kimmel, C. B. & Kimelman, D. (1998). Molecular identification of spadetail: regulation of zebrafish trunk and tail mesoderm formation by T-box genes. *Development*, **125**, 3379–88.

Hadari, Y. R., Gotoh, N., Kouhara, H., Lax, I. & Schlessinger, J. (2001). Critical role for the docking-protein FRS2 alpha in FGF receptor-mediated signal transduction pathways. *Proc. Natl. Acad. Sci. U.S.A.*, **98**, 8578–83.

Hadjantonakis, A.K., Gertsenstein, M., Ikawa, M., Okabe, M. & Nagy, A. (1998). Generating green fluorescent mice by germline transmission of green fluorescent ES cells. *Mech. Dev.*, **76**, 79–90.

Haffner-Krausz, R., Gorivodsky, M., Chen, Y. & Lonai, P. (1999). Expression of Fgfr2 in the early mouse embryo indicates its involvement in pre-implantation development. *Mech. Dev.*, **85**, 167–72.

Hattori, N., Nishino, K., Ko, Y.G. *et al.* (2004). Epigenetic control of mouse Oct-4 gene expression in embryonic stem cells and trophoblast stem cells. *J. Biol. Chem.*, **279**, 17063–9.

Hay, D.C., Sutherland, L., Clark, J. & Burdon, T. (2004). Oct-4 knockdown induces similar patterns of endoderm and trophoblast differentiation markers in human and mouse embryonic stem cells. *Stem Cells*, **22**, 225–35.

Ilgren, E.B. (1981). On the control of the trophoblastic giant-cell transformation in the mouse: homotypic cellular interactions and polyploidy. *J. Embryol. Exp. Morphol.*, **62**, 183–202.

Isaacs, H.V., Pownall, M.E. & Slack, J.M. (1998). Regulation of Hox gene expression and posterior development by the Xenopus caudal homologue Xcad3. *EMBO J.*, **17**, 3413–27.

Kunath, T., Strumpf, D., Tanaka, S. & Rossant, J. (2001). Trophoblast stem cells. In D.R. Marshak, R.L. Gardner & D. Gottlieb, eds. *Stem Cell Biology*. New York: Cold Spring Harbor Press, pp. 267–87.

Kunath, T., Strumpf, D. & Rossant, J. (2004). Early trophoblast determination and stem cell maintenance in the mouse – a review. *Placenta*, **25**, S32–8.

Kunath, T., Arnaud, D., Uy, G.D. *et al.* (2005). Imprinted X-inactivation in extra-embryonic endoderm cell lines from mouse blastocyst. *Development*, **132**, 1649–61.

Liu, L. & Roberts, R.M. (1996). Silencing of the gene for the beta subunit of human chorionic gonadotropin by the embryonic transcription factor Oct-3/4. *J. Biol. Chem.*, **271**, 16683–9.

Liu, L., Leaman, D., Villalta, M. & Roberts, R.M. (1997). Silencing of the gene for the alpha-subunit of human chorionic gonadotropin by the embryonic transcription factor Oct-3/4. *Mol. Endocrinol.*, **11**, 1651–8.

Luo, J., Sladek, R., Bader, J.A. *et al.* (1997). Placental abnormalities in mouse embryos lacking the orphan nuclear receptor ERR-beta. *Nature*, **388**, 778–82.

Martin, G.R. (1981). Isolation of a pluripotent cell line from early mouse embryos cultured in medium conditioned by teratocarcinoma stem cells. *Proc. Natl. Acad. Sci. U.S.A.*, **78**, 7634–8.

Matsuda, T., Nakamura, T., Nakao, K. *et al.* (1999). STAT3 activation is sufficient to maintain an undifferentiated state of mouse embryonic stem cells. *EMBO J.*, **18**, 4261–9.

Mitsui, K., Tokuzawa, Y., Itoh, H. *et al.* (2003). The homeoprotein Nanog is required for maintenance of pluripotency in mouse epiblast and ES cells. *Cell*, **113**, 631–42.

Myers, A.P., Corson, L.B., Rossant, J. & Baker, J.C. (2004). Characterization of mouse Rsk4 as an inhibitor of fibroblast growth factor-RAS-extracellular signal-regulated kinase signaling. *Mol. Cell. Biol.*, **24**, 4255–66.

Nichols, J., Zevnik, B., Anastassiadis, K. *et al.* (1998). Formation of pluripotent stem cells in the mammalian embryo depends on the POU transcription factor Oct4. *Cell*, **95**, 379–91.

Niswander, L. & Martin, G.R. (1992). Fgf-4 expression during gastrulation, myogenesis, limb and tooth development in the mouse. *Development*, **114**, 755–68.

Niwa, H. (2003). Analysis of transcription factors in the differentiation of extra-embryonic ecto-derm (in Japanese). Paper presented at: 36th Japanese Society of Developmental Biology (Sapporo, Japan)

Niwa, H., Burdon, T., Chambers, I. & Smith, A. (1998). Self-renewal of pluripotent embryonic stem cells is mediated via activation of STAT3. *Genes Dev.*, **12**, 2048–60.

Niwa, H., Miyazaki, J. & Smith, A.G. (2000). Quantitative expression of Oct-3/4 defines differ-entiation, dedifferentiation or self-renewal of ES cells. *Nat. Genet.*, **24**, 372–6.

Ornitz, D.M., Xu, J., Colvin, J.S. *et al.* (1996). Receptor specificity of the fibroblast growth factor family. *J. Biol. Chem.*, **271**, 15292–7.

Pages, G., Guerin, S., Grall, D. *et al.* (1999). Defective thymocyte maturation in p44 MAP kinase (Erk 1) knockout mice. *Science*, **286**, 1374–7.

Palmieri, S.L., Peter, W., Hess, H. & Scholer, H.R. (1994). Oct-4 transcription factor is differen-tially expressed in the mouse embryo during establishment of the first two extra-embryonic cell lineages involved in implantation. *Dev. Biol.*, **166**, 259–67.

Pesce, M., Gross, M.K. & Scholer, H.R. (1998). In line with our ancestors: Oct-4 and the mam-malian germ. *BioEssays*, **20**, 722–32.

Pownall, M.E., Isaacs, H.V. & Slack, J.M. (1998). Two phases of Hox gene regulation during early Xenopus development. *Curr. Biol.*, **8**, 673–6.

Qi, X., Li, T.G., Hao, J. *et al.* (2004). BMP4 supports self-renewal of embryonic stem cells by inhibi-ting mitogen-activated protein kinase pathways. *Proc. Natl. Acad. Sci. U.S.A.*, **101**, 6027–32.

Rathjen, J. & Rathjen, P.D. (2001). Mouse ES cells: experimental exploitation of pluripotent differentiation potential. *Curr. Opin. Genet. Dev.*, **11**, 587–94.

Rossant, J. & Ofer, L. (1977). Properties of extra-embryonic ectoderm isolated from postimplan-tation mouse embryos. *J. Embryol. Exp. Morphol.*, **39**, 183–94.

Rossant, J. & Tamura-Lis, W. (1981). Effect of culture conditions on diploid to giant-cell trans-formation in postimplantation mouse trophoblast. *J. Embryol. Exp. Morphol.*, **62**, 217–27.

Russ, A.P., Wattler, S., Colledge, W.H. *et al.* (2000). Eomesodermin is required for mouse tro-phoblast development and mesoderm formation. *Nature*, **404**, 95–9.

Saba-El-Leil, M.K., Vella, F.D., Vernay, B. *et al.* (2003). An essential function of the mitogen-activated protein kinase Erk2 in mouse trophoblast development. *EMBO Rep.*, **4**, 964–8.

Saijoh, Y., Fujii, H., Meno, C. *et al.* (1996). Identification of putative downstream genes of Oct-3, a pluripotent cell-specific transcription factor. *Genes Cells*, **1**, 239–52.

Saxton, T.M., Cheng, A.M., Ong, S.H. *et al.* (2001). Gene dosage-dependent functions for phosphotyrosine-Grb2 signaling during mammalian tissue morphogenesis. *Curr. Biol.*, **11**, 662–70.

Smith, A.G. (2001). Embryo-derived stem cells: of mice and men. *Annu. Rev. Cell. Dev. Biol.*, **17**, 435–62.

Smith, A.G., Heath, J.K., Donaldson, D.D. *et al.* (1988). Inhibition of pluripotential embryonic stem cell differentiation by purified polypeptides. *Nature*, **336**, 688–90.

Strumpf, D., Mao, C.-A., Yamanaka, Y. *et al.* (2005). Cdx2 is required for correct cell fate spec-ification and differentiation of trophectoderm in the mouse blastocyst. *Development*, **132**, 2093–102.

Tanaka, S., Kunath, T., Hadjantonakis, A.K., Nagy, A. & Rossant, J. (1998). Promotion of tro-phoblast stem cell proliferation by FGF4. *Science*, **282**, 2072–5.

Tremblay, G.B., Kunath, T., Bergeron, D. *et al.* (2001). Diethylstilbestrol regulates trophoblast stem cell differentiation as a ligand of orphan nuclear receptor ERR beta. *Genes Dev.*, **15**, 833–8.

Uy, G.D., Downs, K.M. & Gardner, R.L. (2002). Inhibition of trophoblast stem cell potential in chorionic ectoderm coincides with occlusion of the ectoplacental cavity in the mouse. *Development*, **129**, 3913–24.

Velkey, J.M. & O'Shea, K.S. (2003). Oct4 RNA interference induces trophectoderm differentiation in mouse embryonic stem cells. *Genesis*, **37**, 18–24.

Verheijen, M.H., Karperien, M., Chung, U. *et al.* (1999). Parathyroid hormone-related peptide (PTHrP) induces parietal endoderm formation exclusively via the type I PTH/PTHrP receptor. *Mech. Dev.*, **81**, 151–61.

Wassarman, P.M. & Keller, G.M. (eds.) (2003). *Methods in Enzymology, Vol. 365, Differentiation of Embryonic Stem Cells.* London: Elsevier Academic Press.

Wilder, P.J., Kelly, D., Brigman, K. *et al.* (1997). Inactivation of the FGF-4 gene in embryonic stem cells alters the growth and/or the survival of their early differentiated progeny. *Dev. Biol.*, **192**, 614–29.

Xu, X., Weinstein, M., Li, C. *et al.* (1998). Fibroblast growth factor receptor 2 (FGFR2)-mediated reciprocal regulation loop between FGF8 and FGF10 is essential for limb induction. *Development*, **125**, 753–65.

Yao, Y., Li, W., Wu, J. *et al.* (2003). Extracellular signal-regulated kinase 2 is necessary for mesoderm differentiation. *Proc. Natl. Acad. Sci. U.S.A.*, **100**, 12759–64.

Ying, Q.L., Nichols, J., Chambers, I. & Smith, A. (2003). BMP induction of Id proteins suppresses differentiation and sustains embryonic stem cell self-renewal in collaboration with STAT3. *Cell*, **115**, 281–92.

Yoshida, K., Chambers, I., Nichols, J. *et al.* (1994). Maintenance of the pluripotential phenotype of embryonic stem cells through direct activation of gp130 signaling pathways. *Mech. Dev.*, **45**, 163–71.

DISCUSSION

Surani   What conditions did you use to derive the XEN cells?

Kunath   We didn't do anything special. They were derived in trophoblast stem cell medium with FGF. They were actually derived by accident in three different labs, with three different conditions. We have been seeing this cell type for a while in culture but had considered them to be nuisance cells and never characterised them. Then I decided to see what markers they expressed. The easiest way to derive them is to plate blastocysts without disaggregating them. These cells migrate away from the periphery, and you can pick them up and then passage them. If you take them off gelatin they differentiate and express other visceral endoderm markers.

Surani   I have a separate question to do with human ES cells. Unlike mouse ES cells, human ES cells can differentiate into trophoblast cells easily with BMP4. Have you tried using BMP4 to differentiate stem cells from human blastocysts?

Kunath   We haven't tried plating human blastocysts in BMP4. We are trying a couple of different factors and ligands, but we haven't tried BMP2 and BMP4.

McLaren   At least in the mouse, I think there are a number of FGF receptors and different forms of each. But presumably you have tried them all on human.

Kunath   The *FGFR3* and *FGFR4* were also checked in the human, and like the *FGFR1* and *FGFR2* data I showed, they weren't present at the blastocyst stage by RT-PCR.

Loke   What kind of markers do you use to identify human trophoblast cells in vitro? How do you know whether you have or haven't got trophoblast?

Kunath   We are measuring things such as SP1 and human chorionic gonadotrophin (HCG) in the medium from the outgrowths. We haven't yet got a cell line to passage and characterise. It seems that the human blastocyst does express *CDX2*: this may be a good marker if we do get a cell line from human blastocysts. Our problem is that we haven't got anything proliferating.

Dey   There are several papers now showing that Wnt signalling could be involved in this. Have you seen any Wnt signalling in trophoblast cells or ES cells?

Kunath   For ES cells there is a recent paper showing that Wnt signalling is useful for maintaining them (Sato *et al.* 2004). For trophoblast I haven't heard anything. There are data showing that Activin and Nodal are important for trophoblast self-renewal.

Cross   Several of the *Wnt* knockouts and one of the *Wnt receptor* knockouts have placental phenotypes, but this is much later than could be interpreted as being a trophoblast stem cell phenotype. If anything, our hypothesis would be that Wnts might be the allantoic factor that promotes syncytiotrophoblast differentiation.

S. Fisher   I'd like to comment about BMP4 and human trophoblast. Those cells are odd in the sense that they make HCG, but they never proliferate. Thinking of using BMP to make a human TS line is a little simplistic.

Kunath   That's true. The trophoblast cells they get in the cultures are post-mitotic (Xu *et al.* 2002).

McLaren   If one goes back to the preblastocyst stage, what is the first differential gene expression that distinguishes the outer cells – the future trophectoderm – from the inner cells?

Kunath   That's a good question. From published data there is only one convincing marker, *Nanog*, which is expressed in the inner cells. We think *Cdx2* is complementary to *Nanog*, and this is expressed in the outer cells. *Nanog* is the first good example of a differentially expressed gene at the morula stage.

Dey   We also found that transforming growth factor (TGF)β2 is expressed only in the outside cells. This was published several years ago (Paria *et al.* 1992).

McLaren   If one isolates small groups of inner or outer cells at the 16- or 32-cell stage, as Martin Johnson and colleagues did (e.g. Johnson & Ziomek 1983), they can change their fates (see also Hillman *et al.* 1972). It would be very interesting to see how rapidly and in what way the gene expression is changed.

Kunath   The knockout of *Cdx2* does form an initial blastocyst at E3.5 but it collapses to a ball of inner cell mass cells. All the cells are Oct4 positive and no trophectoderm is formed (Strumpf *et al.* 2005). This is the opposite of the *Oct4* knockout where everything becomes trophoblast.

Surani   I wanted to ask you about another gene, *Eomes*. Since frogs don't have trophectoderm, what does it do in mouse trophectoderm cells where it is expressed very early on?

Cross   The *Eomes* mutant phenotype is similar to *Fgf4/Fgfr2/Cdx2* early post-implantation phenotype. There is a failure of the polar trophectoderm to proliferate. Did you try to derive cell lines from the *Eomes* knockouts?

Kunath   Dan Strumpf in Janet Rossant's lab did. It was on our list of 'essential' TS cell genes. We tried to derive mutant TS cells from *Eomes* knockouts, but from the numbers of heterozygous and wild-type lines we obtained, we thought it was impossible to get null TS cell lines. The same was the case for *Cdx2* Strumpf. Ian Scott and I showed that it was possible to derive TS cell lines mutant for *Hand1* and *Mosh2*, respectively (unpublished data), while Robin Lovell-Badge published that it was not possible to derive such cell lines mutant for *Sox2* (Avilion *et al.* 2003).

Moffett   One of the most important things from the point of view of the interaction with the mother is the major histocompatibility complex (MHC) expression on the trophoblast cells. Have you looked at the MHC expression in your lines?

Kunath   No, but there's an immunologist in Buffalo (NY), Shawn Murphy, who has looked at this. I can't remember the details, but it fitted the model of what MHCs the trophoblast should express in vivo.

Moffett   As I understand it, in the mouse the literature is extremely confusing on what *MHC* genes are expressed by trophoblast. It is one of the big mysteries.

Sharkey   Coming back to the difficulties of deriving human trophoblast stem cell lines from ES cells, you said it was very successful in the mouse: you could drive it by taking away *Oct4* or adding *Cdx2*. Is this worth trying in the human?

Kunath   It is difficult to knock genes out in human ES cells.

Sharkey   The reason I ask about this is because Austin Smith has made double knockout mouse ES cell lines, so he has the techniques to do this.

Kunath   For human, Jamie Thompson is the only one who has been able to show that he has targeted a gene in human ES cells (Zwaka & Thompson 2003). Targeting a human ES cell is not a trivial matter. Overexpression may be easier.

Sharkey   Or using antisense RNA.

Kunath   Yes, RNA interference has been used with human ES cells. Still, working with human ES cells is not trivial. Deriving TS cells from the blastocyst would be beautiful, because we do have a source of blastocysts. This would be the best option.

Renfree Would you like to speculate on those species that have no ICM? Insectivores such as hedgehogs develop an ICM much later than the stages you are talking about. Marsupials have a unilaminar blastocyst that has no ICM cells. It would be interesting to see which cells, if any, are producing Nanog or Cdx and when they do it. So far, we can't find a single difference between any of the trophoblast cells. They all have the same morphology.

Kunath Have you tried Nanog?

Renfree Not yet.

Kunath This may be a differentially expressed gene. If any two genes were differentially expressed I'd suggest they were *Cdx2* and *Nanog*. *Oct4* expression doesn't look like *Nanog*: it is expressed in all cells of the late morula, whereas *Nanog* is just in the inner cells.

McLaren There is a marsupial *Oct4*, isn't there?

Renfree Yes.

Kunath The *Oct4* gene is even expressed in the trophectoderm of early blastocysts, so it is probably not a good marker.

REFERENCES

Avilion, A. A., Nicolis, S. K., Pevny, L. H. *et al.* (2003). Multipotent cell lineages in early mouse development depend on SOX2 function. *Genes Dev.*, **17**, 126–40.

Hillman, N., Sherman, M. I. & Graham, C. (1972). The effect of spatial arrangement on cell determination during mouse development. *J. Embryol. Exp. Morphol.*, **28**, 263–78.

Johnson, M. H. & Ziomek, C. A. (1983). Cell interactions influence the fate of mouse blastomeres undergoing the transition from the 16- to the 32-cell stage. *Dev. Biol.*, **95**, 211–18.

Paria, B. C., Jones, K. L., Flanders, K. C. & Dey, S. K. (1992). Localization and binding of transforming growth factor-beta isoforms in mouse pre-implantation embryos and in delayed and activated blastocysts. *Dev. Biol.*, **151**, 91–104.

Sato, N., Meijer, L., Skaltsounis, L., Greengard, P. & Brivanlou, A. H. (2004). Maintenance of pluripotency in human and mouse embryonic stem cells through activation of Wnt signaling by a pharmacological GSK-3-specific inhibitor. *Nat. Med.*, **10**, 55–63.

Strumpf, D., Mao, C.-A. Yamanaka, Y. *et al.* (2005). Cdx2 is required for correct cell fate specification and differentiation of trophectoderm in the mouse blastocyst. *Development*, **132**, 2093–102.

Xu, R. H., Chen, X., Li, D. S. *et al.* (2002). BMP4 initiates human embryonic stem cell differentiation to trophoblast. *Nat. Biotechnol.*, **20**, 1261–4.

Zwaka, T. P. & Thomson, J. A. (2003). Homologous recombination in human embryonic stem cells. *Nat. Biotechnol.*, **21**, 319–21.

3

Epigenetic regulation of trophoblast development

P. Hajkova[1], S. E. Erhardt[2], and M. A. Surani[3]

[1] Wellcome Trust/Cancer Research UK, Gurdon Institute of Cancer and Developmental Biology, University of Cambridge
[2] LBNL, USA
[3] Wellcome Trust/Cancer Research UK, Gurdon Institute of Cancer and Developmental Biology, University of Cambridge, UK

Trophectoderm is the first differentiated lineage to be established during development. In the mouse, the founder cells for this lineage are set aside early as a result of asynchronous division of eight-cell-stage blastomeres, the outer cells being the founder cells for the trophectoderm lineage while the inner cells form the inner cell mass (Johnson & Ziomek 1981). The pluripotent epiblast cells in the inner cell mass of blastocysts serve as the precursors of the developing fetus. However, some of the key signalling molecules for early development of the pluripotent epiblast cells originate from the trophectoderm and primary endoderm cells (Beddington & Robertson 1999), including the signals for the specification of germ cells (McLaren 1999). The purpose of this review is to focus on the role of epigenetic mechanisms in the establishment of the trophectoderm lineage and the subsequent development of the placenta. In particular we are interested in how the maternally inherited factors in the oocyte affect development of the trophoblast through their effect on epigenetic modifications. Although this aspect requires detailed investigations, there are already indications that the interactions between maternal factors in the oocytes and the parental genomes may be critical for early development, including development of the trophoblast.

Role of genomic imprinting in development of the trophoblast

At the time of fertilisation, the parental genomes are epigenetically non-equivalent, but additional epigenetic modifications ensue in the early zygote (Ferguson-Smith & Surani 2001). Evidence shows that parental genomes have differential roles

Biology and Pathology of Trophoblast, eds. Ashley Moffett, Charlie Loke and Anne McLaren.
Published by Cambridge University Press © Cambridge University Press 2005.

during mouse development, which have consequences for embryonic and tro-phoblast development. This is because of genomic imprinting, which results in epigenetic modifications of certain genes that cause parent-of-origin-dependent expression of imprinted genes. Androgenetic mouse and human conceptuses show preferential proliferation of the trophoblast, while parthenogenetic/gynogenetic conceptuses are particularly deficient in development of these extraembryonic tis-sues but with a relatively better development of the embryo (Surani *et al.* 1986). Studies have shown that there are some imprinted genes that are particularly impor-tant for development of the trophoblast. Among these is *Mash2*, coding for a tran-scriptional factor that is required for development of trophoblast progenitors and of the spongiotrophoblast (Guillemot *et al.* 1995, Tanaka *et al.* 1999). Another exam-ple is the placenta-specific transcript of the imprinted *Igf2* gene, which has a role in development of labyrinth and the transfer of nutrients to the fetus (Constancia *et al.* 2002). A number of other imprinted genes, such as *Peg1* and *Peg3*, also have an effect on placental development and functions (Lefebvre *et al.* 1998, Li *et al.* 1999).

Development of the trophoblast in the absence of parental imprints

There has been considerable debate about the purpose of genomic imprinting. One view is that imprinting evolved to regulate the maternal supply of nutrients to the developing fetus (Haig & Wilkins 2000). Development of the conceptus in the absence of imprints is therefore of interest. The only time when the parental genomes are epigenetically equivalent is in the germline following erasure of the parental imprints (Surani 2001, Hajkova *et al.* 2002). To test for the developmental potential of an imprint-free genome, nuclei from imprint-free germ cells from E13.5–16.5 embryos were transplanted into enucleated oocytes (Kato *et al.* 1999, Lee *et al.* 2002). In this instance, any interactions between the imprint-free donor nucleus and maternally inherited factors in the oocyte would also influence the outcome. The resulting embryos progressed up to E9.5 of gestation but they were growth retarded. There was a clear and consistent effect on placental development at E9.5. In particular, the chorion seemed to be developmentally arrested. There was also a thick layer of trophoblast giant cells. Most significantly, there was usually only a small and discrete layer of diploid trophoblast with an evident lack of spongiotrophoblast. The allantois was well developed and seemed to be fusing with the chorion but without interacting with it to become labyrinth (Kato *et al.* 1999). The placental development was reminiscent of what is seen in the *Mash2* mutant conceptus. This phenotype is also somewhat similar to that of the androgenetic conceptus, which also lacks expression of the imprinted and maternally expressed *Mash2*. The evidence showed that interactions between the imprint-free germ cell donor nucleus and oocyte cytoplasm did not alter the status of imprints. Deoxyribonucleic acid methylation analysis of several imprinted genes of the resulting conceptus showed erasure, which was in turn consistent with the repression of some imprinted genes. Thus, some of the key genes, *Igf2r*, *Igf2* and *Cdkn1c* (previously called *p57Kip2*) were repressed.

Role of maternally inherited factors

During normal development, the maternally inherited factors in oocytes play a variety of critical roles, including epigenetic modifications of parental genomes that may have specific effects on development of the trophectoderm lineage. An extreme example of such epigenetic modifications is the restoration of totipotency in a donor somatic nucleus when transplanted into the oocyte. Since development of the trophectoderm lineage is the earliest event in mammals, it follows that differentiated somatic nuclei of many types must be reprogrammed or undergo 'transdifferentiation' to form trophectoderm when transplanted into the oocyte. These oocyte factors may also modify certain target loci resulting in their silencing. This phenomenon was observed for some transgenes that undergo DNA methylation in response to strain-specific modifiers (Allen *et al.* 1990).

Development of interspecific hybrid embryos could also be subject to epigenetic modification through interactions between parental genomes and the oocyte cytoplasmic factors. The reciprocal nature of the resulting phenotype that has a marked effect on placental development, depends on the parental origin of the oocyte in such hybrids. A classical example of interspecific hybrids is that between *Peromyscus maniculatus* and *Peromyscus polionotus* (Rogers & Dawson 1970). Reciprocal crosses result in conceptuses that are phenotypically distinct from those seen within either of the two species. With *P. polionotus* as the female in these crosses, the placenta is substantially larger than in either of the two species, while the reciprocal cross results in a much smaller placenta. Recent studies showed widespread disruption of imprinting in reciprocal crosses between these species resulting in loss of imprints and biallelic expression of *Mash2*, *Peg3*, *Mest* and other genes (Vrana *et al.* 1998). However, the molecular mechanism responsible for these effects is largely unknown. Other studies involving reciprocal crosses between *Mus musculus* and *M. spretus* have also resulted in abnormal placental growth. An X-linked locus was shown to segregate with placental dysplasia and the X-linked gene *Esx1* together with *Igf2* probably contribute to this abnormal development (Zechner *et al.* 2002).

Dynamic epigenetic changes in the zygote

Recent studies have shown that there are indeed dynamic epigenetic changes in parental genomes in the zygote (Fig. 3.1). Amongst this is the finding that the

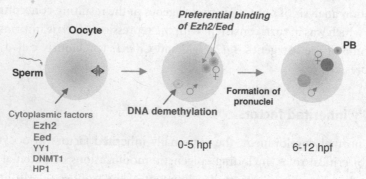

Figure 3.1   Maternal inheritance and epigenetic modifications in the zygote. Hpf, hours post fertilisation; PB polar body.

paternal genome preferentially undergoes extensive and rapid genome-wide DNA demethylation (Mayer *et al.* 2000, Oswald *et al.* 2000, Reik *et al.* 2001). There is also the preferential binding of some proteins in the oocyte to the maternal genome. Amongst these proteins are the Polycomb Group (PcG) proteins, Enhancer of Zeste (Ezh)2 and Eed, which bind preferentially to the maternal genome (Arney *et al.* 2001, 2002, Erhardt *et al.* 2003). The precise role of these early epigenetic changes in parental genomes is not known, nor is it clear how disruption of these early events would affect development. To elucidate how such events may affect development of the conceptus and of the trophectoderm and placenta in particular, we have focused on the role of a key maternally inherited epigenetic modifier Ezh2.

The role of Enhancer of Zeste in trophoblast development

Enhancer of Zeste 2 is a PcG protein with a SET domain, a catalytic domain with activity for methylation of histone H3 lysine 27 (H3meK27) (see Erhardt *et al.* 2003). It usually forms a complex with another PcG protein, Eed, and histone deacetylase 2 (HDAC2). This complex therefore has the capacity to induce epigenetic modifications of target loci. Enhancer of Zeste 2 is essential for early mouse development. Loss of function of this gene results in early post-implantation lethality, and it is not possible to derive pluripotent embryonic stem cells in the absence of Ezh2 (O'Carroll *et al.* 2001). The Ezh2/Eed complex also has a critical role in the initiation of X inactivation in all blastomeres initially, but which is later confined to trophectoderm cells where there is preferential paternal X inactivation (see Brockdorff, Chapter 4, this book).

The primary focus of our ongoing work has been to examine the role of Ezh2 early in development. *Enhancer of Zeste 2* is transcribed in developing oocytes and stored in mature oocytes as a maternally inherited factor (Erhardt *et al.* 2003). The purpose of our investigation was to deplete the oocytes of the maternal inheritance of Ezh2 because this lack of a key epigenetic modifier may perturb the early interactions with parental genomes and the dynamic epigenetic changes that occur in early zygotes (Surani 2001). We therefore used a conditional allele for *Ezh2* with loxP sites that can be deleted in the presence of the Cre enzyme. In our experiments, the Cre enzyme was expressed under the *Zp3* promoter, which occurs specifically when the quiescent oocytes resume growth. Following deletion of *Ezh2* in developing oocytes, the mutant oocytes are essentially devoid of Ezh2 protein. These mutant and control oocytes were then fertilised by wild-type sperm. The paternal allele brought in by the fertilising sperm becomes transcriptionally active and restores the protein level of Ezh2 at about the four-cell stage. Thus, there is loss of Ezh2 during a relatively short duration spanning the period of oocyte growth, zygote and early cleavage divisions.

Analysis of early embryos shows that Ezh2 and Eed bind preferentially to the maternal genome in the early zygote. There is also an apparent epigenetic difference between parental genomes with the maternal genome showing higher global levels of H3meK27. This was not observed in oocytes depleted of Ezh2. The Ezh2 levels in embryos from the maternally depleted oocytes are restored at the four-cell stage and normal H3meK27 levels are restored in late morulae (Erhardt *et al.* 2003).

Despite this very transient loss of Ezh2 from oocytes, there is a marked effect on development. Unlike complete loss of function, which is embryonic lethal (O'Carroll *et al.* 2001), embryos after the transient loss of Ezh2 are viable, but they produce neonates that are substantially smaller than the controls (Erhardt *et al.* 2003). However, these animals eventually catch up with their normal littermates and acquire the appropriate size. This observation indicates that perhaps the effect on fetal growth may be a secondary consequence of an effect of the transient loss of Ezh2 on trophoblast and placental development. Our preliminary results clearly indicate that the placental size is smaller compared to the controls. It is possible that one of the effects may be on development of the spongiotrophoblast, which needs further investigation (P. Hajkova *et al.*, unpublished results).

This preliminary result clearly indicates that the transient loss of Ezh2 has an effect on placental development, particularly on spongiotrophoblast, which could be ascribed to the perturbation of early epigenetic modifications in the developing oocytes and the zygote. Continuing studies should pinpoint the precise molecular effects of loss of Ezh2. Previous work on *Eed*$^{-/-}$ mutant embryos has shown an effect on four imprinted genes where the repression on the paternal allele is alleviated (Ferguson-Smith & Reik 2003, Mager *et al.* 2003). Mutant conceptuses lacking Eed are early embryonic lethal (Mager *et al.* 2003). While this experiment is not comparable to our study on the transient loss of Ezh2 function, it is possible that this may also have an effect on expression of some imprinted genes. Further studies will test this prediction. It is also possible that the major phenotypic effect on placental development that we observed may also be due to aberrant epigenetic modifications and expression of other key extraembryonic-specific gene expression. Our studies in progress should clarify the precise effects, which should lead to an understanding of the underlying mechanism responsible for the effect on placental development.

Ezh2 and MEDEA: an example of parallel evolution in plants and mammals?

The homologue of Ezh2 in Arabidopsis is MEDEA, which has an important role in development of the endosperm. Like the placenta, endosperm is needed for the nourishment of the developing embryo. The MEDEA protein interacts with another PcG protein FIE, a homologue of Eed, illustrating conservation of the PcG genes in plants and mammals (Yadegari et al. 2000). However, in plants, the embryo and the endosperm are the products of double fertilisation by two independent sperm of the egg cell and the central cell, respectively. Thus, while both the embryo and placenta in mammals arise from a single cell, the zygote, the situation in plants allows for epigenetic modifications in the endosperm independently of the embryo. Nevertheless, it is interesting to note that MEDEA has a key role in the regulation of endosperm growth (Dickinson & Scott 2002). The MEDEA gene behaves like an imprinted gene as the paternal copy is silent while the maternal copy is active in the endosperm. This activation of MEDEA in the endosperm is dependent on the activity of another gene, DEMETER, which is active in the endosperm and induces demethylation of MEDEA. In the absence of activation of MEDEA, there is overproliferation of the endosperm and the embryonic growth is retarded. This is an example of parallel evolution of maternal control over development: a PcG gene has an effect on placental development in mammals and endosperm development in plants (Berger 2004). It is important to note the differences in the role of imprinting in development of the placenta and endosperm.

Conclusion

Epigenetic mechanisms apparently have a role in development of the trophoblast and the placenta. The effect is mediated through the activity of imprinted genes, as well as by the maternally inherited epigenetic modifiers in the oocyte. These modifiers may influence development both through their role in maintaining parental imprints, and through their effects on the expression of other key genes that have a critical role in development of the extraembryonic tissues.

REFERENCES

Allen, N.D., Norris, M.L. & Surani, M.A. (1990). Epigenetic control of transgene expression and imprinting by genotype-specific modifiers. *Cell*, **61**, 853–61.

Arney, K.L., Erhardt, S., Drewell, R.A. & Surani, M.A. (2001). Epigenetic reprogramming of the genome – from the germ line to the embryo and back again. *Int. J. Dev. Biol.* **45**, 533–50.

Arney, K.L., Bao, S., Bannister, A.J., Kouzarides, T. & Surani, M.A. (2002). Histone methylation defines epigenetic asymmetry in the mouse zygote. *Int. J. Dev. Biol.* **46**, 317–20.

Beddington, R.S. & Robertson, E.J. (1999). Axis development and early asymmetry in mammals. .*Cell*, **96**, 195–209.

Berger, F. (2004). Plant sciences. Imprinting – a green variation. *Science*, **303**, 483–5.

Constancia, M., Hemberger, M., Hughes, J. *et al.* (2002). Placental-specific IGF-II is a major modulator of placental and fetal growth. *Nature*, **417**, 945–8.

Dickinson, H. & Scott, R. (2002). DEMETER, Goddess of the harvest, activates maternal MEDEA to produce the perfect seed. *Mol. Cell*, **10**, 5–7.

Erhardt, S., Su, I.H., Schneider, R. *et al.* (2003). Consequences of the depletion of zygotic and embryonic Enhancer of Zeste 2 during pre-implantation mouse development. *Development*, **130**, 4235–48.

Ferguson-Smith, A.C. & Reik, W. (2003). The need for Eed. *Nat. Genet.*, **33**, 433–4.

Ferguson-Smith, A.C. & Surani, M.A. (2001). Imprinting and the epigenetic asymmetry between parental genomes. *Science*, **293**, 1086–9.

Guillemot, F., Caspary, T., Tilghman, S.M. *et al.* (1995). Genomic imprinting of Mash2, a mouse gene required for trophoblast development. *Nat. Genet.*, **9**, 235–42.

Haig, D. & Wilkins, J.F. (2000). Genomic imprinting, sibling solidarity and the logic of collective action. *Philos. Trans. R. Soc. Lond. B Biol. Sci.*, **355**, 1593–7.

Hajkova, P., Erhardt, S., Lane, N. *et al.* (2002). Epigenetic reprogramming in mouse primordial germ cells. *Mech. Dev.*, **117**, 15–23.

Johnson, M.H. & Ziomek, C.A. (1981). The foundation of two distinct cell lineages within the mouse morula. *Cell*, **24**, 71–80.

Kato, Y., Rideout, W.M. 3rd, Hilton, K. *et al.* (1999). Developmental potential of mouse primordial germ cells. *Development*, **126**, 1823–32.

Lee, J., Inoue, K., Ono, R. *et al.* (2002). Erasing genomic imprinting memory in mouse clone embryos produced from day 11.5 primordial germ cells. *Development*, **129**, 1807–17.

Lefebvre, L., Viville, S., Barton, S.C. *et al.* (1998). Abnormal maternal behaviour and growth retardation associated with loss of the imprinted gene Mest. *Nat. Genet.*, **20**, 163–9.

Li, L., Keverne, E.B., Aparicio, S.A. *et al.* (1999). Regulation of maternal behavior and offspring growth by paternally expressed Peg3. *Science*, **284**, 330–3.

Mager, J., Montgomery, N.D., de Villena, F.P. & Magnuson, T. (2003). Genome imprinting regulated by the mouse Polycomb group protein Eed. *Nat. Genet.*, **33**, 502–7.

Mayer, W., Niveleau, A., Walter, J., Fundele, R. & Haaf, T. (2000). Demethylation of the zygotic paternal genome. *Nature*, **403**, 501–2.

McLaren, A. (1999). Signaling for germ cells. *Genes Dev.*, **13**, 373–6.

O'Carroll, D., Erhardt, S., Pagani, M. *et al.* (2001). The polycomb-group gene Ezh2 is required for early mouse development. *Mol. Cell. Biol.*, **21**, 4330–6.

Oswald, J., Engemann, S., Lane, N. *et al.* (2000). Active demethylation of the paternal genome in the mouse zygote. *Curr. Biol.*, **10**, 475–8.

Reik, W., Dean, W. & Walter, J. (2001). Epigenetic reprogramming in mammalian development. *Science*, **293**, 1089–93.

Rogers, J. F. & Dawson, W. D. (1970). Foetal and placental size in a *Peromyscus* species cross. *J. Reprod. Fertil.*, **21**, 255–62.

Surani, M. A. (2001). Reprogramming of genome function through epigenetic inheritance. *Nature*, **414**, 122–8.

Surani, M. A., Barton, S. C. & Norris, M. L. (1986). Nuclear transplantation in the mouse: heritable differences between parental genomes after activation of the embryonic genome. *Cell*, **45**, 127–36.

Tanaka, M., Puchyr, M., Gertsenstein, M. *et al.* (1999). Parental origin-specific expression of Mash2 is established at the time of implantation with its imprinting mechanism highly resistant to genome-wide demethylation. *Mech. Dev.*, **87**, 129–42.

Vrana, P. B., Guan, X. J., Ingram, R. S. & Tilghman, S. M. (1998). Genomic imprinting is disrupted in interspecific *Peromyscus* hybrids. *Nat. Genet.*, **20**, 362–5.

Yadegari, R., Kinoshita, T., Lotan, O. *et al.* (2000). Mutations in the FIE and MEA genes that encode interacting polycomb proteins cause parent-of-origin effects on seed development by distinct mechanisms. *Plant Cell*, **12**, 2367–82.

Zechner, U., Hemberger, M., Constancia, M. *et al.* (2002). Proliferation and growth factor expression in abnormally enlarged placentae of mouse interspecific hybrids. *Dev. Dyn.*, **224**, 125–34.

DISCUSSION

McLaren   I have always been intrigued by the similarity between the plant system, where there are imprinted genes and methylation, and the expression in the endosperm, which, like trophoblast, is the initial feeding tissue. It is presumably convergent evolution, but who knows?

Ferguson-Smith   In light of the role of *Ezh2* in X inactivation I was wondering whether in the mutants there was a difference in phenotype between males and females.

Surani   We thought that there could be a difference between males and females, but we can't detect any differences between male and female conceptuses. The ratios of male and female embryos are normal so there is no skewing. It suggests that the effects are on autosomal genes, and possibly on imprinted genes that affect both male and female embryos to the same extent.

Ferguson-Smith   Have you looked at some of the inner/outer markers in the early to mid-preimplantation stages, such as Nanog or Cdx2, to see whether there are any abnormalities?

Surani	We haven't done this, but it would be interesting to look at this aspect. What we do know is that in oocytes depleted of Ezh2, the histone H3meK27 methylation is restored at around the 16-cell stage. This is quite a critical time for the establishment of the inner and outer cells that give rise to the inner cell mass and trophectoderm cells.
Reik	It seems that the most logical thing that could happen in the mutant is that you lose K27 methylation from the maternally imprinted genes, either in the oocyte or perhaps very early after fertilisation. But this would predict the opposite phenotype, namely that you get bigger embryos. Have you looked at *Lit*?
Hajkova	Not yet.
Reik	From the molecular sequence of events that would be the most logical thing to happen, but the phenotype doesn't suggest this.
Surani	There isn't as much histone H3meK27 methylation of the maternal genome in oocytes that are depleted of Ezh2. However, it is possible that this status does not persist for long enough to induce changes in imprints because H3meK27 methylation is restored by the 16-cell stage. This may be too short a time interval for loss of imprints to occur. If we don't find any differences, then I think that this might be an explanation. Further experiments are in progress that might answer this question.
Reik	What you are saying is that Ezh2 is not necessary for the establishment of imprints during oogenesis.
Surani	No, we can't rule out this possibility. The ZP3-Cre that induces deletion of the floxed allele switches on quite soon as the oocyte starts to grow. It is possible therefore that this can affect initiation of imprints as they are being set at this time. We can't exclude this. There is a potential experiment we can do that might get around this problem. We could delay the loss of *Ezh2* to some extent, or reduce the levels of Ezh2 without completely eliminating it.
Reik	If there is altered imprinting or loss of imprinting, do you envisage because of the phenotype that this is limited to the placenta and does not happen in the embryo? If this is the case, how would it work mechanistically? It would be quite a mystery.
Surani	Since the neonates are all right at the end, we can assume that there are no effects on imprinting in the embryo itself. One thing to remember is that the trophectoderm lineage is the first to start differentiating. Enhancer of Zeste is not expressed at the 16-cell stage. There could be a situation in which there is lack of appropriate epigenetic modification which is going to be more critical for the development of the placenta than for the embryo. The embryo has a longer time to recover because it is going to make epiblast and then differentiate later on. This is the only way I can explain it.
Dey	Does transient silencing of Ezh2 have any effect on fertilisation, preimplantation development and implantation timing?

Surani   I don't know about timing, but in terms of numbers of conceptuses we haven't seen any differences between control and experimental ones. We assume that the timing of implantation and the numbers implanting are not affected by this transient loss of Ezh2.

Dey   We have some evidence that if the timing of implantation is changed, there will then be a ripple effect throughout gestation with placental defects and fetal abnormalities.

Surani   When we take out the blastocysts and look at them at a gross level, they look very similar to the control blastocysts. If blastocysts lack Ezh2 completely as is the case when we generate *Ezh2* null embryos, we can't make pluripotent stem cells out of them. We haven't tried making trophectoderm stem cells. We were actually discussing a possibility that we might be able to make male trophectoderm stem cell lines from these blastocysts, but we certainly can't make embryonic stem cell lines.

McLaren   The timing question is interesting because there is a narrow window where implantation in the uterus is possible for a blastocyst, at least in the mouse (McLaren & Michie 1956, McLaren 1965a). If one is towards the end of that window it may well be that the conditions for fetal growth and trophoblast differentiation are not as good.

Keverne   If I remember correctly, David Haig's theory of genomic conflict came from work on endosperm as well as work on *Igf2* and its receptor. But if you are saying that it is polycomb genes that are maternally inherited and that they actually determine methylation or histone deacetylation, does this bring into question which parental genome is doing what in terms of conflict?

Surani   That is a very complicated question, partly because of *MEDEA*, the homologue of *Ezh2* in *Arabidopsis*. This is methylated and it has to be demethylated by another gene called *DEMETER*. This is brought in by sperm and is only active in the endosperm. This causes demethylation of *MEDEA*, which starts to be expressed in the endosperm. Some people have done microarray analysis on endosperm following loss of *MEDEA*. They find that a number of target genes are affected. I am puzzled by the conflict hypothesis and I don't know how to answer that question.

Cross   You showed histological sections of the placenta from a late stage (day 19.5). Have you looked at earlier stages?

Surani   No, we have not done this.

Cross   I would suggest that you do this, only because in the spongiotrophoblast and glycogen cells it looked like there was a change in their normal proportions. This layer often changes as a secondary response to other things going on in the placenta. In particular, the part of the placenta that I would concentrate on is the labyrinth, which represents the major surface area for nutrient transport.

Reik	I was thinking of an answer to my own question that I asked earlier! Both Robert Feil's lab and ours have found that there are histone methylation imprints that do not have DNA methylation imprints to accompany them. These include K27 and they are limited specifically to the placenta. So, if you lost those but maintained the ones that were accompanied by DNA methylation, then you might get an explanation for what you see.
Hajkova	I wanted to make a more general remark. To me it looks very likely that there are different reading systems of imprinting in the placenta and the embryo. There is a difference in general DNA methylation between placenta and embryo. Since the embryo is the one that will pass the imprints on to the next generation, or will erase or re-establish them according to the sex, the imprints must be much more flexible than in the placenta.
Reik	That is probably right, but there is more marking based on histone methylation in the placenta because it is less stable. The placenta is thrown away much earlier than the embryo. You were saying the opposite: they need to be more flexible in the embryo.
S. Fisher	Have you looked at HDAC expression?
Surani	No.
Sharkey	There is quite a bit of concern at the moment about assisted reproductive technology. Richard Schultz has remarked about how in culturing embryos for IVF you can begin to pick up differences between these and normal in vivo embryos. Have you any speculation about whether the expression of some of these factors such as Zest is different? Is anything known about epigenetic modifiers being altered just by culturing?
Surani	This is entirely possible. The impression we get is that epigenetic changes that are occurring post-fertilisation are dynamic and quite extensive. If you are using any kind of manipulation or culture, this is likely to alter it. There is some evidence that there is a higher propensity for Beckwith's Syndrome in procedures called ICSI involving microinjection of sperm into oocytes.
Sharkey	I was wondering whether you have any specific evidence?
Surani	We are not really there yet. We are still looking at this in a rather broad general way. We are still at the level of phenomenology, and we haven't got to the mechanistic levels yet.
McLaren	Just for the record, is the increase of incidence of Beckwith's specifically in ICSI or more generally in IVF? At one time it was thought that it might be the injection of a single sperm that caused this, but it may be a response to culture conditions.
Reik	It is in both. It isn't related to the specific technology that is being used. The other thing to highlight in this regard is that there is an increased incidence of a specific epigenetic defect in those cases, which is the loss of methylation of a maternally methylated gene region. To my mind it is the maintenance of that methylation during manipulation or culture which is the critical event here.

Kunath   Have you looked at the X-inactivation status in fetal embryos?

Surani   In the transient knockouts?

Kunath   Yes. I know you said there wasn't a sex difference.

Surani   We haven't looked at that specifically.

Kunath   Would you predict that the paternal alleles would be expressed normally?

Surani   We are making the assumption that X inactivation proceeds normally in embryos in this case. This is based on the fact that we are getting equal numbers of males and females, but we haven't looked at it directly.

Sibley   Some basic information about the trajectory of fetal growth: it is quite useful to know when the growth restriction starts in relation to when placental restriction starts. Have you looked at those time courses of placental and fetal weights?

Surani   No. So far we have only done our analyses on day 14.5.

Ferguson-Smith   Is the fetal–placental weight ratio the same as normal at that stage? In other words, is your fetus proportionally as small as your placenta?

Surani   I don't think we have numbers on this yet to make a definitive conclusion.

Hajkova   These results are preliminary. We started with comparing the placentas rather than comparing the fetal–placental ratios.

Ferguson-Smith   You have both fetal and placental weights. Calculating the ratio can provide insight about the nutritional supply to the fetus from the placenta. For example, if the placenta is small but the fetus is normal-sized, this means that the fetus is able to get enough nutriment from the small placenta.

Hajkova   The experimental placentas are substantially smaller than the control ones.

Ferguson-Smith   So you get an idea just from looking at it that the placenta is much smaller than you would expect from the size of the fetus.

Sibley   This ratio is particularly important for understanding what is happening in the placenta.

McLaren   One would expect it to be the chorioallantoic placenta that is affected.

Sibley   This was part of my thinking. From the pictures there seems to be a labyrinthine defect. But one should never forget that the yolk sac is really working in these species early on. This is one of the other reasons for asking about conceptus size.

McLaren   The effect of crowding, for instance, on fetal and placental growth in the mouse only happens after the chorioallantoic placenta has formed (Healy *et al.* 1960, McLaren & Michie 1960, McLaren 1965b).

REFERENCES

Healy, M. J. R., McLaren, A. & Michie, D. (1960). Foetal growth in the mouse. *Proc. R. Soc. Ser. B Biol. Sci.*, **153**, 367–79.

McLaren, A. (1965a). Maternal factors in nidation. In W. W. Park, ed., *The Early Conceptus, Normal and Abnormal*. Edinburgh: University of St Andrews Press, pp. 27–33.

(1965b). Genetic and environmental effects on foetal and placental growth in the mouse. *J. Reprod. Fertil.*, **9**, 79–98.

McLaren, A. & Michie, D. (1956). Studies on the transfer of fertilized mouse eggs to uterine foster-mothers. I. Factors affecting the implantation and survival of native and transferred eggs. *J. Exp. Biol.*, **33**, 394–416.

(1960). Control of pre-natal growth in mammals. *Nature*, **187**, 363–5.

4

Regulation of X-chromosome inactivation in relation to lineage allocation in early mouse embryogenesis

Neil Brockdorff

MRC Clinical Sciences Centre, Imperial College Faculty of Medicine, UK

Overview

The X-inactivation hypothesis, put forward by Mary Lyon in 1961, proposed that in mammals a single X chromosome is selected at random and genetically silenced early in embryogenesis. It was further proposed that the inactive state is stably maintained throughout the lifetime of the animal, and therefore that females are comprised of clonal cell populations derived from progenitor cells with either one X chromosome or the other inactive (Lyon 1961). In the intervening years the Lyon hypothesis has been verified on many levels and there has been significant progress towards understanding the molecular mechanisms governing this process (for a recent review see Heard *et al.* 1997). Along the way there have been a number of unanticipated surprises in the form of exceptions to the general pattern. Perhaps of most note is the finding that there is preferential inactivation of the paternally derived X chromosome (Xp), as opposed to random inactivation of either X chromosome, in marsupial mammals (Sharman 1971) and in extraembryonic lineages derived from the trophectoderm (TE) and primitive endoderm (PE) of early mouse embryos (Takagi & Sasaki 1975, Takagi *et al.* 1978).

The quest to understand how the paternally imprinted form of X inactivation is regulated has provided an important impetus that has aided our understanding of the earliest differentiative events in mammalian (eutherian) embryogenesis. Here I will focus on recent studies, which have led to a reappraisal of the classical model for initiation of imprinted X inactivation in mouse embryos. I will discuss how these observations are helping to reshape our understanding of early preimplantation development. I will then discuss the implications of this work for our understanding of somatic cell reprogramming following nuclear transfer or fusion with pluripotent embryonic stem (ES) cells.

Biology and Pathology of Trophoblast, eds. Ashley Moffett, Charlie Loke and Anne McLaren.
Published by Cambridge University Press © Cambridge University Press 2005.

A new model for the initiation of imprinted X inactivation

Classical studies, based on analysis of protein products of X-linked genes indicated that both X chromosomes are active in XX embryos at least up to the morula stage (Epstein *et al.* 1978, Kratzer & Gartler 1978, Monk & Harper 1979). Consistent with this, the earliest stage at which an inactive X chromosome can be detected cytologically is the blastocyst. Importantly, it is always Xp that is inactivated at this time (Takagi *et al.* 1978). Because imprinted X inactivation is seen only in TE and PE derived tissues, it was extrapolated that the inactive Xp originates from these cells. Cells of the inner cell mass (ICM), which gives rise to the embryo proper and are characterised by random X inactivation (initiated in the epiblast of early post-implantation embryos at 5.5–6 days *post coitum* (dpc)), were thought to retain two active X chromosomes. This view was articulated by Monk & Harper (1979) who proposed that imprinted X inactivation is coupled to the onset of cellular differentiation of the TE and PE during blastocyst maturation. In the ICM it was proposed that the imprint governing paternal X inactivation is erased, establishing the ground state for the onset of random X inactivation, coupled to cellular differentiation of the epiblast (see Plate 2A). Initiation of X inactivation could thus be viewed as a marker for cellular differentiation from early totipotent or pluripotent cell types.

The idea that initiation of X inactivation is coupled to cellular differentiation has held sway for a considerable time. However, recent findings are leading to a significant revision. The first discrepancies started to appear following the discovery of the X inactive specific transcript (*Xist*) gene, the master *cis*-acting switch regulating X inactivation. As its name suggests, the *Xist* gene is expressed exclusively from the inactive X chromosome. The gene produces a large non-coding RNA that coats the entire length of the chromosome *in cis*. The *Xist* RNA then triggers chromosome silencing by recruiting factors that modify the chromatin configuration from a euchromatic (active) to a heterochromatic (silent) state (for a recent review see Brockdorff 2002). Consistent with the role of *Xist* in triggering X inactivation, early expression studies, using reverse transcriptase (RT)-PCR, demonstrated that *Xist* expression in preimplantation XX embryos is exclusively from Xp, with expression of the maternal X (Xm) allele only appearing post-implantation when random X inactivation initiates (Kay *et al.* 1993). Surprisingly, Xp *Xist* expression could be detected as early as the two- to four-cell stage, significantly before the time when imprinted X inactivation coupled to TE and PE differentiation was thought to occur (i.e. the morula/blastocyst transition). Moreover, subsequent studies using RNA fluorescent *in situ* hybridisation (FISH) methods demonstrated that coating of Xp with *Xist* RNA could be seen in all cells of XX embryos from the four- to eight-cell stage onwards (Sheardown *et al.* 1997, Nesterova *et al.* 2001, and see

Plate 2B). Thus early *Xist* expression could not be discounted simply as a low level of non-productive transcription. These observations were rationalised by supposing that *Xist* RNA coating is not sufficient to trigger chromosome silencing in undifferentiated cells, and that the critical silencing factors that bind *Xist* RNA are produced only with the onset of cellular differentiation (Sheardown *et al.* 1997).

Further evidence challenging the link between the onset of X inactivation and cellular differentiation came with the development of PCR-based methods for analysing X-linked gene expression in preimplantation embryos. Singer-Sam *et al.* (1992) showed that *Pgk1*, but not *Hprt*, is partially repressed on Xp as early as the eight-cell stage. The authors suggested this could be a proximity effect because *Pgk1* lies closer to the *Xist* locus. Further support for this idea came from a study analysing X-linked gene expression in androgenetic preimplantation embryos bearing only Xp. The *Pgk1* gene was markedly repressed as early as the eight-cell stage. Genes located further away from the *Xist* locus were also repressed but to a lesser extent (Latham & Rambhatla 1995). More recently the gradient of Xp inactivation centred on *Xist* was demonstrated for normal XX embryos at the 8- to 16-cell stage (Huynh & Lee 2003). In considering these findings it should be borne in mind that the disappearance of Xp RNAs, and also their protein products, will lag behind transcriptional silencing to a degree dependent on the stability of individual RNA/protein species. This suggests that Xp inactivation may be initiated prior to specification of TE cells at the morula stage and certainly before overt differentiation of TE cells at the blastocyst stage.

Recent results appear to have resolved these disparate and apparently contradictory findings. Taking advantage of new reagents that allow the detection of chromatin modifications characteristic of the inactive X chromosome (Xi) and/or the enzymes involved in establishing these epigenetic marks, it was demonstrated that Xp inactivation occurs in all cells prior to the morula stage, and that there is a subsequent reactivation event in late blastocysts, specifically in ICM cells that are allocated to the pluripotent epiblast lineage (Mak *et al.* 2004, Okamoto *et al.* 2004; Plate 2C). Thus, differentiation of TE and PE lineages is not required to initiate Xp inactivation but instead serves to fix the imprinted pattern of X inactivation established at or prior to the morula stage.

Although chromosome-wide changes associated with X inactivation can be seen as early as the four- to eight-cell stage, silencing of X-linked genes lags somewhat behind. This is exemplified by the gradient of silencing centred on the *Xist* locus at the morula stage, with near complete silencing seen only for genes close to *Xist* (Singer-Sam *et al.* 1992, Latham & Rambhatla 1995, Huynh & Lee 2003, Mak *et al.* 2004). With this in mind we can explain the biallelic expression of X-linked genes/gene products in preimplantation XX embryos observed in classical studies. At least part of the reason for the delay in gene silencing, as mentioned above, is that disappearance of RNA/protein will lag behind cessation of transcription to an extent determined by the stability of individual RNA/protein species. There is, however, evidence from studies on random X inactivation in differentiating XX ES cells, indicating that establishment of X inactivation occurs in a gradual and progressive manner (Keohane *et al.* 1996, Mermoud *et al.* 1999, Heard *et al.* 2001, Chaumeil *et al.* 2002), and this may also be a factor. Progressive establishment of X inactivation may also account for the fact that classical cytological approaches failed to detect an Xi earlier than the blastocyst stage (Takagi *et al.* 1978).

Time of onset of Xp inactivation

The time of initiation of paternally imprinted X inactivation has been the subject of recent debate. Huynh & Lee (2003) have proposed that the gradient of Xp inactivation observed at the morula stage represents a carry-over of a pre-inactive state established during male meiosis. This idea is predicated on the observation that the XY bivalent is genetically silenced at the pachytene stage of male meiosis (Monesi 1965). To support their contention Huynh & Lee use co-hybridisation of *Xist* and cot1 probes (used to detect nascent RNA transcripts), to show apparent cessation of transcription underlying *Xist* RNA domains in two-cell embryos. Whilst the idea that Xp arrives in the zygote in a pre-inactivated state is attractive, there are both indirect and direct lines of evidence arguing against this hypothesis. The Xi in female soma is characterised by specific chromatin modifications that are not observed in association with the XY bivalent, for example methylation of histone H3-lysine (K) 27 catalysed by the PRC2 Polycomb-group complex (Silva *et al.* 2003). The XY bivalent on the other hand is characterised by tri-methylation of H3-K9 (Cowell *et al.* 2002), localisation of heterochromatin protein 1 (Motzkus *et al.* 1999) and phosphorylation of histone H2AX (Fernandez-Capetillo *et al.* 2003), modifications not seen on Xi in female somatic cells. These differences imply that distinct mechanisms operate in the two situations. Consistent with this, silencing of the XY bivalent does not require *Xist* RNA (McCarrey *et al.* 2002, Turner *et al.* 2002). Given that the gradient of Xp inactivation in morulae is centred on the *Xist* locus, this factor clearly argues against early Xp inactivation being a carry-over of silencing of the XY bivalent.

Direct evidence arguing against the pre-inactivation hypothesis comes from two studies. First, Hendriksen *et al.* (1995) have demonstrated that X- and Y-linked genes inactivated at the pachytene stage of male meiosis, are reactivated during spermiogenesis, indicating that silencing of the XY bivalent is transitory. Second, Okamoto *et al.* (2004) used RNA FISH to demonstrate that the *Brx/chic1* locus is expressed from the Xp allele in two-cell XX embryos. The *Brx/chic1* locus lies very close to the *Xist* locus and is the gene most obviously silenced at the morula stage in the study by Huynh & Lee (2003). In addition, Okamoto *et al.* (2004) observed cessation of transcription underlying *Xist* RNA domains, as measured by absence of RNA polymerase II c-terminal domain (PolII CTD) phosphorylation at the four- to eight-cell stage, but not earlier.

Taken together the data can best be explained by supposing that Xp inactivation is initiated in the zygote, commensurate with the onset of Xp *Xist* expression at the two- to four-cell stage. Gradual spreading of *Xist* RNA and progressive establishment of a fully inactivated chromatin structure would account for the gradient of gene silencing centred on *Xist*, and biallelic expression of X-linked genes in early stage embryos.

Xp inactivation in relation to early lineage allocation

The TE arises from outer cells of morula stage embryos, with the inner cells giving rise to the ICM (Hillman *et al.* 1972). Cell fate is not determined at this time as transplanted cells adopt a fate dependent on their relocation to the inside or outside of the embryo. In the classical model Xp inactivation initiates as TE and subsequently PE cells are determined, and it was therefore envisaged that the inner cells of morulae and the ICM cells of blastocyst never undergo imprinted Xp inactivation. Building on this Huynh and Lee suggested that inner cells of XX morulae may be distinct in having a lower level of Xp *Xist* RNA, providing an early distinguishing feature of cells destined to contribute to ICM versus TE (Huynh & Lee 2003). However, studies by Nesterova *et al.* (2001), and more recently by Okamoto *et al.* (2004), found apparently equivalent Xp *Xist* RNA domains in most cells from four- to eight-cell until late blastocyst stages, regardless of their position in the embryo. Moreover, the recent analysis of chromatin modifications associated with Xi clearly demonstrates that Xp inactivation is initiated in ICM as well as TE cells (Mak *et al.* 2004, Okamoto *et al.* 2004). A possible explanation for Huynh and Lee's observation is that they recorded cells in early G1- or M-phase, which are known to have reduced *Xist* RNA domains. This is because *Xist* RNA dissociates from the X chromosome at mitosis and must be resynthesised in the subsequent G1-phase (Clemson *et al.* 1996, Duthie *et al.* 1999).

As argued above, differentiation of TE is not required to initiate Xp inactivation but instead fixes the Xp inactivation pattern set up in early cleavage stage embryos. A similar argument can be applied to the PE lineage. Nesterova *et al.* (2001) and Okamoto *et al.* (2004) analysed *Xist* expression in cells from isolated ICM. Extinction of Xp *Xist* RNA was observed in approximately 50% of cells but only in the ICM of late stage blastocysts. Mak *et al.* (2004) observed that the homeodomain protein Nanog, a key determinant of the pluripotent epiblast cells (Chambers *et al.* 2003, Mitsui *et al.* 2003), is highly expressed in approximately 50% of cells in the ICM region, and that it is in these cells where Xp *Xist* RNA extinction and loss of Xi heterochromatin marks occurs. This indicates that early ICM cells undergo a bipotential switch giving rise to the PE and pluripotent epiblast lineages. The pluripotent epiblast cells extinguish Xp *Xist* expression with resultant Xp reactivation, whereas cells allocated to PE maintain Xp *Xist* expression, and imprinted X inactivation is therefore fixed.

The study of Mak *et al.* (2004) revealed an unexpected feature of ICM development during separation of PE and pluripotent epiblast lineages. In the ICM region of early- and mid-stage blastocysts Nanog-positive cells (presumptive pluripotent epiblast) and Nanog-negative cells (presumptive PE cells) were randomly distributed (see Plate 3). This contrasts with the organisation of these cells in late-stage blastocysts where the pluripotent epiblast cells are clustered and underlie a single layer of PE cells. These observations indicate that following the bipotential switch to pluripotent epiblast or PE fate, cell sorting and migration is required to establish the prototypical organisation of the ICM.

On the nature of reversible and irreversible heterochromatin

Paternally derived X chromosome reactivation in the pluripotent epiblast provides important insights into the plasticity of cells of the early embryo. X inactivation in XX somatic cells is generally irreversible. Conditional deletion of the *Xist* locus or treatment with drugs known to affect DNA methylation and histone acetylation cause only rare sporadic reactivation of individual genes and never chromosome-wide global reactivation (Mohandas *et al.* 1981, Brown & Willard 1994, Csankovszki *et al.* 1999, 2001). However, X reactivation does occur in XX primordial germ cells around the time that they migrate to the genital ridge (Monk & McLaren 1981), and also in experiments where nuclei from XX somatic cells are exposed to oocyte cytoplasm following nuclear transfer (Eggan *et al.* 2000), or following cell fusion with ES or embryonic germ (EG) cells (Tada *et al.* 1997). It is likely that the mechanisms responsible for reactivating stable heterochromatin on the inactive X in these situations are more generally involved in the erasure of epigenetic marks in somatic cell reprogramming.

An important insight into the mechanism of X reactivation comes from experiments in ES cells using an inducible *Xist* transgene (Wutz & Jaenisch 2000). Switching on the transgene in undifferentiated ES cells leads to chromosome-wide inactivation, but in contrast to the situation in XX somatic cells, inactivation is reversed when transgene expression is then switched off. This reversibility and *Xist* dependence of X inactivation is retained for the first 24–48 hours following differentiation, but is then lost. In a similar timeframe differentiating ES cells lose their ability to respond to *de novo Xist* expression, suggesting that the factors required to establish inactive chromatin structure are only available during a restricted window in early development. This is consistent with results from an earlier study indicating that induction of *Xist* in XX somatic cell lines does not result in chromosome silencing (Clemson *et al.* 1998). The recent observations on reversible Xp inactivation in pluripotent epiblast cells suggest that this may provide an in vivo corollary for the experimental ES cell model.

In differentiated XX somatic cells, where *Xist* is neither necessary to maintain silencing, nor sufficient to induce silencing, the heterochromatin can be considered to be self-maintaining. The mechanisms responsible for this do not appear to operate in ES cells or the pluripotent epiblast. Instead ongoing *Xist* expression and the resulting recruitment of silencing factors maintain Xi heterochromatin through successive cell divisions. From this we can speculate either that a chromatin feature determining self-maintaining heterochromatin is absent in ES/ICM cells, or alternatively that these cells lack a factor(s) that allows Xi chromatin features to be transmitted through S-phase and mitosis. The latter is conceptually similar to the model in which maintenance of centromeric heterochromatin involves recognition of histone H3-K9 methylation by heterochromatin protein 1 (HP1), and direct recruitment of the Suv39 histone methyltransferase, responsible for H3-K9 methylation, by HP1 (Lachner *et al.* 2001). Many, though not necessarily all, chromatin modifications seen on Xi in XX somatic cells have been reported to occur in response to *Xist* RNA in ES/ICM cells (Keohane *et al.* 1996, Mermoud *et al.* 1999, Heard *et al.* 2001, Chaumeil *et al.* 2002, Mak *et al.* 2004, Okamoto *et al.* 2004.) These include hypoacetylation of histones H3 and H4, dimethylation of histone H3-K9, trimethylation of H3-K27, and loss of methylation of histone H3-K4. Incorporation of the variant histone macroH2A, another inactive X feature in XX somatic cells, also occurs in ICM cells (our unpublished results). It follows that none of these modifications in themselves are sufficient to confer irreversibility of X inactivation and *Xist* RNA. Thus, we can conclude that a chromatin modification not yet examined in ICM/ES cells, for example DNA methylation of CpG islands, confers *Xist* independence and irreversibility or, as mentioned above, that a factor with a similar function to HP1 in maintaining centromeric heterochromatin is absent in these cells.

Xist extinction, Xp reactivaton and reprogramming

Studies on inducible *Xist* RNA transgenes demonstrated that switching off *Xist* in ES cells is sufficient for chromosome reactivation. The same appears to be true for pluripotent epiblast cells, as in late blastocysts these cells extinguish *Xist* RNA, and as a result reactivate Xp. A good illustration of this is provided by the sequential extinction of Xp *Xist* RNA, dissociation of the PRC2 Polycomb-group protein Eed, and subsequent loss of H3-K27 methylation, the chromatin modification catalysed by the PRC2 complex (Mak *et al.* 2004).

The importance of *Xist* RNA extinction in X reactivation is interesting to consider in the context of previous studies on the regulation of *Xist* expression. In ES cells *Xist* is transcribed at a low level and in conjunction with an antisense RNA, referred to as *Tsix*, which encompasses the entire *Xist* locus (Debrand *et al.* 1999, Lee *et al.* 1999). This expression pattern occurs at the single *Xist* allele in XY epiblast/ES cells and on both alleles in XX epiblast/ES cells. Upon differentiation *Xist* is up-regulated from a single allele in XX cells and the low level *Xist* and *Tsix* expression is lost from the other allele, or from the single allele in XY cells. *Tsix* is important in the regulation of random X inactivation, as deletion of the major promoter results in non-random X inactivation of the targeted allele in XX cells (Lee & Lu 1999). Current models suggest that *Tsix* represses *Xist* expression at the onset of differentiation. However, deletion of *Tsix* is not sufficient to up-regulate *Xist* in undifferentiated ES cells, suggesting that there is an additional factor involved in *Xist* repression. We can speculate that ES cells, and by extension pluripotent epiblast cells, lack factors required for high level *Xist* expression, or alternatively produce an *Xist* repressor. This scenario would then be reversed when ES/epiblast cells differentiate, allowing high *Xist* expression and consequent random X inactivation. Figure 4.1 illustrates this model in the context of early mouse embryogenesis.

How does the model succeed in accommodating other situations where X reactivation occurs? First, in the female germ line, extinction of *Xist* RNA expression has been shown to occur at around the time primordial germ cells (PGCs) arrive at the genital ridge (Nesterova *et al.* 2002). Our own more recent studies suggest this event is initiated even earlier, in migrating PGCs (our unpublished results). For this to be sufficient to explain reactivation of the inactive X chromosome, we would need to suppose that the nuclear environment in maturing PGCs lacks activities required for *Xist*-independent maintenance of inactive X chromatin structure, similar to the situation in pluripotent epiblast cells. Consistent with this, PGCs, like early epiblast cells, express the key pluripotency associated factors, Oct4 (Scholer *et al.* 1989) and Nanog (Chambers *et al.* 2003). In addition, pluripotent epiblast cells and PGCs both give rise to similar pluripotent cell lines, ES and EG cells respectively, when cultivated in vitro.

X reactivation also occurs in hybrid cells formed by fusion of XX somatic cells with ES/EG cells (Tada *et al.* 1997, 2001). Here too we can invoke a two-step process in which the ES/EG cell contribution establishes a nuclear environment that lacks the factors required for *Xist*-independent maintenance of X inactivation, and additionally results in extinction of *Xist* RNA expression from the somatic cell-derived Xi.

X reactivation following nuclear transfer to unfertilised oocytes provides perhaps the most interesting case to discuss. Here it has been found that genes on Xi in a donor somatic nucleus are reactivated, with expression first seen at around the

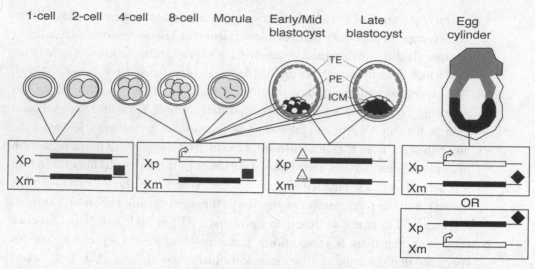

Figure 4.1   The *Xist* gene regulation in early development. This model proposes that the *Xist* promoter is active by default and that specific mechanisms come into play to repress *Xist* at different developmental stages. Up to the two-cell stage absence of embryonic transcription accounts for *Xist* RNA repression. From two-cell until morula stage, Xp *Xist* is expressed in all cells (expression indicated by open rectangle and arrow at 5′ end). X maternal *Xist* is repressed by a maternal imprint (black square), which is thought to be mediated through the *Tsix* promoter located at the 3′ end of the locus (Lee 2000, Sado *et al.* 2001). This pattern is maintained in TE and PE cells and also in their derivative tissues. To account for extinction of *Xist* in the ICM it is proposed that a specific repressor (triangle) is produced in cells allocated to the pluripotent epiblast. It is further proposed that this factor is switched off when epiblast/ES/EG differentiates. It is plausible that the same pathway is responsible for extinction of *Xist* expression in maturing primordial germ cells (PGCs). Re-expression of *Xist* in differentiating XX epiblast cells is monoallelic and random. Current models invoke a blocking factor (filled diamond) that is present in limiting quantities and binds to the 3′ end of one of the two *Xist* alleles (reviewed in Avner & Heard 2001).

8–16-cell stage. However, in post-implantation cloned embryos TE-derived tissues were seen to have the same X chromosome inactive as the original donor nucleus (Eggan *et al.* 2000). This can be explained in the following way. First we can predict that TE cells retain the same X-inactivation pattern as the donor nucleus because the embryos retain donor cell *Xist* expression. The programme leading to erasure of *Xist* expression patterns would however come into play in ICM cells that are allocated to the pluripotent epiblast lineage, as is the case in normal embryos, and this would in turn result in random X inactivation in the embryo proper. The X-inactivation pattern in PE-derived cells should also be the same as in the donor nucleus. This prediction has not been tested as yet.

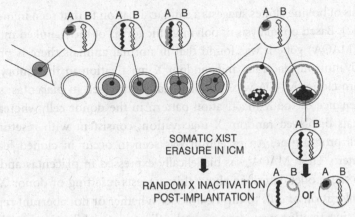

Figure 4.2   A model for regulation of X inactivation in cloned mouse embryos. The figure illustrates an XX donor cell with the inactive X chromosome (A) coated with *Xist* RNA (shaded line). Transcription from the donor nucleus, including *Xist* RNA, is repressed by oocyte factors until the two-cell stage, resulting in X reactivation. Recommencement of *Xist* expression then occurs at the two-cell stage. Retention of the epigenetic marks that regulate *Xist* expression in the donor cell (for example DNA methylation) would result in the chromosome that was inactivated in the donor cell being inactivated again. As in normal embryos this early X inactivation will occur in all cells, accounting for retention of the donor X-inactivation pattern in TE derivatives (Eggan *et al.* 2000, Xue *et al.* 2002). In cells allocated to pluripotent epiblast, however, *Xist* expression will be extinguished, leading to a second reactivation event. Here erasure of the epigenetic marks governing donor *Xist* expression allows for subsequent random X inactivation in the embryo proper.

How does this model account for reactivation of donor Xi genes at the 8 to 16-cell stage? Expression of *Xist* from the donor cell-derived Xi should be ongoing if the factors responsible for *Xist* extinction are only present in pluripotent epiblast cells, and one would expect this to result in maintenance of X inactivation throughout the early stages of preimplantation development. The answer may lie in the fact that the early zygote is transcriptionally inactive. Assuming that the oocyte cytoplasm carries factors required for this genome-wide repression, we could anticipate that *Xist* expression, along with expression of the entire genome of the donor nucleus, would be transiently inhibited. This then could account for early reactivation of genes on Xi. Activation of the donor cell genome and resumption of *Xist* expression should occur at the two-cell stage. If we assume that the marks determining *Xist* expression patterns in the donor nucleus, for example DNA methylation of the *Xist* promoter, remain intact, resumption of *Xist* expression should occur specifically on what was the Xi allele in the donor cell. Thus, during cleavage stages and up until mid-blastocyst stage the embryos will undergo *de novo* X inactivation of the same X chromosome. These ideas are summarised in Figure 4.2.

Analysis of bovine clones suggests a similar situation to that seen in mouse (Xue *et al.* 2002). Based on analysis of polymorphic forms of the X-linked monoamine oxidase (MAOA) gene it was found that in normal animals there is preferential Xp inactivation in placentas and random X inactivation in the embryo proper. In liveborn clones MAOA was monoallelically expressed in placentas, suggestive of maintenance of the X-inactivation pattern in the donor cell, whereas cells of the animals displayed random X inactivation, consistent with resetting of the donor cell programme. An exception was seen to occur in cloned fetuses that died in utero. Here MAOA was biallelically expressed in placentas and embryo. Based on the model described above this suggests resetting of donor *Xist* alleles prior to allocation of cells to the TE lineage. Whether or not aberrant reprogramming of X inactivation provides a general indicator of viability in cloned fetuses is unknown.

Concluding remarks

Analysis of X inactivation in preimplantation mouse embryos has provided valuable insights into early mammalian development. Having said that, regulation of X inactivation in other mammalian species appears to be very different. In marsupials Xp is inactivated in embryonic tissues, suggesting perhaps that the mechanisms for initiating random X inactivation, including *Xist* extinction in epiblast cells, have not evolved. Conversely, in human embryos current evidence argues that random X inactivation occurs both in embryonic and extraembryonic lineages (Daniels *et al.* 1997, Ray *et al.* 1997, Looijenga *et al.* 1999). Here perhaps the imprint governing *Xist* expression is not laid down in the germ line, or alternatively may be erased early, prior to the onset of embryonic genome activation, which occurs at the eight-cell stage in human embryos. These differences highlight that imprinted X inactivation should not be viewed as a defining feature or requirement for the development of the TE and PE lineages in female embryos.

The revised view of regulation of X inactivation during mouse preimplantation embryogenesis has led us to the idea that X reactivation requires extinction of *Xist* RNA expression within a nuclear environment in which Xi heterochromatin is not self-maintaining. This model applies to X reactivation in the pluripotent epiblast lineage but can also be extrapolated to X reactivation in maturing XX PGCs, and in experimentally induced reactivation of Xi in a somatic nucleus following nuclear transfer to an enucleated oocyte, or following fusion with ES/EG cells. Important goals for future research will be to identify the pathway governing *Xist* extinction and to understand what determines reversible versus irreversible Xi heterochromatin.

REFERENCES

Avner, P. & Heard, E. (2001). X-chromosome inactivation: counting, choice and initiation. *Nat. Rev. Genet.*, **2**, 59–67.

Brockdorff, N. (2002). X-chromosome inactivation: closing in on proteins that bind Xist RNA. *Trends Genet.*, **18**, 352–8.

Brown, C. J. & Willard, H. F. (1994). The human X-inactivation centre is not required for maintenance of X-chromosome inactivation. *Nature*, **368**, 154–6.

Chambers, I., Colby, D., Robertson, M. *et al.* (2003). Functional expression cloning of Nanog, a pluripotency sustaining factor in embryonic stem cells. *Cell*, **113**, 643–55.

Chaumeil, J., Okamoto, I., Guggiari, M. & Heard, E. (2002). Integrated kinetics of X chromosome inactivation in differentiating embryonic stem cells. *Cytogenet. Genome Res.*, **99**, 75–84.

Clemson, C. M., McNeil, J. A., Willard, H. F. & Lawrence, J. B. (1996). XIST RNA paints the inactive X chromosome at interphase: Evidence for a novel RNA involved in nuclear chromosome structure. *J. Cell Biol.*, **132**, 259–75.

Clemson, C. M., Chow, J. C., Brown, C. J. & Lawrence, J. B. (1998). Stabilization and localization of Xist RNA are controlled by separate mechanisms and are not sufficient for X inactivation. *J. Cell Biol.*, **142**, 13–23.

Cowell, I. G., Aucott, R., Mahadevaiah, S. K. *et al.* (2002). Heterochromatin, HP1 and methylation at lysine 9 of histone H3 in animals. *Chromosoma*, **111**, 22–36.

Csankovszki, G., Panning, B., Bates, B., Pehrson, J. R. & Jaenisch, R. (1999). Conditional deletion of Xist disrupts histone macroH2A localization but not maintenance of X inactivation. *Nat. Genet.*, **22**, 323–4.

Csankovszki, G., Nagy, A. & Jaenisch, R. (2001). Synergism of Xist RNA, DNA methylation, and histone hypoacetylation in maintaining X chromosome inactivation. *J. Cell Biol.*, **153**, 773–84.

Daniels, R., Zuccotti, M., Kinis, T., Serhal, P. & Monk, M. (1997). XIST expression in human oocytes and pre-implantation embryos. *Am. J. Hum. Genet.*, **61**, 33–9.

Debrand, E., Chureau, C., Arnaud, D., Avner, P. & Heard, E. (1999). Functional analysis of the DXPas34 locus, a 3′ regulator of Xist expression. *Mol. Cell. Biol.*, **19**, 8513–25.

Duthie, S. M., Nesterova, T. B., Formstone, E. J. *et al.* (1999). Xist RNA exhibits a banded localization on the inactive X chromosome and is excluded from autosomal material in cis. *Hum. Mol. Genet.*, **8**, 195–204.

Eggan, K., Akutsu, H., Hochedlinger, K. *et al.* (2000). X-chromosome inactivation in cloned mouse embryos. *Science*, **290**, 1578–81.

Epstein, C. J., Smith, S., Travis, B. & Tucker, G. (1978). Both X chromosomes function before visible X-chromosome inactivation in female mouse embryos. *Nature*, **274**, 500–2.

Fernandez-Capetillo, O., Mahadevaiah, S. K., Celeste, A. *et al.* (2003). H2AX is required for chromatin remodeling and inactivation of sex chromosomes in male mouse meiosis. *Dev. Cell*, **4**, 497–508.

Heard, E., Clerc, P. & Avner, P. (1997). X chromosome inactivation in mammals. *Annu. Rev. Genet.*, **31**, 571–610.

Heard, E., Rougeulle, C., Arnaud, D. *et al.* (2001). Methylation of histone H3 at Lys-9 is an early mark on the X chromosome during X inactivation. *Cell*, **107**, 727–38.

Hendriksen, P. J., Hoogebrugge, J. W., Themmen, A. P. *et al.* (1995). Postmeiotic transcription of X and Y chromosomal genes during spermatogenesis in the mouse. *Dev. Biol.*, **170**, 730–3.

Hillman, N., Sherman, M. I. & Graham, C. F. (1972). The effect of spatial arrangements on cell determination during mouse development. *J. Embryol. Exp. Morphol.*, **28**, 263–78.

Huynh, K. D. & Lee, J. T. (2003). Inheritance of a pre-inactivated paternal X chromosome in early mouse embryos. *Nature*, **426**, 857–62.

Kay, G. F., Penny, G. D., Patel, D. *et al.* (1993). Expression of Xist during mouse development suggests a role in the initiation of X chromosome inactivation. *Cell*, **72**, 171–82.

Keohane, A. M., O'Neill, L. P., Belyaev, N. D., Lavender, J. S. & Turner, B. M. (1996). X inactivation and histone H4 acetylation in embryonic stem cells. *Dev. Biol.*, **180**, 618–30.

Kratzer, P. G. & Gartler, S. M. (1978). HGPRT activity changes in pre-implantation mouse embryos. *Nature*, **274**, 503–4.

Lachner, M., O'Carroll, D., Rea, S., Mechtler, K. & Jenuwein, T. (2001). Methylation of histone H3 lysine 9 creates a binding site for HP1 proteins. *Nature*, **410**, 116–20.

Latham, K. E. & Rambhatla, L. (1995). Expression of X-linked genes in androgenetic, gynogenetic, and normal mouse pre-implantation embryos. *Dev. Genet.*, **17**, 212–22.

Lee, J. T. (2000). Disruption of imprinted X inactivation by parent-of-origin effects at Tsix. *Cell*, **103**, 17–27.

Lee, J. T. & Lu, N. F. (1999). Targeted mutagenesis of Tsix leads to nonrandom X inactivation. *Cell*, **99**, 47–57.

Lee, J. T., Davidow, L. S. & Warshawsky, D. (1999). Tsix, a gene antisense to Xist at the X-inactivation centre. *Nat. Genet.*, **21**, 400–4.

Looijenga, L. H., Gillis, A. J., Verkerk, A. J., van Putten, W. L. & Oosterhuis, J. W. (1999). Heterogeneous X inactivation in trophoblastic cells of human full-term female placentae. *Am. J. Hum. Genet.*, **64**, 1445–52.

Lyon, M. F. (1961). Gene action in the X chromosome of the mouse (*Mus musculus* L). *Nature*, **190**, 372–3.

Mak, W., Nesterova, T. B., de Napoles, M. *et al.* (2004). Reactivation of the paternal X chromosome in early mouse embryos. *Science*, **303**, 666–9.

McCarrey, J. R., Watson, C., Atencio, J. *et al.* (2002). X-chromosome inactivation during spermatogenesis is regulated by an Xist/Tsix-independent mechanism in the mouse. *Genesis*, **34**, 257–66.

Mermoud, J. E., Costanzi, C., Pehrson, J. R. & Brockdorff, N. (1999). Histone macroH2A1.2 relocates to the inactive X chromosome after initiation and propagation of X-inactivation. *J. Cell Biol.*, **147**, 1399–1408.

Mitsui, K., Tokuzawa, Y., Itoh, H. *et al.* (2003). The homeoprotein Nanog is required for maintenance of pluripotency in mouse epiblast and ES cells. *Cell*, **113**, 631–42.

Mohandas, T., Sparkes, R. S. & Shapiro, L. J. (1981). Reactivation of an inactive human X chromosome: evidence for X inactivation by DNA methylation. *Science*, **211**, 393–6.

Monesi, V. (1965). Differential rate of ribonucleic acid synthesis in the autosomes and the sex chromosomes during male meiosis in the mouse. *Chromosoma*, **17**, 11–21.

Monk, M. & Harper, M.I. (1979). Sequential X chromosome inactivation coupled with cellular differentiation in early mouse embryos. *Nature*, 281, 311–13.

Monk, M. & McLaren, A. (1981). X-chromosome activity in foetal germ cells of the mouse. *J. Embryol. Exp. Morphol.*, 63, 75–84.

Motzkus, D., Singh, P.B. & Hoyer Fender, S. (1999). M31, a murine homolog of *Drosophila* HP1, is concentrated in the XY body during spermatogenesis. *Cytogenet. Cell Genet.*, 86, 83–8.

Nesterova, T.B., Barton, S.C., Surani, M.A. & Brockdorff, N. (2001). Loss of Xist imprinting in diploid parthenogenetic pre-implantation embryos. *Dev. Biol.*, 235, 343–50.

Nesterova, T.B., Mermoud, J.E., Hilton, K. *et al.* (2002). Xist expression and macroH2A1.2 localization in mouse primordial and pluripotent embryonic germ cells. *Differentiation*, 69, 216–25.

Okamoto, I., Otte, A.P., Allis, C.D., Reinberg, D. & Heard, E. (2004). Epigenetic dynamics of imprinted X inactivation during early mouse development. *Science*, 303, 644–9.

Ray, P.F., Winston, R.M. & Handyside, A.H. (1997). XIST expression from the maternal X chromosome in human male pre-implantation embryos at the blastocyst stage. *Hum. Mol. Genet.*, 6, 1323–7.

Sado, T., Wang, Z., Sasaki, H. & Li, E. (2001). Regulation of imprinted X-chromosome inactivation in mice by Tsix. *Development*, 128, 1275–86.

Scholer, H.R., Hatzopoulos, A.K., Balling, R., Suzuki, N. & Gruss, P. (1989). A family of octamer-specific proteins present during mouse embryogenesis: evidence for germline-specific expression of an Oct factor. *EMBO J.*, 8, 2543–50.

Sharman, G.B. (1971). Late DNA replication in the paternally derived X chromosome of female kangaroos. *Nature*, 230, 231–2.

Sheardown, S.A., Duthie, S.M., Johnston, C.M. *et al.* (1997). Stabilization of Xist RNA mediates initiation of X chromosome inactivation. *Cell*, 91, 99–107.

Silva, J., Mak, W., Zvetkova, I. *et al.* (2003). Establishment of histone H3 methylation on the inactive X chromosome requires transient recruitment of Eed-Enx1 Polycomb group complexes. *Dev. Cell*, 4, 481–95.

Singer-Sam, J., Chapman, V., LeBon, J.M. & Riggs, A.D. (1992). Parental imprinting studied by allele-specific primer extension after PCR: paternal X chromosome-linked genes are transcribed prior to preferential paternal X chromosome inactivation. *Proc. Natl. Acad. Sci. U.S.A.*, 89, 10469–73.

Tada, M., Tada, T., Lefebvre, L., Barton, S.C. & Surani, M.A. (1997). Embryonic germ cells induce epigenetic reprogramming of somatic nucleus in hybrid cells. *EMBO J.*, 16, 6510–20.

Tada, M., Takahama, Y., Abe, K., Nakatsuji, N. & Tada, T. (2001). Nuclear reprogramming of somatic cells by *in vitro* hybridisation with ES cells. *Curr. Biol.*, 11, 1553–8.

Takagi, N. & Sasaki, M. (1975). Preferential inactivation of the paternally derived X chromosome in the extra-embryonic membranes of the mouse. *Nature*, 256, 640–2.

Takagi, N., Wake, N. & Sasaki, M. (1978). Cytologic evidence for preferential inactivation of the paternally derived X chromosome in XX mouse blastocysts. *Cytogenet. Cell Genet.*, 20, 240–8.

Turner, J.M., Mahadevaiah, S.K., Elliott, D.J. *et al.* (2002). Meiotic sex chromosome inactivation in male mice with targeted disruptions of Xist. *J. Cell Sci.*, 115, 4097–105.

Wutz, A. & Jaenisch, R. (2000). A shift from reversible to irreversible X inactivation is triggered during ES cell differentiation. *Mol. Cell*, **5**, 695–705.

Xue, F., Tian, X. C., Du, F. *et al.* (2002). Aberrant patterns of X chromosome inactivation in bovine clones. *Nat. Genet.*, **31**, 216–20.

DISCUSSION

McLaren   Since Neil Brockdorff is sadly not able to be with us today, I thought it would be useful if we could spend a little time talking among ourselves about X-chromosome inactivation in the early embryo and trophoblast. We have known for many years that both X chromosomes could be expressed during cleavage in the mouse. For an X-coded enzyme such as *Hprt*, Marilyn Monk showed years ago that the level of enzyme expression was bimodal, with one group of embryos (presumably XX) having approximately twice the level of expression of the other group (XO or XY) (Monk 1978, Monk & Harper 1978). So in a sense, you could sex the cleavage stage mouse embryo by *Hprt* levels. We also know that in the extraembryonic membranes, including trophectoderm, the paternal X chromosome was inactivated. So some imprinting must have been retained, even though the paternal X had been expressed in early cleavage. In fetal tissues we knew that X inactivation was random, and it was widely assumed that both X chromosomes were active in the ICM, with one X becoming randomly inactivated in the epiblast. This picture has changed somewhat recently. There were two papers recently in *Science*, one from Neil Brockdorff's lab (Mak *et al.* 2004) and the other from Edith Heard's lab (Okamoto *et al.* 2004). Azim, tell us something of what is known today about X-chromosome inactivation in those early stages.

Surani   This is a story about two Marilyns. Marilyn Monk showed that there is preferential paternal X inactivation in the trophoblast. In the embryo itself, however, there is random X inactivation of either the maternal or the paternal X chromosome. This is an imprinting cycle that goes round and round with each generation. The question is, what is the mechanism by which you get random X inactivation in the embryo derived from epiblast, whereas there is paternal X inactivation in trophectoderm. It turns out that *Enhancer of Zeste* (*Ezh2*) and *Eed* complex are involved initially in the initiation of X inactivation, especially through histone H3-K27 methylation. This is the work that was done by Neil Brockdorff's and other groups. If we look at a blastocyst we can see accumulation of *Ezh2* and *Eed* on one of the two X chromosomes. If we use antibody against histone H3-K27 we get these two spots co-localised. This shows that the same complex that I was telling you about previously, is involved in this initiation process. The sequence of events taking place early on is as follows. There is the initial expression of *Xist* starting at around the two- to four-cell stage. This expression seems to be important for the recruitment of the Ezh2/Eed complex to the site of *Xist* expression. It turns out that all the cells show this including the histone H3meK27 methylation. Later on, at the 32-cell stage, there is another histone modification, an H3meK9 methylation. As far as the trophectoderm/primitive endoderm are concerned, there is a preferential inactivation of the paternal X chromosome. What happens in the ICM is that there is a loss of H3meK27 methylation. Somehow, the epiblast cells lose all these markings. This is important, because it then allows for random X inactivation to take place in the embryo itself. What is interesting is that this is where the *Nanog* connection comes in. This loss of modifications and *Xist* expression is seen exclusively in the epiblast cells in the late blastocyst. It is not seen in either the trophectoderm or the primary endoderm cells. This ties up with the expression of *Nanog*, which starts at the late morula stage and then is seen only in the epiblast. But this isn't seen in the trophectoderm or the primary endoderm cells. These epiblast cells are the cells from which all the marks are lost. When they develop subsequently after implantation, there is random X inactivation. This brings us to marsupials, and the second Marilyn: Marilyn Renfree. Marsupials have paternal X inactivation in all tissues. As far as I know there is no evidence for *Xist* expression. Marsupials lack an *Xist* homologue and there are other epigenetic differences between eutherian mammals and marsupials. One explanation might be that somehow when these epiblast cells develop in eutherians, it creates a special niche which may be necessary for the reversal of these markings. In marsupial embryos such a niche might be lacking. There is no special environment, which might be necessary for this erasure and then subsequent random X inactivation.

McLaren   There are two things about the Edith Heard/Neil Brockdorff story that puzzle me. The *Xist* RNA coats the inactive X chromosome, so when *Xist* is turned off both X chromosomes are presumably active. Is there a time in the epiblast when one can show that both X chromosomes in a female embryo are expressed? This should follow, but I have never heard this discussed.

Surani   In the embryo itself this period might be very short, during the late blastocyst stage. If you looked at blastocysts cultured in vitro you might be able to see it.

McLaren   The other thing that puzzled me was that Edith Heard showed that *Xist* is coating the inactive X already at the four-cell stage. This presumably prevents transcription. Would this mean that the expression of isoenzymes, e.g. HPRT, is all post-transcriptional at the 8- to 16-cell stage, which is when you can show that both X chromosomes are being expressed?

Ferguson-Smith   I think the work by her and also by Jeannie Lee has shown that it is probably a progressive process along the X that initiates very early and then progressively becomes more inactivated during the preimplantation stages.

McLaren   Do you that mean some blastomeres in the embryo but not others are affected, or that in each blastomere the inactivation proceeds gradually along the X chromosome?

Ferguson-Smith   Both, as far as I understand it. Yes, it is suggested that not all blastomeres are inactivating at the same time, but also that the X is inactivating in a gradient along its length. The gradient is bidirectional from *Xist* so not all genes are inactivating at the same time.

McLaren   Certainly, the *Hprt* gene in the mouse is located quite near the end of the X chromosome, so rather far from the X-inactivation centre.

Kunath   The primitive endoderm stuff is bewildering to me. Does the ICM lose the paternally imprinted X and then reactivate it again when the primary endoderm forms?

Surani   As I understand it this reversal starts relatively late in the blastocyst, and probably after the primary endoderm is already formed. It is only occurring in the epiblast cells that are Nanog positive.

Kunath   But the Nanog-positive cells appear quite early, prior to blastocyst formation.

Surani   Nanog is just a marker in this case. If you look in the blastocyst it is only in the epiblast cells but not the primary endoderm or the trophectoderm cells.

Kunath   So there isn't an erasure and then a re-imprinting of the inactive X chromosome in the primary endoderm.

Surani   I don't think so. The reactivation of the paternal X occurs after the primary endoderm is formed and then the marks are erased in the epiblast cells.

Kunath   What do Edith Heard and Neil Brockdorff think is the original imprint that is coming in from the fertilising sperm that causes *Xist* to accumulate on the paternal X at the four-cell stage?

Surani   I suppose it is lack of maternal *Xist* expression. The paternal *Xist* is therefore permissive for expression. There is some kind of parental-origin-dependent difference. It is quite controversial: many people have tried to see whether there were methylation differences between maternal and paternal *Xist* and this issue has not yet been resolved.

Ferguson-Smith   It is probably fair to mention in the context of the Heard and Brockdorff work a paper in *Nature* by Jeannie Lee (Huynh & Lee 2003). She says that the paternal X chromosome comes in pre-inactivated. One model for this is that the male meiotic germ-cell sex-chromosome inactivation has been carried through into the early embryo. This is a controversial area because there is an element of inconsistency between the two-cell embryo data of Edith Heard and the two-cell data from Jeannie Lee. Heard sees biallelic expression from both Xs at the two-cell stage and Lee doesn't. These are technically difficult questions to address so we need to wait to find out exactly what is going on.

Surani   This relates to the experiment that Rudi Jaenisch did with somatic nuclear transplantation (Eggan *et al.* 2000). In this case, what happens is that the original

X that is inactive is the one that becomes inactivated in trophectoderm, but in the embryo itself, X inactivation becomes random. This suggests that there is some signal there that is picked up when you do somatic nuclear transplantation which stays and then continues as inactivated X in the trophectoderm, but which is erased in the epiblast.

McLaren   Whatever the imprint is, it means that the inactive X status is remembered. It could well be the same in the somatic cell XX nucleus as it is in the sperm. In both cases there is an imprint that is being remembered and then comes on again. According to the Brockdorff/Heard model this must be true in the ICM of the blastocyst as well as in the trophectoderm. There is an initial paternal imprint, which is then switched off and then there is random inactivation. I see no suggestion as to what the imprint is.

Reik   The intriguing facet of this is the reprogramming that goes on in the epiblast cell. Presumably this starts with down-regulation of *Xist*. But then what happens to all the histone modifications? How quickly are they lost and by what mechanism are they lost? Are there histone demethylases involved? This should happen quite quickly.

Surani   I think that the mechanism is completely unknown. The chronology is that *Xist* is first down-regulated and then histone modifications are lost slightly later on.

McLaren   It is happening at a time when the cells are still dividing relatively slowly, with a doubling time of some 12 hours, before the rapid, explosive 5 hours doubling time sets in. Going back to the primary endoderm, as I understand it Janet Rossant's recent hypothesis (Rossant *et al.* 2003) is that the cells in the ICM that go to form the primary endoderm are actually cells that have come in from the trophectoderm. In other words, they were originally designed as trophectoderm – they were the last ones to come into the interior of the morula – and they are the ones that migrate to the border of the ICM to become primary endoderm. In both cases there is paternal imprinting.

Kunath   I was speaking with Edith Heard recently, and that is why I was asking about the primary endoderm. Janet Rossant thinks that primary endoderm cells may be mixed in with the ICM before this is seen morphologically. Part of the reason is because they see speckled GATA6 expression in the ICM. Oct4 is in all the cells, but GATA6 is in some of them, and not at the surface of the ICM. Edith Heard also sees some of these epigenetic markers at embryonic day 3.5 (E3.5) in some of the ICMs. Some of the cells appear to be starting to lose their imprint before the primary endoderm forms. I asked Edith whether these are the same cells that are GATA6 positive, but she hasn't checked this yet. Are the ICM cells, between E3.5 and E4.5, that are losing *Xist* and all the other epigenetic markers of an inactive X also the cells that are GATA6 negative? This would be interesting to investigate. It could be that the GATA6-negative/Oct4-positive cells are the ones losing these markers and the imprint, while those that maintain GATA6 continue to keep stabilised *Xist*, sort themselves out and come to the surface of the ICM as opposed to the cells at the surface differentiating. In the morula, the model is that the GATA6-positive cells derive from outside cells that divide to give inside cells at the late morula stage.

McLaren This links up with Martin Johnson's inside–outside model of how the blastocyst forms.

Kunath We were speculating that perhaps the inside cells were losing this *Xist* painting. Neil Brockdorff published quite a while ago (Sheardown *et al.* 1997) that all eight cells in the eight-cell embryo had *Xist* painting. We were wondering what happens with the inside cells of the late morula (E2.5–3.0): we thought they are probably losing *Xist* painting. But they are not losing it (Mak *et al.* 2004, Okamoto *et al.* 2004). The Nanog-positive cells in the inner morula still have all the epigenetic marks and the *Xist* painting. So they are not losing it until a day later (E3.5–4.0).

REFERENCES

Eggan, K., Akutsu, H., Hochedlinger, K. *et al.* (2000). X-chromosome inactivation in cloned mouse embryos. *Science*, **290**, 1578–81.

Huynh, K.D. & Lee, J.T. (2003). Inheritance of a pre-inactivated paternal X chromosome in early mouse embryos. *Nature*, **426**, 857–62.

Mak, W., Nesterova, T.B., de Napoles, M. *et al.* (2004). Reactivation of the paternal X chromosome in early mouse embryos. *Science*, **303**, 666–9.

Monk, M. (1978). Biochemical studies on mammalian X-chromosome activity. In M.H. Johnson, ed., *Development in Mammals*, vol. 3. Amsterdam: Elsevier, pp. 189–223.

Monk, M. & Harper, M.I. (1978). X-chromosome activity in pre-implantation mouse embryos from XX and XO mothers. *J. Embryol. Exp. Morphol.*, **46**, 53–64.

Okamoto, I., Otte, A.P., Allis, C.D., Reinberg, D. & Heard, E. (2004). Epigenetic dynamics of imprinted X inactivation during early mouse development. *Science*, **303**, 644–9.

Rossant, J., Chazaud, C. & Yamanaka, Y. (2003). Lineage allocation and asymmetries in the early mouse embryo. *Philos. Trans. R. Soc. Lond. B Biol. Sci.*, **358**, 1341–49.

Sheardown, S.A., Duthie, S.M., Johnston, C.M. *et al.* (1997). Stabilization of Xist RNA mediates initiation of X chromosome inactivation. *Cell*, **91**, 99–107.

General discussion I

McLaren   We set aside some time for general discussion, so please feel free to raise any points the previous speakers have raised. I would like to go back to marsupials. Some of you may not remember Marilyn Renfree's justified indignation at a number of international conferences, when people talked about marsupials versus placental mammals. I think she has now succeeded in erasing this latter terminology from the scientific literature.

Renfree   Not quite!

McLaren   Do marsupials have placentas? We think they do. Do they have trophoblast? If so, where does this trophoblast come from?

Renfree   Absolutely. Marsupials certainly have placentas. The use of the term 'placental mammals' to refer only to eutherians sadly does persist in the literature. This is partly because, as my good friend and close colleague Michael Archer, who is one of Australia's eminent palaeontologists, points out, Placentalia is a taxonomic term and has precedence over Eutheria as a term. His comment is why do you want to call them 'Eutheria' (true animal) versus 'Metatheria' (middle animal)? 'Marsupialia' lacks connotations like this but, *sensu strictu*, it is not consistent with 'Eutheria'. Placental mammal has been a very persuasive term, so textbooks still exist saying that marsupials are 'aplacental'. However, as we have shown (Renfree 1973, Freyer *et al.* 2003), they have a fully functional placenta, which in most cases is formed by the yolk sac, making a choriovitelline placenta that persists through pregnancy. Some species do have a chorioallantoic placenta. In the bandicoot there is probably the most invasive placenta of all mammals, because the fetal and maternal tissues actually form a syncytiotrophoblast (Padykula & Taylor 1977). The syncytium is not just a syncytium of trophoblast cells within itself, but consists of fetal and maternal cells. Fetal and maternal nuclei are sitting next to each other within the same cell. This really needs a lot more investigation. This is

Biology and Pathology of Trophoblast, eds. Ashley Moffett, Charlie Loke and Anne McLaren. Published by Cambridge University Press © Cambridge University Press 2005.

something that is up there for grabs. The bandicoot also has one of the shortest gestations of any mammal, at 12.5 days. This is only just longer than that of the stripe-faced dunnart, a small carnivorous marsupial. The syncytium forms just in the last couple of days. We still have an awful lot to learn about marsupial placentas, and most of the work has been done on the yolk sac placenta. In a little bit of reverse engineering, we are now starting to look at the human yolk sac because this has been a tissue that has largely been ignored. It has the first and very important placental function in humans, and it is there very early on. The question must be raised: are some of those early abortions we see in humans – and there are a lot of them – to do with failure of the yolk sac, rather than failure of the later placenta? This is where marsupials are likely to come into their own.

McLaren   Do marsupials have trophoblast giant cells?

Renfree   I think so. I haven't directly compared a mouse placenta with a marsupial one, but the trophectoderm cells are very large compared with the endoderm cells, which are thin and pale-looking by comparison. They look bigger than the early germ cells and have very large nuclei. I presume they perform the same function.

Reik   To continue on the comparative theme, when people begin to define the regulatory changes in the genes that make a placenta, we want to know what the switch is. Is there a simple switch that can make a placenta or that doesn't make a placenta? Comparative studies with these genes in hand should go some way to address this. There are also placental sharks and snakes: do they use the same genes to make their placentas?

McLaren   And do monotremes have placentas?

Renfree   Yes, they do. The monotreme egg is about 3 mm in diameter at ovulation, so it is considerably larger than a marsupial or eutherian oocyte. It forms both a yolk sac and an allantois, and obtains a vast array of nutrients from the uterus across these fetal membranes (fulfilling true placental function) before the shell coat is laid down. We call it a shell, but it is more like a reptile egg, with keratin as the key component. By the time the shell coat has formed and the egg is 'laid' the conceptus has grown to a 15-somite-stage embryo, and is about 17–18 mm in diameter (Griffiths 1978). It has accumulated quite an additional resource, which then must supply it for the next 10 days while it completes that development.

Burton   I want to echo support for the idea that the human yolk sac is important in the earliest stages of pregnancy. We have recently demonstrated receptor proteins on the surface of the yolk sac such as alpha tocopherol transfer protein (Jauniaux *et al.* 2004). We put forward the idea that the yolk sac is very important in taking up nutrients and materials from the coelomic fluid and transporting them to the fetus in the earliest stages (Burton *et al.* 2001). Although the human isn't morphologically a choriovitelline placenta, it might be functioning as such before the fetal circulation to the placenta is established.

McLaren   I know there was a lot of early work on the yolk sac placenta in rabbits, showing selective transport (e.g. Brambell *et al.* 1950, Brambell 1966).

Renfree   In the rabbit, the inverted yolk sac is the primary source of transfer of immunoglobulins.

McLaren   Colin Sibley, I have always been unclear about how transport differs in the yolk sac placenta and the chorioallantoic placenta. Is the transport system similar or are they quite different?

Sibley   The problem is that in terms of functional transport measurements, the yolk sac has hardly been studied at all. Certainly, it is very difficult to do functional measurements with the human yolk sac. I once tried to invent a way to do this with David Abramovich, but we weren't able to do it. All we use are techniques such as immunocytochemistry. I don't think even this has been done for the full range of transport proteins. There is a study by Kent Thornburg some years ago in the guinea pig where he ablated the vitelline vessels and looked at what was transferred (Thornburg & Faber 1977). The major difference between the ablated and non-ablated was the transfer of albumin, which does fit with these sorts of functions. There is a high degree of endocytosis/exocytosis transport, with larger things getting across in the yolk sac compared with chorioallantoic placenta. We did a similar study in the rat looking at Ca^{2+} transport. Calcium ion is reduced about 10% if the yolk sac is ablated. Overall, the yolk sac might be very important early on, but for the total mass of fetal growth I suspect it doesn't make a major contribution once you get beyond the first trimester. In the first trimester it could be very important.

McLaren   You have got to get far enough to get that allantois meeting the chorion, though.

Sibley   The other thing to remember is that the human fetus isn't growing much in the first trimester. It is laying down systems. You don't need a lot of nutrient; it is only important once growth starts kicking in.

Burton   Can I expand on this? What we have seen is that the receptors are on the exocoelomic surface, on the mesothelial layer forming the outer surface of the yolk sac, facing the coelomic fluid, rather than on the inner endodermal layer. When Barry King did some experiments with the rhesus monkey and uptake of horseradish peroxidase, it was the outer surface that took up the substrate much more avidly than the endodermal cells on the inside of the yolk sac (King & Wilson 1983). It is not strictly comparable to the mouse therefore, since it is the mesothelial layer that is taking up the nutrients rather than the actual endodermal side.

McLaren   Surely in any yolk sac, materials have to be taken up from the maternal tissue by the outer layer and passed through to the cavity of the yolk sac and the fetus.

Burton   In the inverted yolk sac it would be the endoderm layer that is exposed to the nutrients. There is a functional analogy but not a histological analogy.

Kunath   Does the human have something analogous to the trophoblast giant cell/parietal endoderm membrane?

Burton   The yolk sac never makes physical contact with the extraembryonic mesoderm or the chorion, and so there is no physical choriovitelline placenta as such. This is why the yolk sac has been ruled out in terms of transport in the human because it never does make that physical contact which it does in other species. What we are suggesting is that materials might diffuse through the placenta into the coelomic fluid, and then be taken up from that fluid by the yolk sac.

Kunath   The XEN (extraembryonic endoderm) cells that I have express a lot of Rab proteins important for vesicle transport. These cells are very vacuolated when cultured without gelatin.

McLaren   I thought I saw Ashley shuddering at the thought that the bandicoot has a maternal nucleus and a fetal nucleus actually in a single syncytium (i.e. in a single body of cytoplasm). From the immunological point of view this is really rather extraordinary. Could this be linked with the very short gestation period of the bandicoot? If it only has to survive that condition for 48 hours, is it being actively rejected by the mother?

Renfree   There is no evidence for that, although it has been proposed as a reason for the uniformly short gestation of all marsupials. Hugh Tyndale-Biscoe subsequently tried to test this out by a variety of experiments, including repeated matings of the same female with the same male, and looking at various antigen responses (Walker & Tyndale-Biscoe 1978). There is no evidence that parturition in a marsupial is an immunological rejection. From our work (Renfree & Shaw 1996), it has a typically mammalian physiology: the signals come from the fetus and the hormones are the same, although they are a bit more like the sheep than human. However, the idea that it's an immunological rejection still rears its head in the literature.

Cross   In ruminant species it is typical for trophoblast cells to fuse with uterine epithelium as well.

McLaren   So this is not confined to marsupials. I hadn't realised that in some eutherian placentas the syncytium actually has a maternal component.

Loke   Why is there selective paternal X inactivation in trophoblast?

Renfree   I have no idea. Paternal X inactivation was first described by Geoff Sharman in marsupials, and this was really the first description of an imprinted gene (Cooper *et al.* 1971, Sharman 1971).

Loke   As an immunologist, my first reaction would be that this is one way of getting rid of any paternal allogeneic signals in the maternal–trophoblast interface. However, I don't know what signals there will be from the X chromosome. I am not clear what the X chromosomes actually produce. They must produce enzymes, and if these are isoenzymes then one would expect that the mother would react against the paternal allotype.

Renfree We don't have any evidence from marsupials. The X contains lots of genes that are important for males, including all the spermatogenesis genes.

McLaren It includes human leukocyte antigen (*HLA*) genes.

Jacobs It was my understanding that not all eutherians have paternal X inactivation in the trophoblast. Surely humans don't? I don't think there is any convincing evidence for this.

S. Fisher We have some evidence. Wilfred Mak who did this work that has been mentioned has come to our lab. It is far from complete, but our initial results show that it is true. We have been doing the experiments for about two months now.

McLaren The earlier literature was conflicting. I'm interested that there is now new evidence for this. What about other eutherian species? I don't know how many have been looked at. I haven't seen any papers that have said that there isn't paternal X inactivation, but that is not the same thing as not saying that there is.

Moffett Azim Surani, do you have a view on the biology of this? Why has paternal X inactivation been retained in the trophoblast?

Surani No, I do not know the answer to this question.

Renfree I'd like to ask you to go a bit further with the discussion on the Haig hypothesis and the 'parental tug of war' hypothesis. I was talking to Marilyn Monk the other day. Her view is that imprinting was just a mistake that happened at random, and there has been nothing to select against it so it has been retained. Azim, could you comment on Marilyn Monk's theory versus the other hypotheses?

Surani The only comment that comes to mind is one from Rudi Jaenisch (1997). He published a paper in 1997 titled 'DNA methylation and imprinting: why bother?' The problem is that these questions concerning imprinting are here to stay. Every time people do experiments and start looking at functions of imprinted genes and try to think that it is not that important, it comes back with results that are difficult to dismiss. I don't think we have reached a point where we can say anything conclusively about why it is there and what it is doing. One of the problems is that as far as the functions of imprinted genes are concerned, we still know very little about the functions of most of them. Until we have this, we won't be able to assemble a clearer picture.

McLaren Isn't there another factor here? During spermatogenesis, there are rather good reasons for silencing the X chromosome. Single unpaired bits of chromosomes in meiosis are not happy. There has been published evidence of this quite recently in *Caenorhabditis elegans* (Hynes & Todd 2003). Paul Burgoyne has also shown that there are problems with unpaired chromosomes during male meiosis in the mouse (Odorisio *et al.* 1998). If the X chromosome has to be silenced and it is contained in the XY body during spermatogenesis, perhaps it takes time for that silencing to wear off.

Reik   That is what Jeannie Lee is trying to show (Huynh & Lee 2003). Her model is that part of the X chromosome comes in pre-inactivated, as a sort of carry-over from spermatogenic inactivation. This could then be reinforced by *Xist* expression.

McLaren   This makes sense to me. If there is anything in that, then the question to answer is why (in eutherians at least) it becomes random in the fetus? Why shouldn't it be paternal throughout?

Burton   Linked to this is the question of why paternal mitochondria are excluded. One of the theories is that they are subjected to more oxidative stress during spermatogenesis and sperm transport. If you are going to keep a clean sheet of mitochondrial DNA it is better to rely on the maternal rather than the paternal. Would this theory support the idea of the single X in the male being more vulnerable?

McLaren   I have never heard that the nuclear genes from one's father are of poor quality because they have been subjected to oxidative stress. I know this is a suggestion for mitochondrial genes.

Burton   You were saying that a single unpaired chromosome is more vulnerable.

McLaren   That is rather different. If a chromosome isn't paired at meiosis when recombination happens, then the cell tends to be done away with, as a form of quality control.

Ferguson-Smith   This comes back to the point you were making about why paternal X inactivation is retained in the trophoblast whereas it is random in the inner cell mass (ICM) derivatives. One possibility might be that the earliest blastomeres need to be activated in some way to become embryonic stem cells. Their default state might be trophectoderm, and in order to generate pluripotent lineages in embryonic derivatives you need to reverse or reprogramme that state in some way. In the ICM there is a general reprogramming type of event and X-chromosome inactivation is being reprogrammed at the same time. This links with the idea expressed earlier about how trophectoderm development needs to be inhibited in order to obtain a stem cell population: if you have a group of blastomeres that are going down that potential lineage to become trophoblast, they need to be reprogrammed to form embryonic lineages.

McLaren   Marsupials wouldn't need to do that because they don't have an ICM. That's a thought.

Kunath   So everything starts off as trophectoderm, and the first thing to differentiate is the ICM. We have always thought that the first cell type to differentiate is trophectoderm, but that is there all the time. This is a different way of thinking.

Surani   The founder cells in mammals for ICM and trophectoderm start to form when eight-cell blastomeres divide. The eight-cell blastomeres are apparently totipotent.

There is asymmetric division at this point. This is the first time when distinct populations of inner and outer cells of a morula are formed. It looks like at that time Nanog starts to be transcribed in the inner cells. The asymmetric division is important here.

Kunath Before that, everything is trophectoderm.

Surani No, before that the blastomeres are totipotent.

Renfree That is really the same in marsupials. It just happens further down the line. Eventually you are still going to get an endoderm forming from the trophectoderm, but the initial segregation of endoderm mother cells just starts off at a place that doesn't look any different from any other place on the blastocyst. Once the bilaminar blastocyst is formed, then and only then do you get the trilaminar layer forming in the embryonic disk in one region of the conceptus.

McLaren Just to stick up for the ICM, it is able to make more different kinds of cells than trophectoderm. Indeed, in the human it can even make trophectoderm. Trophectoderm can't make all the things that ICM can.

Reik Would non-placental mammals also start off as trophectoderm?

Renfree Yes.

Cross I'm not sure that I buy the argument that those primitive blastomeres are trophectoderm. They are trophectoderm with Oct4, which makes them multipotential. I think you go from a primitive state into three cell states just by flipping on a few transcription factors.

Surani Also there are very old experiments that Chris Graham and others did in which they took early morulae and surrounded them with other embryos (Hillman *et al.* 1972). This forces all of the cells present inside to become ICM. This shows that they are not trophectoderm.

Kunath If you separate blastomere at late stages the cells usually make trophoblast vesicles.

Moffett What are the first species where trophoblast might be considered to be a unique cell? Although you say there are placental lizards and snakes, they have membranes but they don't really have a trophoblast cell as such, do they?

McLaren From what we have heard today, perhaps it is the monotremes.

Renfree The reptile placenta is mainly made out of the yolk sac. Of course, reptiles are mainly oviparous (they lay eggs) but the viviparous ones have placentas. Reptiles also have both chromosomal and temperature-sensitive sex determination.

McLaren What about that reptile yolk sac placenta, because mammals can't make a yolk sac placenta without trophoblast? So reptiles may have some form of trophoblast.

Renfree I think they do, yes.

McLaren What does it look like?

Renfree It looks like a mammalian placenta. In the 1930s Elizabeth Weekes (Weekes 1935) did a whole range of beautiful studies on the reptilian placenta in Australian viviparous lizards. They look just like any other placentas. I can't say whether or not there is a true trophoblast but it looks like it. Selachian sharks, seahorses and scorpions all have a variety of placental-type attachments (Amoroso *et al.* 1980). There is a whole range across viviparous species. This brings us back to the Haig hypothesis: do all these viviparous species have imprinting? Birds don't, as far as we know.

REFERENCES

Amoroso, E.C., Heap, R.B. & Renfree, M.B. (1980). Hormones and the evolution of viviparity. In E.J.W. Barrington, ed., *Hormones and Evolution*, vol. 2. London: Academic Press, pp. 925–89.

Brambell, F.W.R. (1966). The transmission of immunity from mother to young and the catabolism of immunoglobulins. *Lancet*, II, 1087–93.

Brambell, F.W.R., Hemmings, W.A., Henderson, M. & Rowlands, M.T. (1950). The selective admission of antibodies to the fetus by the yolk sac splanchnopleur in rabbits. *Proc. Roy. Soc. B*, **137**, 239–52.

Burton, G.J., Hempstock, J. & Jauniaux, E. (2001). Nutrition of the early human fetus – a review. *Placenta*, **22**[A], S70–6.

Cooper, D.W., Vandeberg, J.L., Sharman, G.B. & Poole, W.E. (1971). Phosphoglycerate kinase polymorphism in kangaroos provides further evidence for paternal X-inactivation. *Nat. New Biol.*, **230**, 155–7.

Freyer, C., Zeller, U. & Renfree, M.B. (2003). The marsupial placenta: a phylogenetic analysis. *J. Exp. Zool.*, **299**, 59–77.

Griffiths, M.E. (1978). *The Biology of Monotremes*. London: Academic Press.

Hillman, N., Sherman, M.I. & Graham, C. (1972). The effect of spatial arrangement on cell determination during mouse development. *J. Embryol. Exp. Morphol.*, **28**, 263–78.

Huynh, K.D. & Lee, J.T. (2003). Inheritance of a pre-inactivated paternal X chromosome in early mouse embryos. *Nature*, **426**, 857–62.

Hynes, M.J. & Todd, R.B. (2003). Detection of paired DNA at meiosis results in RNA-mediated silencing. *BioEssays*, **25**, 99–103.

Jaenisch, R. (1997). DNA methylation and imprinting: why bother? *Trends Genet.* **13**, 323–9.

Jauniaux, E., Cindrova-Davies, T., Johns, J. *et al.* (2004). Distribution and transfer pathways of antioxidant molecules inside the first trimester human gestational sac. *J. Clin. Endocrinol. Metab.* **89**, 1452–8.

King, B.F. & Wilson, A.M. (1983). A fine structural and cytochemical study of the rhesus monkey yolk sac: endoderm and mesothelium. *Anat. Rec.*, **205**, 143–58.

Odorisio, T., Rodriguez, T.A., Evans, E.P., Clark, A.R. & Burgoyne, P.S. (1998). The meiotic checkpoint monitoring synapsis eliminates spermatocytes via p53-independent apoptosis. *Nat. Genet.*, **18**, 257–61.

Padykula, H.A. & Taylor, J.M. (1977). Uniqueness of the bandicoot chorioallantoic placenta (Marsupialia: Peramelidae). Cytological and evolutionary interpretations. In J.H. Calaby, & C.H. Tyndale-Biscoe, eds., *Reproduction and Evolution*. Canberra: Australian Academy of Science, pp. 303–24.

Renfree, M.B. (1973). The composition of fetal fluids of the marsupial, *Macropus eugenii*. *Dev. Biol.*, **33**, 62–79.

Renfree, M.B. & Shaw, G. (1996). Reproduction of a marsupial: from uterus to pouch. *Anim. Reprod. Sci.*, **42**, 393–404.

Sharman, G.B. (1971). Late DNA replication in the paternally derived X chromosome of female kangaroos. *Nature*, **230**, 231–2.

Thornburg, K.L. & Faber, J.J. (1977). Transfer of hydrophilic molecules by placenta and yolk sac of the guinea pig. *Am. J. Physiol. Cell. Physiol.*, **233**, C111–24.

Walker, K.Z. & Tyndale-Biscoe, C.H. (1978). Immunological aspects of gestation in the tammar wallaby, *Macropus eugenii*. *Aust. J. Biol. Sci.*, **31**, 173–82.

Weekes, H.C. (1935). A review of placentation among reptiles, with particular regard to the function and evolution of the placenta. *Proc. Zool. Soc. Lond.*, **2**, 625–46.

5

Gestational trophoblastic disease

R. A. Fisher[1] and N. J. Sebire[2]

[1] Imperial College London, UK
[2] Charing Cross Hospital, UK

Introduction

Gestational trophoblastic diseases (GTD) are a group of diseases involving abnormal proliferation of trophoblastic tissue. They include the benign condition hydatidiform mole (HM), both partial (PHM) and complete (CHM), invasive mole (IM) and the overtly malignant tumours, choriocarcinoma (CC) and placental site trophoblastic tumour (PSTT). Complete hydatidiform mole and PHM are unique in having two copies of the paternal genome. Gestational trophoblastic tumours (GTT) are unusual malignancies in that they are allografts, derived from a conceptus and not from host tissue and are potentially curable even when widely disseminated.

Hydatidiform moles

The abnormal pregnancy HM is characterised by placental overgrowth and abnormal fetal development. In the UK approximately 1 in 700 pregnancies develop as a HM (Bagshawe *et al.* 1986). The incidence of GTD varies widely and has been reported to be considerably higher in some parts of Asia and South America (Bracken 1987, Palmer 1994). Interestingly, recent evidence suggests that the incidence of HM may now be declining in some areas (Kim *et al.* 1998, Matsui *et al.* 2003). Molar pregnancies may be classified on the basis of both pathology and genetics as CHM or PHM (Vassilakos & Kajii 1976, Vassilakos *et al.* 1977, Szulman & Surti 1978a, b). Both are more common in young women and in women over 45 years of age (Sebire *et al.* 2002). Clinically, CHM usually present with first trimester bleeding, an absence of fetal parts on ultrasound and abnormally elevated levels of human chorionic gonadotrophin (HCG), whereas PHM are more likely to

Biology and Pathology of Trophoblast, eds. Ashley Moffett, Charlie Loke and Anne McLaren.
Published by Cambridge University Press © Cambridge University Press 2005.

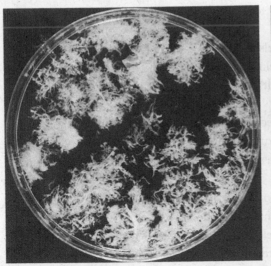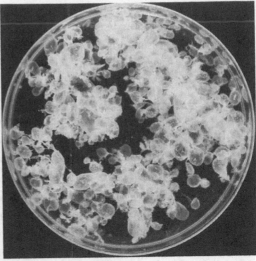

Figure 5.1   Macroscopic photographs demonstrating dissected and cleaned early second trimester chorionic villi from a non-molar miscarriage (left) and CHM (right); the macroscopic vesicles are easily seen.

present as spontaneous abortions and may in fact go undiagnosed (Jeffers *et al.* 1993, Paradinas 1994).

Pathology of hydatidiform moles

Complete hydatidiform moles

In the classical, fully developed CHM evacuated in the second trimester, pathological examination usually demonstrates markedly hydropic villi (Fig. 5.1) with extensive circumferential trophoblastic hyperplasia, often with nuclear pleomorphism. Clumps of extravillous trophoblast are often also present. Acellular 'cisterns' form centrally in the villi, which demonstrate few or no blood vessels. However, since the introduction of routine ultrasound examination in early pregnancy, HM are now evacuated much earlier than previously (Paradinas *et al.* 1996), at an average of 12 weeks' gestational age. The most useful features by which to recognise these more immature CHM differ from the above description of second trimester CHM and include (Plate 4):

(1) Circumferential trophoblast hyperplasia, a prerequisite for diagnosis, although the extent is unrelated to clinical behaviour (Hertig & Sheldon 1947, Hertig & Mansell 1956, Elston & Bagshawe 1967, Genest *et al.* 1991, Paradinas *et al.* 1996).

(2) Mild villus hydrops, often only focal in nature in the first trimester, with only occasional cisterns.

(3) Presence of stromal blood vessels, usually seen in first trimester CHM, in most cases collapsed and empty (Szulman & Surti 1978b, Kajii *et al.* 1984, Paradinas 1994, Paradinas *et al.* 1996), although occasionally containing nucleated red cells (see below).

(4) Presence of stromal karyorrhectic debris in otherwise well-preserved villi, almost always seen in CHM (Szulman & Surti 1978b).

(5) Prominent 'clubbed' villi with a secondary 'budding' architecture (Szulman & Surti 1978b, Kajii *et al.* 1984).

(6) Oval or irregular pseudoinclusions of trophoblast.

(7) Presence of 'mucoid' villus stroma with little fibrosis.

(8) No evidence of embryonic development in most CHM; rarely nucleated fetal red cells or amnion may be present (Jacobs *et al.* 1982a, Fisher *et al.* 1997, Paradinas *et al.* 1997, Zaragoza *et al.* 1997, Weaver *et al.* 2000).

Partial hydatidiform moles

Confusion between the pathological diagnoses of CHM and PHM has resulted from the failure to update diagnostic criteria for HM evacuated at the earlier gestations seen in current practice. A diagnosis of PHM based exclusively on the presence of villus blood vessels or partial as opposed to complete hydrops is often wrong. The main features useful in positively diagnosing PHM are as follows (Plate 4):

(1) Trophoblastic hyperplasia, which is required for definitive diagnosis, but is often patchy in nature and less extensive than observed with CHM. Extensive sampling is therefore important in this regard as changes may be highly focal and the abnormal distribution and vacuolated appearance of trophoblast may be more striking than the degree of excess.

(2) Hydrops and cisterns, which characteristically involve only some villi although in some PHM, hydrops is mild and cisterns may be absent, with prominent fibrosis of villi rather than hydrops (Berkowitz *et al.* 1985). A common pitfall is to interpret fragments of a gestational sac in a non-molar abortion as villi with large cisterns, but as a rule the wall of the gestational sac contains more collagen than surrounding villi and the possibility of this should always be considered when the suspected cisterns are few and surrounded by smaller villi with no trophoblastic hyperplasia.

(3) Villus vessels, often containing nucleated fetal red cells, are common in PHM although some PHM are apparently avascular. In a minority of PHM some villi may show characteristic angiomatoid vascular change (Szulman & Surti 1978b).

(4) Karyorrhexis in villous stroma is seldom present or intense in PHM in contrast to CHM.
(5) Partial hydatidiform moles have abnormally shaped villi often described as scalloped or dentate with invaginations of trophoblast resulting in rounded inclusions.
(6) In PHM the villous stroma appears fibrotic, which increases with gestation.
(7) Embryonic tissue may be identifiable in the specimen, although fetal tissue may only be identified in about 20% due to sampling (Paradinas *et al.* 1996). Similarly, numerous nucleated fetal red cells may be present in villus vessels.

Due to their differences in clinical behaviour and risk of persistent trophoblastic disease (PTD), distinction between CHM and PHM is required for accurate patient counselling and interpretation of epidemiological and research studies. However, from a practical standpoint, all patients with a diagnosis of molar pregnancy, CHM or PHM, are initially managed in a similar manner, with serial HCG estimations. In this setting, treatment is almost always based on failure of HCG levels to fall to normal, or rising HCG concentrations (Newlands 1997).

Genetics of hydatidiform moles

Partial hydatidiform moles and CHM are genetically distinct in that PHM are generally triploid while CHM have a normal diploid number of chromosomes (Szulman & Surti 1978a, b). Despite this, they are similar in that both have two paternally derived sets of chromosomes and as such are one of a small group of diseases in which the pathology results from deregulation of imprinted genes.

Partial hydatidiform moles

Triploid conceptions may result from failure at the first or second meiotic division in either gamete followed by normal fertilisation or fertilisation of an ovum by two sperm (Jacobs *et al.* 1978a). Genetic polymorphisms have shown that PHM are almost invariably diandric, the additional chromosome set being paternally derived (Jacobs *et al.* 1982b, Lawler *et al.* 1982a, Zaragoza *et al.* 2000). Occasional cases of PHM have been reported in which the most likely origin is fertilization of an egg by a diploid sperm (Zaragoza *et al.* 2000). However, most PHM have been shown to arise by dispermy (Jacobs *et al.* 1982a, Lawler *et al.* 1982a, 1991) and to have a 69,XXX, 69,XXY or 69,XYY karyotype.

Complete hydatidiform moles

In contrast to PHM, CHM are generally diploid with no maternal contribution to the nuclear genome, all 46 chromosomes being of paternal origin (Kajii & Ohama 1977, Jacobs *et al.* 1978b, Wake *et al.* 1978). Like PHM, 20%–25% of CHM arise by dispermy although in CHM the egg is anucleate resulting in an androgenetic conceptus that may be 46,XX or 46,XY (Ohama *et al.* 1981, Fisher *et al.* 1989, Kovacs *et al.* 1991). However, most CHM are monospermic and result from fertilization of an anucleate egg by a single haploid sperm which then undergoes reduplication to restore the diploid number of chromosomes (Lawler *et al.* 1979, 1982b, Jacobs *et al.* 1980, 1982a). These monospermic CHM have a 46,XX karyotype. Complete hydatidiform moles with a 46,YY karyotype have not been reported and are presumably non-viable. The fate of the maternal chromosomes in CHM is unknown although one likely origin of an anucleate ovum is non-disjunction, with loss of chromosomal material to one of the polar bodies, during meiosis. Despite loss of the nuclear genome, the cytoplasm of the ovum, giving rise to CHM, appears to be intact since the mitochondrial DNA, as in normal pregnancies, is maternal in origin (Wallace *et al.* 1982, Edwards *et al.* 1984).

Diploid, biparental hydatidiform moles

Although almost all CHM are androgenetic, occasional HM have been described which are CHM on the basis of pathology and genetically diploid but have both a maternal and paternal contribution to the nuclear genome (Jacobs *et al.* 1982a, Ko *et al.* 1991, Kovacs *et al.* 1991, Fisher *et al.* 1997, Repiska *et al.* 2003). Although rare, these biparental CHM (BiCHM) are of interest because of their association with families in which two or more individuals have recurrent molar pregnancies (Helwani *et al.* 1999, Sensi *et al.* 2000, Fisher *et al.* 2002, Hodges *et al.* 2003). To date 14 families with familial recurrent HM have been reported in the literature (Ambani *et al.* 1980, La Vecchia *et al.* 1982, Parazzini *et al.* 1984, Mangili *et al.* 1993, Sunde *et al.* 1993, Kircheisen & Ried 1994, Seoud *et al.* 1995, Helwani *et al.* 1999, Sensi *et al.* 2000, Fisher *et al.* 2002, Judson *et al.* 2002, Al-Hussaini *et al.* 2003, Fallahian 2003, Hodges *et al.* 2003). In most cases the recurrent HM have the pathological features of CHM although a small number have been described as PHM. In addition to frequent molar pregnancies, affected individuals have a high incidence of miscarriage while normal pregnancies are rare. Where the genetic origin of the recurrent HM has been examined, irrespective of whether they are described as CHM or PHM, they have been shown to be diploid and of biparental origin (Vejerslev *et al.* 1991, Sunde *et al.* 1993, Helwani *et al.* 1999, Sensi *et al.* 2000, Fisher *et al.* 2002, Judson *et al.* 2002, Hodges *et al.* 2003). Thus, diploid, biparental HM appears to represent a familial form of HM. The high degree of consanguinity in some families with recurrent HM, together with the pattern of inheritance, suggests an autosomal recessive condition, predisposing to molar pregnancies.

Although families with recurrent HM are rare, a number of sporadic cases have been reported in the literature, some women having as many as nine or ten consecutive moles (Wu 1973). These women rarely have normal pregnancies, have been found to have HM with more than one partner and, where examined, have been shown to have CHM of biparental origin (Fisher *et al.* 2000). It is hypothesised that these women are likely to represent single affected members of families with the same inherited predisposition to molar pregnancies.

Genetically unusual hydatidiform moles

Occasional HM may not have regular diploid or triploid karyotypes but may be tetraploid, aneuploid or mosaic. Both tetraploid PHM and CHM usually have an excess of paternal contributions to the genome with three or four paternal genomes respectively (Sheppard *et al.* 1982, Surti *et al.* 1986, Vejerslev *et al.* 1987b). The pathology of aneuploid HM reflects their basic karyotype. Hyperdiploid HM are morphologically CHM while hypo- or hypertriploid HM are PHM (Berkowitz *et al.* 1982, Jacobs *et al.* 1982a, Lawler *et al.* 1982a, Vejerslev *et al.* 1987a). Areas of molar change in the placenta of an otherwise normal pregnancy can occasionally represent a mosaic (Ford *et al.* 1986, Sarno *et al.* 1993, Ikeda *et al.* 1996, Zhang *et al.* 2000, Makrydimas *et al.* 2002). Care must be taken to distinguish these rare mosaics from PHM since, unlike PHM, they may result in a normal live birth (Sarno *et al.* 1993, Makrydimas *et al.* 2002).

Differential diagnosis of hydatidiform mole

The greatest risk factor for the development of PTD, which may be IM, CC or PSTT, is a pregnancy with a CHM. It is estimated that the risk of CC following a HM is in the order of 1000 times more likely than after a normal conception (Bagshawe & Lawler 1982). In the UK approximately 1 in 12 patients with CHM require treatment for PTD (Bagshawe *et al.* 1986). The risk of PTD following PHM is considerably lower, ranging from 0.5% (Bagshawe *et al.* 1990) to 5% (Rice *et al.* 1990), although even the lower of these figures is likely to be an overestimate due to the large number of PHM that go undiagnosed (Jeffers *et al.* 1993, Paradinas 1994). It is therefore important to distinguish between CHM, PHM and non-molar abortions.

Although CHM and PHM can usually be distinguished by the pathologist, earlier termination of suspected molar pregnancies, when the distinction between CHM and PHM is less marked, can present diagnostic problems (Paradinas 1994). The differential diagnosis of CHM has been greatly facilitated by the recent introduction of immunostaining for p57[KIP2], a protein that is expressed in the villous trophoblast and stromal cells of all pregnancies except CHM (Chilosi *et al.* 1998, Castrillon *et al.* 2001, Fisher *et al.* 2002, Fukunaga *et al.* 2002, Crisp *et al.* 2003, Jun *et al.* 2003) so enabling CHM to be distinguished from other types of abnormal placental development (Plate 5).

Rare genetic disorders such as Beckwith–Weidemann syndrome (BWS) and placental angiomatoid malformation, known collectively as placental mesenchymal dysplasia, may exhibit placental hydrops similar to that seen in PHM (Sander 1993, Jauniaux *et al.* 1997, Genest 2001, Paradinas *et al.* 2001). Since these conditions will be essentially diploid, PHM may be distinguished from these and other hydropic abortions, with some features of PHM, by studies of cell ploidy. Determination of cell ploidy by flow cytometry (Fisher *et al.* 1987, Hemming *et al.* 1987, Lage *et al.* 1988, Fukunaga *et al.* 1993, Paradinas *et al.* 1996, Genest 2001) or *in situ* hybridization with chromosome-specific probes (Van de Kaa *et al.* 1993, Cheville *et al.* 1995, Chew *et al.* 2000, Lai *et al.* 2004) has been used to distinguish CHM from PHM, and diploid hydropic abortions from triploid tissue. However, the differential diagnosis between maternal triploidy and PHM requires the origin of the additional chromosome set to be determined.

Molecular genetic techniques have been useful in confirming a diagnosis of androgenetic CHM or diandric PHM (Fisher *et al.* 1989, Saji *et al.* 1989, Takahashi *et al.* 1990, Fukuyama *et al.* 1991, Ko *et al.* 1991, Kovacs *et al.* 1991, Lawler *et al.* 1991, Cho & Kim 1993, Fisher & Newlands 1993, Fujita *et al.* 1994), differentiating twin, or multiple, pregnancies with CHM and coexisting normal fetus(es) from PHM (Azuma *et al.* 1992, Hsu *et al.* 1993, Hoshi *et al.* 1994, Osada *et al.* 1995, Higashino *et al.* 1999) and to differentiate recurrent HM, i.e. a new conceptus, from PTD originating in a previous HM. Parental origin of tissue can now be easily identified, even in archival samples, by comparing highly polymorphic microsatellite repeats in DNA from parental and placental tissue (Lane *et al.* 1993, Bell *et al.* 1999, Lai *et al.* 2004) (Fig. 5.2).

Molecular genetic diagnosis can also be used to differentiate between CHM of different origin (Fisher *et al.* 1989, 2000, Kovacs *et al.* 1991, Helwani *et al.* 1999), a distinction that cannot be made on the basis of morphology alone. The relative malignant potential and hence the significance of differentiating between monospermic (homozygous) and dispermic (heterozygous) CHM remains controversial (Fisher & Lawler 1984, Wake *et al.* 1984, 1987, Lawler *et al.* 1991, Mutter *et al.* 1993a, Cheung *et al.* 1994a, Shahib *et al.* 2001). However, the ability to differentiate BiCHM from CHM of androgenetic origin (AnCHM) (Fig. 5.2) is clinically important.

Women with HM are concerned about the risk of PTD and that subsequent pregnancies may be further HM. The overall risk of HM in a subsequent pregnancy, following a single CHM or PHM, is about 2% (Lorigan *et al.* 2000, Matsui *et al.* 2001, Sebire *et al.* 2003a, b) increasing to approximately 20% (Bagshawe *et al.* 1986, Berkowitz *et al.* 1998, Shapter & McLellan 2001) after two or more consecutive CHM. The most likely outcome in subsequent pregnancies is still a full-term normal delivery for most women. However, for women with familial recurrent mole

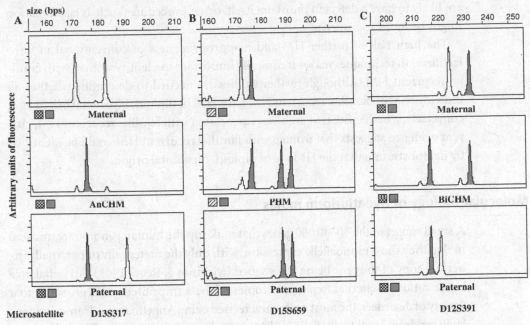

Figure 5.2   Fluorescently labelled PCR products identified following amplification of polymorphic microsatellite markers from DNA prepared from parental blood and HM tissue, microdissected from fixed sections. A single informative marker is shown in each vertical panel with sizes of the DNA fragments generated (in base pairs) represented by the X-axis. (A) A CHM, homozygous for a single allele from the father (shaded), but inheriting neither of the maternal alleles and therefore androgenetic in origin. (B) A trisomic locus in a PHM with two paternally derived and a single maternally derived allele (shaded). Trisomy for this and other markers (not shown) is consistent with a diandric, triploid conception. (C) A CHM from a patient with recurrent HM. The HM is disomic, with one allele from each parent (shaded), consistent with a biparental conception.

the chance of a successful pregnancy is likely to be very much lower. In 14 families described in the literature, 37 affected individuals had a total of 152 pregnancies of which 113 (74%) were CHM, 26 miscarriages, 6 PHM and only 7 normal pregnancies (Ambani *et al.* 1980, La Vecchia *et al.* 1982, Parazzini *et al.* 1984, Mangili *et al.* 1993, Sunde *et al.* 1993, Kircheisen & Ried 1994, Seoud *et al.* 1995, Helwani *et al.* 1999, Sensi *et al.* 2000, Fisher *et al.* 2002, Judson *et al.* 2002, Al-Hussaini *et al.* 2003, Fallahian 2003, Hodges *et al.* 2003).

Women who have experienced two or more molar pregnancies may wish to consider artificial reproductive technologies to avoid further HM. While intracytoplasmic sperm injection followed by preimplantation genetic diagnosis can be used to prevent further PHM and AnCHM (Reubinoff *et al.* 1997) it is unlikely to benefit women with recurrent HM of diploid, biparental origin. For these women, who are likely to have a defect in the ovum itself, other procedures such as egg donation might be more appropriate.

The high risk of further HM and inappropriateness of conventional in vitro fertilization techniques makes it clinically important to identify women with familial recurrent HM. Although further studies are needed to determine whether all individuals with familial recurrent HM have HM of diploid, biparental origin and, conversely, whether BiCHM are always associated with familial recurrent HM, current evidence suggests that women with familial recurrent HM could be identified by demonstrating that the HM are of diploid, biparental origin.

Molecular biology of hydatidiform moles

A small subset of the 30–40 000 genes that make up the human genome are unusual in that they show monoallelic expression, with only the maternally or paternally inherited copy of the gene being transcribed (Morison & Reeve 1998). An imbalance in the ratio of maternal to paternal copies of these imprinted genes gives rise to a variety of disorders, the most well characterised being Angelman syndrome, Prader–Willi syndrome and BWS (Falls et al. 1999, Walter & Paulsen 2003). These disorders result from a parental imbalance of a small region of the genome. Hydatidiform moles represent an extreme example of unbalanced parental contribution to the genome in that the whole nuclear genome is paternal in origin in CHM and in PHM the paternal contribution is twice that of the maternal contribution.

There is strong evidence that the pathological features shared by CHM and PHM, in particular the trophoblastic hyperplasia, are associated with an excess of paternal genomes. Digynic triploids, which have two maternal contributions to the nuclear genome, are not associated with molar pathology (Jacobs et al. 1982b, Zaragoza et al. 2000) but have an abnormally small placenta and growth-retarded fetus (McFadden et al. 1993). Similarly, ovarian teratomas, genetically analogous to CHM, but with a maternally derived diploid genome (Parrington et al. 1984), are very different to CHM in terms of their biology. In ovarian teratomas no development of extraembryonic tissues occurs while mature tissues, such as hair and teeth, can be clearly identified. These observations suggest that loss of embryonic development in CHM is associated with loss of the maternal genome. These hypotheses are supported by experimentally generated androgenetic and parthenogenetic mouse models, which demonstrated the need for both male and female genomes in normal development (Barton et al. 1984, McGrath & Solter 1984, Surani et al. 1984). In these models good trophoblast differentiation occurred only in androgenetic, not gynogenetic, embryos (Barton et al. 1984), thus demonstrating an association between extraembryonic development and the paternal genome analogous to that seen in CHM.

In both PHM and CHM extraembryonic proliferation is associated with an excess of paternal genomes and likely to involve overexpression of paternally transcribed genes. In CHM the loss of maternally transcribed genes is also likely to play a role in their pathology, in particular the lack of fetal development associated with CHM.

Most diploid, biparental HM are pathologically indistinguishable from AnCHM. Therefore deregulation of normal imprinting is also likely to be the underlying mechanism in BiCHM. By analogy with AnCHM, in which all paternally transcribed genes are potentially overexpressed and all maternally transcribed gene products absent, the defective gene that gives rise to BiCHM is likely to regulate the expression of several imprinted genes.

Approximately 50 imprinted genes have been identified in mammals to date (http://www.otago.ac.nz/IGC). Expression or methylation status of some of these genes has now been examined in both AnCHM and BiCHM. Expression of two maternally transcribed genes, *CDKN1C* and *IPL/TSSC3*, both highly expressed in normal placenta (Lee *et al.* 1995, Frank *et al.* 1999), has been shown to be abnormal in CHM. Immunohistochemical staining with p57^{KIP2}, the product of *CDKN1C*, and IPL has shown that expression is lost in the cytotrophoblast and villous mesenchyme of CHM in contrast to normal pregnancies and PHM in which these cells are strongly positive (Chilosi *et al.* 1998, Castrillon *et al.* 2001, Saxena *et al.* 2003). Although expression of IPL has not been examined in BiCHM, p57^{KIP2} shows the same loss of gene expression in BiCHM as seen in AnCHM (Fisher *et al.* 2002). In mice *Ipl* appears to limit placental growth (Frank *et al.* 2002). Loss of IPL may therefore play a role in the placental overgrowth seen in HM. In mice, embryos lacking p57^{KIP2} expression also exhibit trophoblastic hyperplasia (Takahashi *et al.* 2000). However, the role of p57^{KIP2} expression in CHM is less clear given that an unusual case of CHM, which expressed p57^{KIP2} due to retention of a maternal chromosome 11, was pathologically indistinguishable from CHM in which p57^{KIP2} expression was lost (Fisher *at al.* 2004b). Studies of the maternally transcribed gene *H19* have been inconclusive but generally suggest that *H19* is expressed in some cells of CHM (Mutter *et al.* 1993b, Ariel *et al.* 1994, Walsh *et al.* 1995, Wake *et al.* 1998).

Imprinted genes are typically marked by differentially methylated regions dependent on the parent of origin (Reik & Walter 2001, Walter & Paulsen 2003). Several genes that would normally have a maternal methylation imprint have been shown to have only a paternal, i.e. unmethylated, epigenetic pattern in CHM (Mowery-Rushton *et al.* 1996, Arima *et al.* 2000, Kamiya *et al.* 2000, Judson *et al.* 2002, El-Maarri *et al.* 2003). Where paternally expressed genes have been examined in BiCHM, the same methylation patterns have been found in both AnCHM and

BiCHM (Judson *et al.* 2002, El-Maarri *et al.* 2003) supporting the hypothesis that the mutation in women with BiCHM results in failure to set maternal imprints within the ovum.

The status of maternally expressed genes in BiCHM is less well defined. In most CHM, maternally transcribed gene products are absent as a consequence of their androgenetic origin. In BiCHM, which have a maternal genome, these genes might be expected to show normal expression. Although expression of the maternally transcribed p57^{KIP2} has been shown to be deregulated in CHM (Fisher *et al.* 2002), this is likely to be secondary to loss of maternal-specific methylation at *KvDMR1*, an imprinting control region in *KCNQ1* that regulates expression of other genes in the 11p15.5 region including *CDKN1C* (Fitzpatrick *et al.* 2002). In one study, the maternally expressed gene *H19* was reported to remain unmethylated in a BiCHM, in contrast to AnCHM in which both alleles were methylated (Judson *et al.* 2002). However, a subsequent investigation found hypermethylation of the maternally derived *H19* allele in two of four BiCHM (El-Maarri *et al.* 2003), a methylation pattern closer to that of AnCHM. In the same study imprinted genes in a normal offspring, of an affected woman, were shown to have no abnormalities in relation to methylation status for either the maternally or paternally transcribed genes examined (El-Maarri *et al.* 2003). Thus, deregulation of imprinting appears to occur to a variable degree in different pregnancies of affected women. This variation provides an explanation for the occurrence of occasional PHM, non-molar miscarriages and normal pregnancies in affected individuals. Further investigation of imprinted genes in BiCHM may help identify those genes that are deregulated as a consequence of the androgenetic origin of CHM and those that contribute to the pathology of the condition.

Mapping of the gene for familial recurrent hydatidiform mole

The function of the gene mutated in women with BiCHM has not been formally proven. However, it is clearly an important regulator of imprinting in early development. As such there has been considerable interest in identifying the gene involved (Moglabey *et al.* 1999, Sensi *et al.* 2000, Hodges *et al.* 2003). Linkage and homozygosity mapping in a large consanguineous family (Helwani *et al.* 1999) enabled the gene for familial recurrent HM to be mapped to a 15.2 cM interval on 19q13.3–13.4 flanked by the markers *D19S924* and *D19S890* (Moglabey *et al.* 1999). This region was further refined at the centromeric (Sensi *et al.* 2000) and telomeric end (Hodges *et al.* 2003) to give a minimal overlap of 1.1 Mb containing approximately 60 genes (The International Human Genome Sequencing Consortium 2001). However, not all women with familial recurrent HM are homozygous for the 19q13.4 region (Judson *et al.* 2002, Hodges *et al.* 2003). The predisposition to familial recurrent

HM may therefore show genetic heterogeneity and involve other regions in some families.

Recently it has been shown that establishment of the maternal imprint in mice requires the methyltransferase-related gene product, Dnmt3L (Bourc'his *et al.* 2001). Progeny of mice, homozygous for disruption of the *Dnmt3L* gene, die early in gestation and show abnormalities of the extraembryonic tissue that make the human orthologue, *DNMT3L*, an attractive candidate for the familial recurrent HM locus. However, *DNMT3L* is unlikely to be the gene responsible for familial recurrent HM since it maps to chromosome 21q22.3 in humans (Aapola *et al.* 2000) and was not found to be mutated in a family in which the gene did not map to chromosome 19q13.4 (Judson *et al.* 2002). The *DNMT3L* gene has been shown to act as a general stimulatory factor for *de novo* methylation by Dnmt3a in human cells (Chedin *et al.* 2002). Other factors, including the normal product of the gene mutated in familial recurrent HM, may be important in correct targeting of these methyl transferases to maternally methylated regions. Further narrowing of the critical region on chromosome 19, clarification of other familial recurrent HM loci and the isolation of the causative gene(s) require further investigation of novel families with this condition.

Gestational trophoblastic tumours

Trophoblastic tumours are fetal allografts in maternal tissues and present unique biological, immunological and pathological problems. One of the main functions of trophoblast is to gain access to the maternal circulation, and normal trophoblast infiltrates, invades vessels and can even be transported to the lungs in a fashion that is otherwise only seen in malignant neoplasms. Invasion and metastases are criteria used to diagnose and stage malignancy in other neoplasms but are not easily applicable to trophoblastic disease. Gestational trophoblastic tumours (GTT) include IM, CC and PSTT. Invasive moles generally derive from CHM and have a correspondingly similar pathology. Choriocarcinoma may occur following CHM, PHM, non-molar abortion, stillbirth, ectopic pregnancy or an apparently normal term pregnancy. Approximately half of all CC reportedly follow HM and half non-molar pregnancies (Bagshawe *et al.* 1986), although this may represent an underestimate since with improved recognition of early CHM in recent years it is clear that many historical cases thought to be subsequent to 'hydropic abortion' actually followed early CHM. Further, the incidence of CC derived from HM is likely to be higher than that reported, since it is now recognised that the clinically antecedent pregnancy may not be the pregnancy in which the tumour originated, particularly in patients with a history of HM (Fisher *et al.* 1992a, 1995, Suzuki *et al.* 1993, Roberts & Mutter 1994, Arima *et al.* 1995, Shahib 2001). The much rarer PSTT are more likely to occur after non-molar pregnancies (Feltmate *et al.* 2001, Papadopoulos *et al.* 2002).

Pathology of gestational trophoblastic tumours

Invasive mole

This entity represents a CHM with deep villous invasion of the myometrium resulting in uterine perforation and/or extension to adjacent organs (Hertig & Mansell 1956, Park 1971, Elston 1976). Histologically, the appearance of the chorionic villi is similar to that of other CHM. Since hysterectomy is nowadays rarely necessary in the treatment of CHM, few specimens are now seen. Invasive mole after PHM is very rare.

Choriocarcinoma

This is a malignant neoplasm with differentiation towards villus cytotrophoblast and syncytiotrophoblast. It can occur after any type of pregnancy but the incidence of CC after CHM is about 1000 times greater than after a normal pregnancy (World Health Organization Scientific Group 1983). Uterine CC usually appears as a haemorrhagic nodule, in contact with the endometrium or deep in the myometrium. Microscopically, viable tumour is usually seen only at the periphery and within vascular spaces in the adjacent myometrium; no intrinsic vasculature can be demonstrated. The characteristic bilaminar trophoblast structure is usually easily identifiable although some cases may appear to be composed predominantly of syncytiotrophoblast or mononuclear cytotrophoblast. Furthermore, the morphology of CC may be changed after chemotherapy, with therapy-resistant metastases often composed of mononuclear cells (Mazur 1989). Choriocarcinoma metastasises readily and the cervix, vagina, lungs, brain and liver are organs most often involved (Bagshawe & Noble 1966, Magrath *et al.* 1971). Unexplained intracerebral haemorrhage or acute cor pulmonale in a woman of childbearing age should prompt suspicions of CC. Choriocarcinoma following a normal term pregnancy is sometimes the result of malignant transformation in an otherwise normal placenta but the primary tumour may be microscopical and may not be detected, since pathological examination of apparently normal placentas from normal births is seldom carried out. It should be remembered that placental CC can metastasize to the infant as well as the mother (Emery 1952, Buckell & Owen 1954). Choriocarcinoma should be diagnosed with caution in uterine curettage specimens. The pleomorphic trophoblast from a mole, particularly a CHM, can be morphologically indistinguishable from that of CC, although it has a different biological behaviour.

Selective sampling of a second curettage after evacuation of a CHM may yield trophoblast without villous stroma, when a diagnosis of persistent trophoblast should be made and its significance judged together with clinical, ultrasound and serological data. As a rule, the longer the period between evacuation of a known pregnancy and the finding of trophoblast in curettings, the more likely its pathological significance, provided a new pregnancy can be ruled out (Elston & Bagshawe 1972).

Placental site trophoblastic tumour

This is the neoplasmic counterpart of the non-villous implantation site intermediate trophoblast, which infiltrates the placental site in normal pregnancy (Kurman *et al.* 1976, Shih & Kurman 2001a). Placental site trophoblastic tumours usually present with amenorrhea or irregular vaginal bleeding months or years after a normal pregnancy, an abortion or HM (Eckstein *et al.* 1982, 1985, Young & Scully 1984). Their origin from both HM and normal pregnancy has been demonstrated genetically (Fisher *et al.* 1992b, Bower *et al.* 1996). The uterus in PSTT is usually enlarged and serum proteins such as HCG and human placental lactogen (HPL) may be elevated although HCG is seldom as high as in CC. A curettage may yield decidua or myometrium infiltrated by trophoblastic cells with dense eosinophilic cytoplasm and pleomorphic nuclei; they can be mononuclear or multinucleated and they often form clusters or cords and separate smooth muscle fibres (Plate 6). It may be difficult, or even impossible, to differentiate between an exaggerated placental site reaction and PSTT in endometrial curettings, since there may be scanty material or this may be extensively necrotic (Paradinas 1992). Confluent sheets of predominantly monomorphic cells, unequivocal mitoses, an elevated Ki67 index and an absence of chorionic villi are all in favour of a PSTT (Shih & Kurman 1998a, 2001a, b). In hysterectomy specimens, PSTT forms masses in which necrosis is marked, but haemorrhage is less conspicuous with a lesser tendency to destructive vascular invasion, infiltration being predominantly interstitial. Placental site trophoblastic tumour can infiltrate locally into adjacent organs such as ovary, parametrium, rectum or bladder and distant metastases can occur. The importance of recognising PSTT lies in its lesser metastasising potential, which makes it amenable to surgery, but its higher resistance to chemotherapy. Immunocytochemistry for HCG and HPL is helpful in diagnosis since PSTT contains more positive cells for HPL than HCG, in contrast to CC. Tumours are also reported with morphology of PSTT in the uterus and CC in metastases, as well as tumours with areas indistinguishable between PSTT and cytotrophoblastic CC. The differential diagnosis of PSTT from non-neoplastic placental site nodules (Lee & Chan 1990, Young *et al.* 1990, Silva *et al.* 1993, Huettner & Gersell 1994, Shitabata & Rutgers 1994) relies on the presence, in regressing lesions, of marked hyalinisation, normal urinary or serum HCG levels and a low proliferation index.

Epithelioid trophoblastic tumours

This is the most recently described and rarest GTT. It is composed of chorionic-type intermediate trophoblast and is distinct from both CC and PSTT although mixed tumours have been reported (Shih & Kurman 1998b). Epithelioid trophoblastic tumour (ETT) usually presents as a discrete uterine mass, often occurring several years after the last known pregnancy. Microscopically, there is a characteristic nodular, expansive growth pattern rather than the infiltrative pattern seen with PSTT, the tumour being composed of sheets and nests of mononuclear trophoblast with clear, eosinophilic and vacuolated cytoplasm resembling 'chorionic' type intermediate trophoblast (Shih & Kurman 1998a, b, Hamazaki *et al.* 1999). Epithelioid trophoblastic tumours usually immunostain diffusely positive with placental alkaline phosphatase (PLAP) and cytokeratin, whereas HCG and HPL positivity is weak and scattered, in contrast to CC and PSTT (Shih & Kurman 1998b, Hamazaki *et al.* 1999, Ohira *et al.* 1999).

Differential diagnosis of gestational trophoblastic tumours

Gestational trophoblastic tumours are characterised by trophoblastic differentiation and HCG production, features that can sometimes occur in non-gestational CC (Braunstein *et al.* 1973). Molecular genetic techniques can be used to distinguish gestational from non-gestational trophoblastic tumours and, in cases of GTT, identify the causative pregnancy. Since the genome of a GTT reflects that of the pregnancy in which it arose, it will have paternal and maternal genes if it derives from a normal pregnancy or spontaneous abortion, or paternal genes if it originates in a CHM. In any case the presence of paternal genes will distinguish it from a non-gestational carcinoma that will have a genome that reflects that of the host (Fisher *et al.* 1988, 1992a, b, Azuma 1990, Osada *et al.* 1991, Arima *et al.* 1995, Bower *et al.* 1995, Suryanarayan *et al.* 1998, Shigematsu *et al.* 2000, Shahib *et al.* 2001) (Fig. 5.3).

Tumours that arise in a molar pregnancy have a more favourable prognosis than tumours arising from a spontaneous abortion or term pregnancy (Bagshawe 1976). The nature of the pregnancy from which a tumour derived is therefore clinically important as is the time interval between pregnancy and diagnosis. In GTT the clinically antecedent pregnancy is not always the causative pregnancy (Fisher *et al.* 1992a, 1995, Suzuki *et al.* 1993, Roberts & Mutter 1994, Arima *et al.* 1995, Shahib

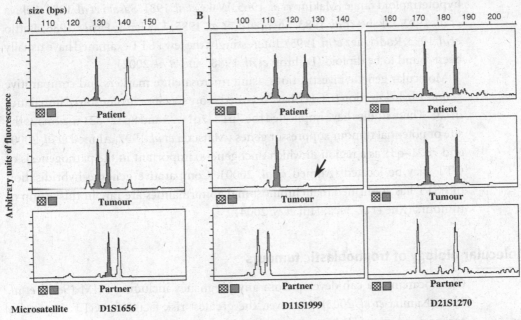

Figure 5.3   Fluorescently labelled PCR products identified following amplification of polymorphic microsatellite markers from DNA prepared from parental blood and tumour tissue, microdissected from fixed sections. (A) A GTT with two alleles, one derived from each parent (shaded). (B) A non-gestational tumour in which both alleles (shaded) are maternally derived (right panel). Loss of one of the two maternal alleles (arrowed) confirms that the tissue examined is tumour and not contaminating host cells (left panel).

et al. 2001) and in fact women may have more than one intervening pregnancy before developing a GTD (Fisher *et al.*, unpublished observations).

Genetics of gestational trophoblastic tumours

Development of most solid tumours results from a multistep process involving oncogenes, tumour suppressor genes and epigenetic modification. Although these pathways are becoming unravelled in some tumours, the steps involved in the development of GTT are poorly understood. This is in part due to the limited availability of GTT tissue resulting from successful treatment with chemotherapy without surgical intervention. A small number of cytogenetic studies have described chromosomal abnormalities in GTT (Wake *et al.* 1981, Sheppard *et al.* 1985, Lawler & Fisher 1986, Bettio *et al.* 1993, Rodriguez *et al.* 1995). However, these studies have not identified any specific chromosome rearrangements associated with either CC or PSTT. Karyotyping has shown that IM are generally diploid (Wake *et al.* 1984, Yang *et al.* 1986) while most CC are aneuploid with modes in the hyperdiploid and hypotetraploid range (Makino *et al.* 1965, Wake *et al.* 1981, Sasaki *et al.* 1982, Sekiya *et al.* 1983, Okabe *et al.* 1983, Sheppard *et al.* 1985, Lawler & Fisher 1986, Bettio *et al.* 1993, Rodriguez *et al.* 1995). Interestingly, the few PSTT examined have usually been found to be diploid (Lathrop *et al.* 1988, Xue *et al.* 2002).

Molecular genetic investigations using microsatellite markers and comparative genome hybridization (CGH), have revealed more specific chromosomal imbalance in CC. These studies have implicated the 7p12–7q11.23 and 8p12–p21 regions as the site of potential tumour suppressor genes (Matsuda *et al.* 1997, Ahmed *et al.* 2000) and 7q21–q31 as a region in which oncogene(s) important in the pathogenesis of GTT may be located (Ahmed *et al.* 2000). Comparative genome hybridisation of PSTT has confirmed that chromosomal abnormalities are rare in this group of tumours (Xue *et al.* 2002, Hui *et al.* 2004).

Molecular biology of trophoblastic tumours

Choriocarcinoma can develop from any pregnancy including PHM (Seckl *et al.* 2000, Namba *et al.* 2003). However, the greatest risk factor for GTT, even with earlier diagnosis of HM, is a pregnancy with CHM. In the UK approximately 10% of women with CHM require subsequent chemotherapy for a GTT (Bagshawe *et al.* 1986). Since histopathological features of HM lack prognostic significance (Genest 2001), a number of studies have been initiated to identify molecular markers that may be related to the subsequent development of PTD.

Overexpression of several growth factors including epidermal growth factor receptor (EGFR), ERBB2, and BCL2 has been found in CHM, CC and PSTT compared to normal placenta and PHM (Muller-Hocker *et al.* 1997, Fulop *et al.* 1998b, Tuncer *et al.* 2000), suggesting a role for these proteins in tumorigenesis. The significance of up-regulation of these growth factors is unclear given that the HM is a rapidly proliferating tissue. However, a small number of studies have suggested that increased expression of ERBB2, EGFR and BCL2 may be correlated with the development of PTD (Wong *et al.* 1999, Tuncer *et al.* 2000, Yang *et al.* 2002). Data relating to other oncogenes such as *MYC* and *FMS* remains controversial (Fulop *et al.* 1998b, Cheung *et al.* 1993).

The tumour suppressor genes *p53*, *p21* and *RB* are also overexpressed in CHM, CC and PSTT compared to normal placenta and PHM (Cheung *et al.* 1994b, 1998, Lee 1995, Muller-Hocker *et al.* 1997, Fulop *et al.* 1998c). However, mutations in *p53* are uncommon in GTD (Shi *et al.* 1996, Fulop *et al.* 1998c, Cheung *et al.* 1999a) and no correlation has been found between p53 expression and prognosis (Cheung *et al.* 1999a), suggesting that increased expression may simply reflect proliferative activity.

A novel candidate tumour suppressor gene *NECC1* (not expressed in CC clone 1) has recently been identified in CC by means of subtractive hybridisation. This gene has been shown to be ubiquitously expressed in tissues including the placenta but is absent in CC tissue and cell lines (Asanoma *et al.* 2003). Transfection of *NECC1* into CC cell lines suppressed tumorigenesis suggesting a role in the development of GTT. The *DOC-2/hDab* gene, originally identified as down-regulated, or absent, in ovarian tumours, may also play a role in the development of GTT. It also shows low levels of expression in the trophoblast cells of CHM and CC compared to normal placenta and is able to reduce growth when transfected into CC cell lines (Fulop *et al.* 1998a). Further investigations are required to determine the exact role of these tumour suppressor genes in GTT.

Increased telomerase activity has been suggested as a factor that may play a role in development of post-mole CC. Telomerase, which is expressed in all IM and CC, has been found in only 16% of those HM that resolved spontaneously compared to approximately 80% of those that progressed to PTD (Bae & Kim 1999, Cheung *et al.* 1999b). More specifically, expression of human telomerase reverse transcriptase (hTERT) has been shown to be associated with the development of GTT in that no cases of CHM negative for hTERT expression have failed to resolve spontaneously (Amezcua *et al.* 2001).

Techniques using cDNA microarrays and protein chip analysis to compare CHM and normal chorionic villi have revealed up-regulation of molecules involved in cell signalling, apoptosis and cell attachment (Kato *et al.* 2002) and reduced expression of a small number of proteins (Batorfi *et al.* 2003). These techniques have future potential for identifying differences between those CHM that resolve spontaneously and those that progress to PTD.

Demonstration that HM were homozygous (Kajii & Ohama 1977) provided an explanation for the high incidence of PTD following CHM, since any heterozygous recessive mutation in the sperm could potentially become homozygous on doubling of the paternal genome. However, since CHM have been shown to be an imprinted condition, deregulation of imprinted genes might be the more important factor in the development of post-mole tumours. Several observations support this hypothesis. First, monospermic CHM, which have a greater degree of homozygosity than dispermic CHM, have a similar, or lesser, risk of progressing to PTD than dispermic CHM (Fisher & Lawler 1984, Lawler *et al.* 1991, Mutter *et al.* 1993a, Cheung *et al.* 1994a). Second, women with familial recurrent HM, in whom the CHM are likely to be biparental and therefore heterozygous in origin, also have a significant incidence of PTD. Within the 37 women with familial recurrent HM described in the literature, 2 developed CC, 7 had a single episode of PTD and 2 patients had courses of treatment following 2 different molar pregnancies (reviewed in Fisher *et al.* 2004a). In total, 12 of 113 CHM (11%) failed to resolve spontaneously, a risk of PTD similar to that following AnCHM.

A role for deregulation of imprinted genes in tumorigenesis is now well recognised (Feinberg & Tycko 2004). The preferential loss of specific parental alleles in several childhood tumours has been recognised for some time (Schroeder *et al.* 1987, Toguchida *et al.* 1989). An association between excess paternal genes and tumorigenesis is also present in BWS. Individuals with BWS, which may result from unipaternal disomy or paternal duplication of part of chromosome 11, have been shown to have a predisposition to embryonal tumours (Henry *et al.* 1991). Loss of heterozygosity for imprinted regions may lead to loss of the only functional copy of a gene, while uniparental diosmy for an imprinted region is likely to result in overexpression of imprinted genes within that domain. Direct evidence of a role for imprinted genes in tumorigenesis came from the demonstration of biallelic expression of the maternally imprinted *IGF2* gene in Wilms' tumour (Ogawa *et al.* 1993, Rainier *et al.* 1993).

In CHM loss of maternally transcribed genes or overexpression of paternally transcribed genes might be expected to play a role. Relaxation of both *H19* and *IGF2* has been shown to be a frequent event in GTT. Most CC following either HM or non-molar pregnancies show biallelic expression of one or both genes (Hashimoto *et al.* 1995, Lustig-Yariv *et al.* 1997, Wake *et al.* 1998). In addition, we have recently shown re-expression of p57^{KIP2} to be a frequent event in CC and PSTT originating in CHM (Sebire *et al.* 2004). Complete hydatidiform moles that progress to PTD are likely to show deregulation of a large number of imprinted genes. Identification of specific genes that play a role in the development of post-mole tumours may well result from studies of those GTT that follow non-molar pregnancies in which fewer genes are abnormally expressed.

Summary

Gestational trophoblastic diseases include the abnormal pregnancy HM, IM and the overtly malignant CC and PSTT. Hydatidiform moles are characterised by trophoblastic hyperplasia and abnormal or absent fetal development. They can be classified as CHM or PHM on the basis of histopathological features and genetic origin. Partial hydatidiform moles are diandric triploids whereas CHM are diploid and usually androgenetic in origin. In both PHM and AnCHM trophoblastic proliferation is associated with two copies of the paternal genome while in PHM the presence of a maternal contribution to the genome is associated with greater fetal development. Occasional diploid, biparental HM have been reported. These unusual HM are associated with a rare autosomal recessive condition predisposing affected women to recurrent molar pregnancies. Despite having a maternal genome, most of these diploid, biparental HM are pathologically indistinguishable from AnCHM and show similar deregulation of imprinted genes. Gestational trophoblastic tumours may originate from the trophoblast cells of any type of pregnancy. However, the greatest risk factor for the development of these tumours is a pregnancy with a CHM, suggesting that the development of GTT is also associated with overexpression of paternally transcribed genes and/or loss of the maternal genome. Deregulation of imprinted genes is clearly an important underlying mechanism in this group of diseases. Further investigations are required to identify the specific genes involved and elucidate their role in embryonic development and tumorigenesis.

REFERENCES

Aapola, U., Kawasaki, K., Scott, H. S. *et al.* (2000). Isolation and initial characterization of a novel zinc finger gene, DNMT3L, on 21q22.3, related to the cytosine-5-methyltransferase 3 gene family, *Genomics,* **65**, 293–8.

Ahmed, M.N., Kim, K., Haddad, B., Berchuck, A. & Qumsiyeh, M.B. (2000). Comparative genomic hybridization studies in hydatidiform moles and choriocarcinoma: amplification of 7q21-q31 and loss of 8p12-p21 in choriocarcinoma. *Cancer Genet. Cytogenet.,* **116**, 10–15.

Al-Hussaini, T.K., Abd El Aal, D.M. & Van den Veyver, I.B. (2003). Recurrent pregnancy loss due to familial and non-familial habitual molar pregnancy. *Int. J. Gynaecol. Obstet.,* **83**, 179–86.

Ambani, L.M., Vaidya, R.A., Rao, C.S., Daftary, S.D. & Motashaw, N.D. (1980). Familial occurrence of trophoblastic disease – report of recurrent molar pregnancies in sisters in three families. *Clin. Genet.,* **18**, 27–9.

Amezcua, C.A., Bahador, A., Naidu, Y.M. & Felix, J.C. (2001). Expression of human telomerase reverse transcriptase, the catalytic subunit of telomerase, is associated with the development of persistent disease in complete hydatidiform moles. *Am. J. Obstet. Gynecol.,* **184**, 1441–6.

Ariel, I., Lustig, O., Oyer, C.E. *et al.* (1994). Relaxation of imprinting in trophoblastic disease. *Gynecol. Oncol.,* **53**, 211–19.

Arima, T., Imamura, T., Sakuragi, N. *et al.* (1995). Malignant trophoblastic neoplasms with different mode of origin. *Cancer Genet. Cytogenet.,* **85**, 5–15.

Arima, T., Drewell, R.A., Oshimura, M., Wake, N. & Surani, M.A. (2000). A novel imprinted gene, HYMAI, is located within an imprinted domain on human chromosome 6 containing ZAC. *Genomics,* **67**, 248–55.

Asanoma, K., Matsuda, T., Kondo, H. *et al.* (2003). NECC1, a candidate choriocarcinoma suppressor gene that encodes a homeodomain consensus motif. *Genomics,* **81**, 15–25.

Azuma, C., Saji, F., Nobunaga, T. *et al.* (1990). Studies of the pathogenesis of choriocarcinoma by analysis of restriction fragment length polymorphisms. *Cancer Res.,* **50**, 488–91.

Azuma, C., Saji, F., Takemura, M. *et al.* (1992). Triplet pregnancy involving complete hydatidiform mole and two foetuses: Genetic analysis by deoxyribonucleic acid fingerprint. *Am. J. Obstet. Gynecol.,* **166**, 664–7.

Bae, S.N. & Kim, S.J. (1999). Telomerase activity in complete hydatidiform mole. *Am. J. Obstet. Gynecol.*, **180**, 328–33.

Bagshawe, K.D. (1976). Risk and prognostic factors in trophoblastic neoplasia. *Cancer*, **38**, 1373–85.

Bagshawe, K.D. & Lawler, S.D. (1982). Choriocarcinoma. In D. Schottenfeld & J.F. Fraumeni, eds. *Cancer Epidemiology and Prevention.* Philadelphia: W.B. Saunders, pp.909–24.

Bagshawe, K.D. & Noble, M.I.M. (1966). Cardio-respiratory aspects of trophoblastic tumors. *Q. J. Med.*, **35**, 39–54.

Bagshawe, K.D., Dent, J. & Webb, J. (1986). Hydatidiform mole in England and Wales 1973–83. *Lancet*, **2**, 673–7.

Bagshawe, K.D., Lawler, S.D., Paradinas, F.J. *et al.* (1990). Gestational trophoblastic tumors following initial diagnosis of partial hydatidiform mole. *Lancet*, **335**, 1074–6.

Barton, S.C., Surani, M.A.H. & Norris, M.L. (1984). Role of maternal and paternal genomes in mouse development. *Nature*, **311**, 374–6.

Batorfi, J., Ye, B., Mok, S.C. *et al.* (2003). Protein profiling of complete mole and normal placenta using ProteinChip analysis on laser capture microdissected cells. *Gynecol. Oncol.*, **88**, 424–8.

Bell, K.A., Van Deerlin, V., Addya, K. *et al.* (1999). Molecular genetic testing from paraffin-embedded tissue distinguishes nonmolar hydropic abortion from hydatidiform mole. *Mol. Diagn.*, **4**, 11–19.

Berkowitz, R.S., Sandstrom, M., Goldstein, D.P. & Driscoll, S.G. (1982). 45,X complete hydatidiform mole. *Gynecol. Oncol.*, **14**, 279–83.

Berkowitz, R.S., Goldstein, D.P. & Bernstein, M.R. (1985). Natural history of partial molar pregnancy. *Obstet. Gynecol.*, **66**, 677–81.

Berkowitz, R.S., Im, S.S., Bernstein, M.R. & Goldstein, D.P. (1998). Gestational trophoblastic disease. Subsequent pregnancy outcome, including repeat molar pregnancy. *J. Reprod. Med.*, **43**, 81–6.

Bettio, D., Giardino, D., Rizzi, N. & Simoni, G. (1993) Cytogenetic abnormalities detected by direct analysis in a case of choriocarcinoma. *Cancer Genet. Cytogenet.*, **68**, 149–51.

Bourc'his, D., Xu, G.L., Lin, C.S., Bollman, B. & Bestor, T.H. (2001). Dnmt3L and the establishment of maternal genomic imprints. *Science*, **294**, 2536–9.

Bower, M., Brock, C., Fisher, R.A., Newlands, E.S.N. & Rustin, G.J.S. (1995). Gestational choriocarcinoma. *Ann. Oncol.*, **6**, 503–8.

Bower, M., Paradinas, F.J., Fisher, R.A. *et al.* (1996). Placental site trophoblastic tumor: clinical experience and genetic origin. *Clin. Cancer Res.*, **2**, 897–902.

Bracken, M.B. (1987). Incidence and aetiology of hydatidiform mole: an epidemiological review. *Br. J. Obstet. Gynaecol.*, **94**, 1123–35.

Braunstein, G.D., Vaitukaitis, J.L., Carbone, P.P. & Ross, G.T. (1973). Ectopic production of human chorionic gonadotropin by neoplasms. *Ann. Intern. Med.*, **78**, 39–45.

Buckell, E.W.C. & Owen, T.K. (1954). Chorionepithelioma in mother and infant. *Br. J. Obstet. Gynaecol.*, **61**, 329–30.

Castrillon, D.H., Sun, D., Weremowicz, S. *et al.* (2001). Discrimination of complete hydatidiform mole from its mimics by immunohistochemistry of the paternally imprinted gene product p57KIP2. *Am. J. Surg. Pathol.*, **25**, 1225–30.

Chedin, F., Lieber, M.R. & Hsieh, C.L. (2002). The DNA methyltransferase-like protein DNMT3L stimulates de novo methylation by Dnmt3a. *Proc. Natl. Acad. Sci. U.S.A.*, **99**, 16916–21.

Cheung, A.N., Srivastava, G., Pittaluga S. *et al.* (1993). Expression of c-myc and c-fms oncogenes in trophoblastic cells in hydatidiform mole and normal human placenta. *J. Clin. Pathol.*, **46**, 204–7.

Cheung, A.N., Sit, A.S., Chung, L.P. *et al.* (1994a). Detection of heterozygous XY complete hydatidiform mole by chromosome in situ hybridization. *Gynecol. Oncol.*, **55**, 386–92.

Cheung, A.N., Srivastava, G., Chung, L.P. *et al.* (1994b). Expression of the p53 gene in trophoblastic cells in hydatidiform moles and normal human placentae. *J. Reprod. Med.*, **39**, 223–7.

Cheung, A.N., Shen, D.H., Khoo, U.S., Wong, L.C. & Ngan, H.Y. (1998). p21WAF1/CIP1 expression in gestational trophoblastic disease: correlation with clinicopathological parameters, and Ki67 and p53 gene expression. *J. Clin. Pathol.*, **51**, 159–62.

Cheung, A.N., Shen, D.H., Khoo, U.S. *et al.* (1999a). Immunohistochemical and mutational analysis of p53 tumor suppressor gene in gestational trophoblastic disease: correlation with mdm2, proliferation index, and clinicopathologic parameters. *Int. J. Gynecol. Cancer*, **9**, 123–30.

Cheung, A.N., Zhang, D.K., Liu, Y. *et al.* (1999b). Telomerase activity in gestational trophoblastic disease. *J. Clin. Pathol.*, **52**, 588–92.

Cheville, J.C., Greiner, T., Robinson, R.A. & Benda, J.A. (1995). Ploidy analysis by flow cytometry and fluorescence in situ hybridization in hydropic placentae and gestational trophoblastic disease. *Hum. Pathol.*, **26**, 753–7.

Chew, S.H., Perlman, E.J., Williams, R., Kurman, R.J. & Ronnett, B.M. (2000). Morphology and DNA content analysis in the evaluation of first trimester placentae for partial hydatidiform mole (PHM). *Hum. Pathol.*, **31**, 914–24.

Chilosi, M., Piazzola, E., Lestani, M. *et al.* (1998). Differential expression of p57kip2, a maternally imprinted cdk inhibitor, in normal human placenta and gestational trophoblastic disease. *Lab. Invest.*, **78**, 269–76.

Cho. S. & Kim, S.J. (1993). Genetic study of hydatidiform moles by restriction fragment length polymorphisms (RFLPs) analysis. *J. Korean Med. Sci.*, **8**, 446–52.

Crisp, H., Burton, J.L., Stewart, R. & Wells, M. (2003) Refining the diagnosis of hydatidiform mole: image ploidy analysis and p57KIP2 immunohistochemistry. *Histopathology*, **43**, 363–73.

Eckstein, R.P., Paradinas, F.J. & Bagshawe, K.D. (1982). Placental site trophoblastic tumor (trophoblastic pseudotumour): a study of four cases requiring hysterectomy including one fatal case. *Histopathology*, **6**, 211–26.

Eckstein, R.P., Russell, P., Friedlander, M.L., Tattersall, M.H. & Bradfield, A. (1985). Metastasizing placental site trophoblastic tumor: a case study. *Hum. Pathol.*, **16**, 632–6.

Edwards, Y.H., Jeremiah, S.J., McMillan, S.L. *et al.* (1984). Complete hydatidiform moles combine maternal mitochondria with a paternal nuclear genome. *Ann. Hum. Genet.*, **48**, 119–27.

El-Maarri, O., Seoud, M., Coullin, P. *et al.* (2003). Maternal alleles acquiring paternal methylation patterns in biparental complete hydatidiform moles. *Hum. Mol. Genet.*, **12**, 1405–13.

Elston, C. W. (1976). The histopathology of trophoblastic tumors. *J. Clin. Pathol.*, **29**, 111–31.

Elston, C. W. & Bagshawe, K. D. (1967). The value of histological grading in the management of hydatidiform mole. *Br. J. Obstet. Gynaecol.*, **79**, 717–24.

Elston, C. W. & Bagshawe, K. D. (1972). The diagnosis of trophoblastic tumors from uterine curettings. *J. Clin. Pathol.*, **25**, 111–18.

Emery, J. L. (1952). Chorionepithelioma in new-born male child with hyperplasia of interstitial cells of testis. *J. Pathol. Bacteriol.*, **64**, 735–9.

Fallahian, M. (2003). Familial gestational trophoblastic disease. *Placenta*, **24**, 797–9.

Falls, J. G., Pulford, D. J., Wylie, A. A. & Jirtle, R. L. (1999). Genomic imprinting: implications for human disease. *Am. J. Pathol.*, **154**, 635–47.

Feinberg, A. P. & Tycko, B. (2004). The history of cancer epigenetics. *Nat. Rev. Cancer.*, **4**, 143–53.

Feltmate, C. M., Genest, D. R., Wise, L. *et al.* (2001). Placental site trophoblastic tumor: a 17-year experience at the New England Trophoblastic Disease Center. *Gynecol. Oncol.*, **82**, 415–19.

Fisher, R. A. & Lawler, S. D. (1984). Heterozygous complete hydatidiform moles: do they have a worse prognosis than homozygous complete moles? *Lancet*, **ii**, 51

Fisher, R. A. & Newlands, E. S. (1993). Rapid diagnosis and classification of hydatidiform moles using the polymerase chain reaction. *Am. J. Obstet. Gynecol.*, **168**, 563–9.

Fisher, R. A., Lawler, S. D., Ormerod, M. G., Imrie, P. & Povey, S. (1987). Flow cytometry used to distinguish between complete and partial hydatidiform moles. *Placenta*, **8**, 249–56.

Fisher, R. A., Lawler, S. D., Povey, S. & Bagshawe, K. D. (1988). Genetically homozygous choriocarcinoma following pregnancy with hydatidiform mole. *Br. J. Cancer*, **58**, 788–92.

Fisher, R. A., Povey, S., Jeffreys, A. J. *et al.* (1989). Frequency of heterozygous complete hydatidiform moles, estimated by locus-specific minisatellite and Y chromosome-specific probes. *Hum. Genet.*, **8**, 259–63.

Fisher, R. A., Newlands, E. S., Jeffreys, A. J. *et al.* (1992a). Gestational and non-gestational trophoblastic tumors distinguished by DNA analysis. *Cancer*, **69**, 839–45.

Fisher, R. A., Paradinas, F. J., Newlands, E. S. & Boxer, G. M. (1992b). Genetic evidence that placental site trophoblastic tumors can originate from a hydatidiform mole or a normal conceptus. *Br. J. Cancer*, **65**, 355–8.

Fisher, R. A., Soteriou, B., Meredith, L., Paradinas, F. J. & Newlands, E. S. (1995). Previous hydatidiform mole identified as the causative pregnancy of choriocarcinoma following birth of normal twins. *Int. J. Gynecol. Cancer*, **5**, 64–70.

Fisher, R. A., Paradinas, F. J., Soteriou, B. A., Foskett, M. & Newlands, E. S. (1997). Diploid hydatidiform moles with fetal red blood cells in molar villi. 2 – Genetics. *J. Pathol*, **181**, 189–95.

Fisher, R. A., Khatoon, R., Paradinas, F. J., Roberts, A. P. & Newlands, E. S. (2000). Repetitive complete hydatidiform mole can be biparental in origin and either male or female. *Hum. Reprod.*, **15**, 594–8.

Fisher, R. A., Hodges, M. D., Rees, H. C. *et al.* (2002). The maternally transcribed gene p57KIP2 (CDNK1C) is abnormally expressed in both androgenetic and biparental complete hydatidiform moles. *Hum. Mol. Genet.*, **11**, 3267–72.

Fisher, R. A., Hodges, M. D. & Newlands, E. S. (2004a). Familial recurrent hydatidiform mole: a review. *J. Reprod. Med.*, **49**, 595–601.

Fisher, R.A., Nucci, M.R., Thaker, H.M. *et al.* (2004b). Complete hydatidiform mole retaining a chromosome 11 of maternal origin: molecular genetic analysis of a case. *Mod. Pathol.*, **17**, 1155–60.

Fitzpatrick, G.V., Soloway, P.D. & Higgins, M.J. (2002). Regional loss of imprinting and growth deficiency in mice with a targeted deletion of KvDMR1. *Nat. Genet.*, **32**, 426–31.

Ford, J.H., Brown, J.K., Lew, W.Y. & Peters, G.B. (1986). Diploid complete hydatidiform mole, mosaic for normally fertilized cells and androgenetic homozygous cells. Case report. *Br. J. Obstet. Gynaecol.*, **93**, 1181–6.

Frank, D., Mendelsohn, C.L., Ciccone, E. *et al.* (1999). A novel pleckstrin homology-related gene family defined by Ipl/Tssc3, TDAG51, and Tih1: tissue-specific expression, chromosomal location, and parental imprinting. *Mamm. Genome*, **10**, 1150–9.

Frank, D., Fortino, W., Clark, L. *et al.* (2002). Placental overgrowth in mice lacking the imprinted gene Ipl. *Proc. Natl. Acad. Sci. U.S.A.*, **99**, 7490–5.

Fujita, N., Tamura, S., Shimizu, N. & Nozawa, S. (1994). Genetic analysis of hydatidiform mole and non-molar abortion using the polymerase chain reaction method. *Acta Obstet. Gynecol. Scand.*, **73**, 719–25.

Fukunaga, M. (2002). Immunohistochemical characterization of p57(KIP2) expression in early hydatidiform moles. *Hum. Pathol.*, **33**, 1188–92.

Fukunaga, M., Ushigome, S., Fukunaga, M. & Sugishita, M. (1993). Methods in pathology: application of flow cytometry in diagnosis of hydatidiform moles. *Mod. Pathol.*, **6**, 353–9.

Fukuyama, R., Takata, M., Kudoh, J. *et al.* (1991). DNA diagnosis of hydatidiform mole using the polymerase chain reaction. *Hum. Genet.*, **87**, 216–18.

Fulop, V., Colitti, C.V., Genest, D. *et al.* (1998a). DOC-2/hDab2, a candidate tumor suppressor gene involved in the development of gestational trophoblastic diseases. *Oncogene*, **17**, 419–24.

Fulop, V., Mok, S.C., Genest, D.R. *et al.* (1998b). p53, p21, Rb and mdm2 oncoproteins. Expression in normal placenta, partial and complete mole, and choriocarcinoma. *J. Reprod. Med.*, **43**, 119–27.

Fulop, V., Mok, S.C., Genest, D.R. *et al.* (1998c). c-myc, c-erbB-2, c-fms and bcl-2 oncoproteins. Expression in normal placenta, partial and complete mole, and choriocarcinoma. *J. Reprod. Med.*, **43**, 101–10.

Genest, D.R. (2001). Partial hydatidiform mole: clinicopathological features, differential diagnosis, ploidy and molecular studies, and gold standards for diagnosis. *Int. J. Gynecol. Pathol.*, **20**, 315–22.

Genest, D.R., Laborde, O., Berkowitz, R.S. *et al.* (1991). A clinicopathologic study of 153 cases of complete hydatidiform mole (1980–1990): histologic grade lacks prognostic significance. *Obstet. Gynecol.*, **78**, 402–9.

Hamazaki, S., Nakamoto, S., Okino, T. *et al.* (1999). Epithelioid trophoblastic tumor: morphological and immunohistochemical study of three lung lesions. *Hum. Pathol.*, **30**, 1321–7.

Hashimoto, K., Azuma, C., Koyama, M. *et al.* (1995). Loss of imprinting in choriocarcinoma. *Nat. Genet.*, **9**, 109–10.

Helwani, M.N., Seoud, M., Zahed, L. *et al.* (1999). A familial case of recurrent hydatidiform molar pregnancies with biparental genomic contribution. *Hum. Genet.*, **105**, 112–15.

Hemming, J. D., Quirke, P., Womack, C., Wells, M. & Elston, C. W. (1987). Diagnosis of molar pregnancy and persistent trophoblastic disease by flow cytometry. *J. Clin. Pathol.*, **40**, 615–20.

Henry, I., Bonaiti-Pellie, C., Chehensse, V. *et al.* (1991). Uniparental paternal disomy in a genetic cancer-predisposing syndrome. *Nature*, **351**, 665–7.

Hertig, A. T. & Mansell, H. (1956). Tumors of the female sex organs. Part 1. Hydatidiform mole and choriocarcinoma. In *Atlas of Tumor Pathology*, Sect. 9, Fasc. 33, 1956, Armed Forces Institute of Pathology, Washington, DC

Hertig, A. T. & Sheldon, W. H. (1947). Hydatidiform mole: a pathologico-clinical correlation of 200 cases. *Am. J. Obstet. Gynecol.*, **53**, 1–36.

Higashino, M., Harada, N., Hataya, I. *et al.* (1999). Trizygotic pregnancy consisting of two foetuses and a complete hydatidiform mole with dispermic androgenesis. *Am. J. Med. Genet.*, **82**, 67–9.

Hodges, M. D., Rees, H. C., Seckl, M. J. Newlands, E. S. & Fisher, R. A. (2003). Genetic refinement and physical mapping of a biparental complete hydatidiform mole locus on chromosome 19q13.4. *J. Med. Genet.*, **40**, e95.

Hoshi, K., Morimura, Y., Azuma, C. *et al.* (1994). A case of quadruplet pregnancy containing complete mole and three foetuses. *Am. J. Obstet. Gynecol.*, **170**, 1372–3.

Hsu, C. C., McConnell, J., Ko, T. M. & Braude, P. R. (1993). Twin pregnancy consisting of a complete hydatidiform mole and a foetus: genetic origin determined by DNA typing. *Am. J. Obstet. Gynecol.*, **100**, 867–9.

Huettner, P. C. & Gersell, D. J. (1994). Placental site nodule: a clinicopathologic study of 38 cases. *Int. J. Gynecol. Pathol.*, **13**, 191–8.

Hui, P., Riba, A., Pejovic, T. *et al.* (2004). Comparative genomic hybridization study of placental site trophoblastic tumor: a report of four cases. *Mod. Pathol.*, **17**, 248–51.

Ikeda, Y., Jinno, Y., Masuzaki, H., Niikawa, N. & Ishimaru, T. (1996). A partial hydatidiform mole with 2N/3N mosaicism identified by molecular analysis. *J. Assist. Reprod. Genet.*, **13**, 739–44.

Jacobs, P. A., Angell, R. R., Buchanan, I. M. *et al.* (1978a). The origin of human triploids. *Ann. Hum. Genet.*, **42**, 49–57.

Jacobs, P. A., Hassold, T. J., Matsuyama, A. M. & Newlands, I. M. (1978b). Chromosome constitution of gestational trophoblastic disease. *Lancet*, **ii**, 49.

Jacobs, P. A., Wilson, C. M., Sprenkle, J. A., Rosenshein, N. B. & Migeon, B. R. (1980). Mechanism of origin of complete hydatidiform moles. *Nature*, **286**, 714–16.

Jacobs, P. A., Hunt, P. A., Matsuura, J. S., Wilson, C. C. & Szulman, A. E. (1982a). Complete and partial hydatidiform mole in Hawaii: cytogenetics, morphology and epidemiology. *Br. J. Obstet. Gynaecol.*, **89**, 258–66.

Jacobs, P. A., Szulman, A. E., Funkhouser, J., Matsuura, J. S. & Wilson, C. C. (1982b). Human triploidy: relationship between parental origin of the additional haploid complement and development of partial hydatidiform mole. *Ann. Hum. Genet.*, **46**, 223–31.

Jauniaux, E., Nicolaides, K. H. & Hustin, J. (1997). Perinatal features associated with placental mesenchymal dysplasia. *Placenta*, **18**, 701–6.

Jeffers, M. D., O'Dwyer, P., Curran, B., Leader, M. & Gillan, J. E. (1993). Partial hydatidiform mole: a common but underdiagnosed condition. A 3-year retrospective clinicopathological and DNA flow cytometric analysis. *Int. J. Gynecol. Pathol.*, **12**, 315–23.

Judson, H., Hayward, B. E., Sheridan, E. & Bonthron, D. T. (2002). A global disorder of imprinting in the human female germ line. *Nature*, **416**, 539–42.

Jun, S. Y., Ro, J. Y. & Kim, K. R. (2003). p57kip2 is useful in the classification and differential diagnosis of complete and partial hydatidiform moles. *Histopathology*, **43**, 17–25.

Kajii, T. & Ohama, K. (1977). Androgenetic origin of hydatidiform mole. *Nature*, **268**, 633–4.

Kajii, T., Kurashige, H., Ohama, K. & Uchino, F. (1984). XY and XX complete moles: clinical and morphological correlations. *Am. J. Obstet. Gynecol.*, **150**, 57–64.

Kamiya, M., Judson, H., Okazaki, Y. *et al.* (2000). The cell cycle control gene ZAC/PLAGL1 is imprinted – a strong candidate gene for transient neonatal diabetes. *Hum. Mol. Genet.*, **9**, 453–60.

Kato, H. D., Terao, Y., Ogawa, M. *et al.* (2002). Growth-associated gene expression profiles by microarray analysis of trophoblast of molar pregnancies and normal villi. *Int. J. Gynecol. Pathol.*, **21**, 255–60.

Kim, S. J., Bae, S. N. & Kim, J. H. (1998). Epidemiology and time trends of gestational trophoblastic disease in Korea. *Int. J. Gynaecol. Obstet.*, **60** (Suppl 1), S33–8.

Kircheisen, R. & Ried, T. (1994). Hydatidiform moles. *Hum. Reprod.*, **9**, 1783–5.

Ko, T.-M., Hsieh, C.-Y., Ho, H.-N., Hsieh, F.-J. & Lee, T.-Y. (1991). Restriction fragment length polymorphism analysis to study the genetic origin of hydatidiform mole. *Am. J. Obstet. Gynecol.*, **164**, 901–6.

Kovacs, B. W., Shahbahrami, B., Tast, D. E. & Curtin, J. P. (1991). Molecular genetic analysis of complete hydatidiform moles. *Cancer Genet. Cytogenet.*, **54**, 143–52.

Kurman, R. J., Scully, R. E. & Norris, H. J. (1976). Trophoblastic pseudotumour of the uterus: an exaggerated form of 'syncytial endometritis' simulating a malignant tumor. *Cancer*, **38**, 1214–26.

La Vecchia, C., Franceschi, S., Fasoli, M. & Mangioni, C. (1982). Gestational trophoblastic neoplasms in homozygous twins. *Obstet. Gynecol.*, **60**, 250–2.

Lai, C. Y., Chan, K. Y., Khoo, U. S. *et al.* (2004). Analysis of gestational trophoblastic disease by genotyping and chromosome in situ hybridization. *Mod. Pathol.*, **17**, 40–8.

Lage, J. M., Driscoll, S. G., Yavner, D. L. *et al.* (1988). Hydatidiform moles; application of flow cytometry in diagnosis. *Am. J. Clin. Pathol.*, **89**, 596–600.

Lane, S. A., Taylor, G. R., Ozols, B. & Quirke, P. (1993). Diagnosis of complete molar pregnancy by microsatellites in archival material. *J. Clin. Pathol.*, **46**, 346–8.

Lathrop, J. C., Lauchlan, S., Nayak, R. & Ambler, M. (1988). Clinical characteristics of placental site trophoblastic tumor (PSST). *Gynecol. Oncol.*, **31**, 32–42.

Lawler, S. & Fisher, R. A. (1986). Genetic aspects of gestational trophoblastic tumors. In K. Ichinoe, ed., *Trophoblastic Diseases*. New York: Igaku-Shoin, pp. 23–33.

Lawler, S. D., Pickthall, V. J., Fisher, R. A. *et al.* (1979). Genetic studies of complete and partial hydatidiform moles. *Lancet*, **2**, 580.

Lawler, S. D., Fisher, R. A., Pickthall, V. J., Povey, S. & Evans, M. W. (1982a). Genetic studies on hydatidiform moles. I. The origin of partial moles. *Cancer Genet. Cytogenet.*, **5**, 309–20.

Lawler, S. D., Povey, S., Fisher, R. A. & Pickthall, V. J. (1982b). Genetic studies on hydatidiform moles. II. The origin of complete moles. *Ann. Hum. Genet.*, **46**, 209–22.

Lawler, S. D., Fisher, R. A. & Dent, J. (1991). A prospective study of hydatidiform mole. *Am. J. Obstet. Gynecol.*, **164**, 1270–7.

Lee, Y. S. (1995). p53 expression in gestational trophoblastic disease. *Int. J. Gynecol. Pathol.*, **14**, 119–24.

Lee, K.C. & Chan, J. K. (1990). Placental site nodule. *Histopathology*, **16**, 193–5.

Lee, M. H., Reynisdottir, I. & Massague, J. (1995). Cloning of p57KIP2, a cyclin-dependent kinase inhibitor with unique domain structure and tissue distribution. *Genes Dev.*, **9**, 639–49.

Lorigan, P. C., Sharma, S., Bright, N., Coleman, R. E. & Hancock, B. W. (2000). Characteristics of women with recurrent molar pregnancies. *Gynecol. Oncol.*, **78**, 288–92.

Lustig-Yariv, O., Schulze, E. & Komitowski, D. (1997). The expression of the imprinted genes H19 and IGF-2 in choriocarcinoma cell lines. Is H19 a tumor suppressor gene? *Oncogene*, **15**, 169–77.

Magrath, I. T., Golding, P. R. & Bagshawe, K. D. (1971). Medical presentations of choriocarcinoma. *Br. Med. J.*, **ii**, 633–7.

Makino, S., Sasaki, M. S. & Fukuschima, T. (1965). Cytological studies of tumors XLI, chromosomal instability in human chorionic lesions. *Okajimas Folia Anat. Jpn.*, **40**, 439–65.

Makrydimas, G., Sebire, N. J., Thornton, S. E. *et al.* (2002). Complete hydatidiform mole and normal live birth: a novel case of confined placental mosaicism: case report. *Hum. Reprod.*, **17**, 2459–63.

Mangili, G., Parazzini, F., Maggi, R. & Spolti, N. (1993). Repeated gestational trophoblastic disease after natural and heterologous assisted conception. A case report. *J. Reprod. Med.*, **38**, 405–6.

Matsuda, T., Sasaki, M. & Kato, H. (1997). Human chromosome 7 carries a putative tumor suppressor gene(s) involved in choriocarcinoma. *Oncogene*, **15**, 2773–81.

Matsui, H., Iitsuka, Y., Suzuka, K., Seki, K. & Sekiya, S. (2001). Subsequent pregnancy outcome in patients with spontaneous resolution of hCG after evacuation of hydatidiform mole: comparison between complete and partial mole. *Hum. Reprod.*, **16**, 1274–7.

Matsui, H., Iitsuka, Y., Yamazawa, K. *et al.* (2003). Changes in the incidence of molar pregnancies. A population-based study in Chiba Prefecture and Japan between 1974 and 2000. *Hum. Reprod.*, **18**, 172–5.

Mazur, M. T. (1989). Metastatic gestational choriocarcinoma: unusual pathological variant following therapy. *Cancer*, **50**, 1370–7.

McFadden, D. E., Kwong, L. C., Yam, I. Y. & Langlois, S. (1993). Parental origin of triploidy in human foetuses: evidence for genomic imprinting. *Hum. Genet.*, **92**, 465–9.

McGrath, J. & Solter, D. (1984). Completion of mouse embryogenesis requires both the maternal and paternal genomes. *Cell*, **37**, 179–83.

Moglabey, Y. B., Kircheisen, R., Seoud, M. *et al.* (1999). Genetic mapping of a maternal locus responsible for familial hydatidiform moles. *Hum. Mol. Genet.*, **8**, 667–71.

Morison, I. M. & Reeve, A. E. (1998). A catalogue of imprinted genes and parent-of-origin effects in humans and animals. *Hum. Mol. Genet.*, **7**, 1599–1609.

Mowery-Rushton, P. A., Driscoll, D. J., Nicholls, R. D., Locker, J. & Surti, U. (1996). DNA methylation patterns in human tissues of uniparental origin using a zinc-finger gene (ZNF127) from the Angelman/Prader–Willi region. *Am. J. Med. Genet.*, **61**, 140–6.

Muller-Hocker, J., Obernitz, N., Johannes, A. & Lohrs, U. (1997). p53 gene product and EGF-receptor are highly expressed in placental site trophoblastic tumor. *Hum. Pathol.*, **28**, 1302–6.

Mutter, G. L., Pomponio, R. J., Berkowitz, R. S. & Genest, D. R. (1993a). Sex chromosome compo-
    sition of complete hydatidiform moles: Relationship to metastasis. *Am. J. Obstet. Gynecol.*,
    168, 1547–51.

Mutter, G. L., Stewart, C. L., Chaponot, M. L. & Pomponio, R. J. (1993b). Oppositely imprinted
    genes H19 and insulin-like growth factor 2 are coexpressed in human androgenetic tro-
    phoblast. *Am. J. Hum. Genet.*, **53**, 1096–102.

Namba, A., Nakagawa, S., Nakamura, N. *et al.* (2003). Ovarian choriocarcinoma arising from
    partial mole as evidenced by deoxyribonucleic acid microsatellite analysis. *Obstet. Gynecol.*,
    102, 991–4.

Newlands, E. S. (1997). Presentation and management of persistent gestational trophoblastic dis-
    ease and gestational trophoblastic tumors in the UK. In B. W. Hancock, E. S. Newlands
    & R. S. Berkowitz, eds., *Gestational Trophoblastic Disease*. London: Chapman and Hall,
    pp. 5–26.

Ogawa, O., Eccles, M. R., Szeto, J. *et al.* (1993). Relaxation of insulin-like growth factor II gene
    imprinting implicated in Wilms' tumor. *Nature*, **362**, 749–51.

Ohama, K., Kajii, T., Okamoto, E. *et al.* (1981). Dispermic origin of XY hydatidiform moles.
    Nature, **29**, 551–2.

Ohira, S., Yamazaki, T., Hatano, H. *et al.* (1999). Trophoblastic tumor metastatic to the
    vagina: an immunohistochemical and ultrastructural study. *Int. J. Gynecol. Pathol.*, **19**,
    381–6.

Okabe, T., Sasaki, N., Matsuzaki, M. *et al.* (1983). Establishment and characterization of a new
    human functional cell line from a choriocarcinoma. *Cancer Res.*, **43**, 4920–6.

Osada, H., Kawata, M., Yamada, M., Okumura, K. & Takamizawa, H. (1991). Genetic iden-
    tification of pregnancies responsible for choriocarcinomas after multiple pregnancies
    by restriction fragment length polymorphism analysis. *Am. J. Obstet. Gynecol.*, **165**,
    682–8.

Osada, H., Iitsuka, Y., Matsui, H. & Sekiya, S. (1995). A complete hydatidiform mole co-existing
    with a normal foetus was confirmed by variable number tandem repeat (VNTR) polymor-
    phism analysis using polymerase chain reaction. *Gynecol. Oncol.*, **56**, 90–3.

Palmer, J. R. (1994). Advances in the epidemiology of gestational trophoblastic disease. *J. Reprod.
    Med.*, **39**, 155–62.

Papadopoulos, A. J., Foskett, M., Seckl, M. J. *et al.* (2002). Twenty-five years' clinical experience
    with placental site trophoblastic tumors. *J. Reprod. Med.*, **47**, 460–4.

Paradinas, F. J. (1992). Pathology and classification of trophoblastic tumors. In: M. Coppleson,
    J. M. Monaghan, C. P. Morrow and M. H. N. Tattersall, eds., *Gynecologic Oncology*. Edinburgh:
    Churchill Livingstone, pp. 1013–26.

    (1994). The histological diagnosis of hydatidiform moles. *Curr. Diag. Pathol.*, **1**, 24–31.

Paradinas, F. J., Browne, P., Fisher, R. A. *et al.* (1996). A clinical, histopathological and flow
    cytometric study of 149 complete moles, 146 partial moles and 107 non-molar hydropic
    abortions. *Histopathology*, **28**, 101–9.

Paradinas, F. J., Fisher, R. A., Browne, P. & Newlands, E. S. (1997). Diploid hydatidiform moles
    with fetal red blood cells in molar villi: 1 – Pathology, Incidence and Prognosis. *J. Pathol.*,
    181, 183–8.

Paradinas, F. J., Sebire, N. J., Fisher, R. A. *et al.* (2001). Pseudo-partial moles; placental stem vessel hydrops and the association with Beckwith–Wiedemann syndrome and complete moles. *Histopathology*, **39**, 447–54.

Parazzini, F., La Vecchia, C., Franceschi, S. & Mangili, G. (1984). Familial trophoblastic disease: case report. *Am. J. Obstet. Gynecol.*, **149**, 382–3.

Park, W. W. (1971). *Choriocarcinoma: A Study of its Pathology.* London: Heinemann.

Parrington, J. M., West, L. F. & Povey, S. (1984). The origin of ovarian teratomas. *J. Med. Genet.*, **21**, 4–12.

Rainier, S., Johnson, L. A., Dobry, C. J. *et al.* (1993). Relaxation of imprinted genes in human cancer. *Nature*, **362**, 747–9.

Reik, W. & Walter, J. (2001). Genomic imprinting: Parental influence on the genome. *Nat. Rev. Genet.*, **2**, 21–32.

Repiska, V., Vojtassak, J., Danihel, L. *et al.* (2003). Application of DNA polymorphism analysis to detection of complete hydatidiform mole origin. *Biologia*, **58**, 403–8.

Reubinoff, B. E., Lewin, A., Verner, M. *et al.* (1997). Intracytoplasmic sperm injection combined with pre-implantation genetic diagnosis for the prevention of recurrent gestational trophoblastic disease. *Hum. Reprod.*, **12**, 805–8.

Rice, L. W., Berkowitz, R. S., Lage, J. M., Goldstein, D. P. & Bernstein, M. R. (1990). Persistent gestational trophoblastic tumor after partial hydatidiform mole. *Gynecol. Oncol.*, **36**, 358–62.

Roberts, D. J. & Mutter, G. L. (1994). Advances in the molecular biology of gestational trophoblastic disease. *J. Reprod. Med.*, **39**, 201–8.

Rodriguez, E., Melamed, J., Reuter, V. & Chaganti, R. S. (1995). Chromosomal abnormalities in choriocarcinomas of the female. *Cancer Genet. Cytogenet.*, **80**, 9–12.

Saji, F., Tokugawa, Y., Kimura, T. *et al.* (1989). A new approach using DNA fingerprinting for the determination of androgenesis as a cause of hydatidiform mole. *Placenta*, **10**, 399–405.

Sander, C. M. (1993). Angiomatous malformation of placental chorionic stem vessels and pseudo-partial molar placentae: report of five cases. *Pediatr. Pathol.*, **13**, 621–33.

Sarno, A. P. & Jr, Moorman, A. J. Kalousek, D. K. (1993). Partial molar pregnancy with fetal survival: an unusual example of confined placental mosaicism. *Obstet. Gynecol.*, **82**, 716–19.

Sasaki, S., Katayama, P. K., Roesler, M. *et al.* (1982). Cytogenetic analysis of choriocarcinoma cell lines. *Acta Obstet. Gynaecol. Jpn.*, **34**, 2253–6.

Saxena, A., Frank, D., Panichkul, P. *et al.* (2003). The product of the imprinted gene IPL marks human villous cytotrophoblast and is lost in complete hydatidiform mole. *Placenta*, **24**, 835–42.

Schroeder, W. T., Chao, L. Y., Dao, D. D. *et al.* (1987). Nonrandom loss of maternal chromosome 11 alleles in Wilms' tumor. *Am. J. Hum. Genet.*, **40**, 413–20.

Sebire, N. J., Foskett, M., Fisher, R. A. *et al.* (2002). Risk of partial and complete hydatidiform molar pregnancy in relation to maternal age. *Br. J. Obstet. Gynaecol.*, **109**, 99–102.

Sebire, N. J., Fisher, R. A., Foskett, M. *et al.* (2003a). Risk of recurrent hydatidiform mole and subsequent pregnancy outcome following complete or partial hydatidiform molar pregnancy. *Br. J. Obstet. Gynaecol.*, **110**, 22–6.

Sebire, N.J., Fisher, R.A. & Rees, H. (2003b). Histopathological diagnosis of partial and complete hydatidiform mole in the first trimester of pregnancy. *Pediatr. Dev. Pathol.*, **6**, 69–77.

Sebire, N.J., Rees, H.C., Peston, D. *et al.* (2004). P57^{KIP2} immunohistochemical staining of gestational trophoblastic tumors does not identify the type of the causative pregnancy. *Histopathology*, **45**, 135–41.

Seckl, M.J., Fisher, R.A., Salerno, G. *et al.* (2000). Choriocarcinoma and partial hydatidiform moles. *Lancet*, **356**, 36–9.

Sekiya, S., Shirotake, S., Kaiho, T. *et al.* (1983). A newly established human gestational choriocarcinoma cell line and its characterization. *Gynecol. Oncol.*, **15**, 413–21.

Sensi, A., Gualandi, F., Pittalis, M. C. *et al.* (2000). Mole maker phenotype: possible narrowing of the candidate region. *Eur. J. Hum. Genet.*, **8**, 641–4.

Seoud, M., Khalil, A., Frangieh, A. *et al.* (1995). Recurrent molar pregnancies in a family with extensive intermarriage: report of a family and review of the literature. *Obstet. Gynecol.*, **86**, 692–5.

Shahib, N., Martaadisoebrata, D., Kondo, H. *et al.* (2001). Genetic origin of malignant trophoblastic neoplasms analyzed by sequence tag site polymorphic markers. *Gynecol. Oncol.*, **81**, 247–53.

Shapter, A.P. & McLellan, R. (2001). Gestational trophoblastic disease. *Obstet. Gynecol. Clin. North Am.*, **28**, 805–17.

Sheppard, D.M., Fisher, R.A., Lawler, S.D. & Povey, S. (1982). Tetraploid conceptus with three paternal contributions. *Hum. Genet.*, **62**, 371–4.

Sheppard, D.M., Fisher, R.A. & Lawler, S.D. (1985). Karyotypic analysis and chromosome polymorphisms in four choriocarcinoma cell lines. *Cancer Genet. Cytogenet.*, **16**, 251–9.

Shi, Y.F., Xie, X., Zhao, C.L. *et al.* (1996). Lack of mutation in tumor-suppressor gene p53 in gestational trophoblastic tumors. *Br. J. Cancer*, **73**, 1216–19.

Shigematsu, T., Kamura, T., Arima, T., Wake, N. & Nakano, H. (2000). DNA polymorphism analysis of a pure non-gestational choriocarcinoma of the ovary: case report. *Eur. J. Gynaecol. Oncol.*, **21**, 153–4.

Shih, I.M. & Kurman, R. (1998a). Ki67 labelling in the differential diagnosis of exaggerated placental site reaction, placental site trophoblastic tumor and choriocarcinoma. *Hum. Pathol.*, **29**, 27–33.

(1998b). Epithelioid trophoblastic tumor: a neoplasm distinct from choriocarcinoma and placental site trophoblastic tumor simulating carcinoma. *Am. J. Surg. Pathol.*, **22**, 1393–1403.

(2001a). The pathology of intermediate trophoblast, tumors and tumor-like lesions. *Int. J. Gynecol. Pathol.*, **20**, 31–47.

(2001b). Placental site trophoblastic tumor. Past as prologue. *Gynecol. Oncol.*, **82**, 413–14.

Shitabata, P.K. & Rutgers, J.L. (1994). The placental site nodule: an immunohistochemical study. *Hum. Pathol.*, **25**, 1295–30.

Silva, E.G., Tornos, C., Lage, J. *et al.* (1993). Multiple nodules of intermediate trophoblast following hydatidiform moles. *Int. J. Gynecol. Pathol.*, **12**, 324–32.

Sunde, L., Vejerslev, L.O., Jensen, M.P. *et al.* (1993). Genetic analysis of repeated, biparental, diploid, hydatidiform moles. *Cancer Genet. Cytogenet.*, **66**, 16–22.

Surani, M. A. H., Barton, S. C. & Norris, M. L. (1984). Development of reconstituted mouse eggs suggests imprinting of the genome during gametogenesis. *Nature*, **308**, 548–50.

Surti, U., Szulman, A. E., Wagner, K., Leppert, M. & O'Brien, S. J. (1986). Tetraploid partial hydatidiform moles: two cases with a triple paternal contribution and a 92,XXXY karyotype. *Hum. Genet.*, **72**, 15–21.

Suryanarayan, K., O'Hanlan, K. A., Surti, U. *et al.* (1998). Nongestational choriocarcinoma in the postpartum period: a case report. *J. Pediatr. Hematol. Oncol*, **20**, 169–73.

Suzuki, T., Goto, S., Nawa, A. *et al.* (1993). Identification of the pregnancy responsible for gestational trophoblastic disease by DNA analysis. *Obstet. Gynecol.*, **82**, 629–34.

Szulman, A. E. & Surti, U. (1978a). The syndromes of hydatidiform mole. I. Cytogenetic and morphological correlations. *Am. J. Obstet. Gynecol.*, **131**, 665–71.

(1978b). The syndromes of hydatidiform mole. II. Morphologic evolution of the complete and partial mole. *Am. J. Obstet. Gynecol.*, **132**, 20–7.

Takahashi, H., Kanazawa, K., Ikarashi, T., Sudo, N. & Tanaka, K. (1990). Discrepancy in the diagnoses of hydatidiform mole by macroscopic findings and the deoxyribonucleic acid fingerprint method. *Am. J. Obstet. Gynecol.*, **163**, 112–13.

Takahashi, K., Kobayashi, T. & Kanayama, N. (2000). p57 KIP2 regulates the proper development of labyrinthine spongiotrophoblasts. *Mol. Hum. Reprod.*, **6**, 1019–25.

The International Human Genome Sequencing Consortium. (2001). Initial Sequencing and analysis of the human genome. *Nature*, **409**, 860–921.

Toguchida, J., Ishizaki, K., Sasaki, M. S. *et al.* (1989). Preferential mutation of paternally derived RB gene as the initial event in sporadic osteosarcoma. *Nature*, **338**, 156–8.

Tuncer, Z. S., Vegh, G. L., Fulop, V. *et al.* (2000). Expression of epidermal growth factor receptor-related family products in gestational trophoblastic diseases and normal placenta and its relationship with development of postmolar tumor. *Gynecol. Oncol.*, **77**, 389–93.

Van de Kaa, C. A., Hanselaar, A. G. J. M, Hopman, A. H. N. *et al.* (1993). DNA cytometric and interphase cytogenetic analyses of paraffin-embedded hydatidiform moles and hydropic abortions. *J. Pathol.*, **170**, 229–38.

Vassilakos, P. & Kajii, T. (1976). Hydatidiform mole: two entities. *Lancet*, **i**, 259.

Vassilakos, P., Riotton, G. & Kajii, T. (1977). Hydatidiform mole: a morphological and cytogenetic study with some clinical considerations. *Am. J. Obstet. Gynecol.*, **127**, 167–70.

Vejerslev, L. O., Dissing, J., Hansen, H. E. & Poulsen, H. (1987a). Hydatidiform mole: genetic origin in polyploid conceptuses. *Hum. Genet.*, **76**, 11–19.

Vejerslev, L. O., Fisher, R. A., Surti, U. & Wake, N. (1987b). Hydatidiform mole: cytogenetically unusual cases and their implications for the present classification. *Am. J. Obstet. Gynecol.*, **157**, 180–4.

Vejerslev, L., Sunde, L., Hansen, B. F. *et al.* (1991). Hydatidiform mole and foetus with normal karyotype: support of a separate entity. *Obstet. Gynecol.*, **77**, 868–74.

Wake, N., Takagi, N. & Sasaki, M. (1978). Androgenesis as a cause of hydatidiform mole. *J. Natl. Cancer Inst.*, **60**, 51–7.

Wake, N., Tanaka, K.-I., Chapman, V., Matsui, S. & Sandberg, A. A. (1981). Chromosomes and cellular origin of choriocarcinoma. *Cancer Res.*, **41**, 3137–43.

Wake, N., Seki, T., Fujita, H. *et al.* (1984). Malignant potential of homozygous and heterozygous complete moles. *Cancer Res.*, **44**, 1226–30.

Wake, N., Fujino, T., Hoshi, S. *et al.* (1987). The propensity to malignancy of dispermic heterozygous moles. *Placenta*, **8**, 319–26.

Wake, N., Arima, T. & Matsuda, T. (1998). Involvement of IGF2 and H19 imprinting in choriocarcinoma development. *Int. J. Gynaecol. Obstet.*, **60**, S1–8.

Wallace, D.C., Surti, U., Adams, C.W. & Szulman, A.E. (1982). Complete moles have paternal chromosomes but maternal mitochondrial DNA. *Hum. Genet.*, **61**, 145–7.

Walsh, C., Miller, S.J., Flam, F., Fisher, R.A. & Ohlsson, R. (1995). Paternally-derived H19 is differentially expressed in malignant and non-malignant trophoblast. *Cancer Res.*, **55**, 1111–16.

Walter, J. & Paulsen, M. (2003). Imprinting and disease. *Semin. Cell. Dev. Biol.*, **14**, 101–10.

Weaver, D.T., Fisher, R.A., Newlands, E.S. & Paradinas, F.J. (2000). Amniotic tissue in complete moles can be androgenetic. *J. Pathol.*, **191**, 67–70.

Wong, S.Y., Ngan, H.Y., Chan, C.C. & Cheung, A.N. (1999). Apoptosis in gestational trophoblastic disease is correlated with clinical outcome and Bcl-2 expression but not Bax expression. *Mod. Pathol.*, **12**, 1025–33.

World Health Organization Scientific Group (1983). *Gestational trophoblastic diseases.* Technical Report Series 692.

Wu, F.Y. (1973). Recurrent hydatidiform mole. A case report of nine consecutive molar pregnancies. *Obstet. Gynecol.*, **41**, 200–4.

Xue, W.C., Guan, X.Y., Ngan, H.Y. *et al.* (2002). Malignant placental site trophoblastic tumor: a cytogenetic study using comparative genomic hybridization and chromosome in situ hybridization. *Cancer*, **94**, 2288–94.

Yang, Y.H., Kwak, H.M., Park, T.K., Kim, C.K. & Lee, Y.B. (1986). Comparative cytogenetic and clinicopathologic studies on gestational trophoblastic neoplasia, especially hydatidiform mole. *Yonsei Med. J.*, **27**, 250–60.

Yang, X., Zhang, Z., Jia, C. *et al.* (2002). The relationship between expression of c-ras, c-erbB-2, nm23, and p53 gene products and development of trophoblastic tumor and their predictive significance for the malignant transformation of complete hydatidiform mole. *Gynecol. Oncol.*, **85**, 438–44.

Young, R.H. & Scully, R.E. (1984). Placental-site trophoblastic tumor: current status. *Clin. Obstet. Gynecol.*, **27**, 248–58.

Young, R.H., Kurman, R.J. & Scully, R.E. (1990). Placental site nodules and plaques: a clinicopathologic analysis of 20 cases. *Am. J. Surg. Pathol.*, **14**, 1001–9.

Zaragoza, M.V., Keep, D., Genest, D.R., Hassold, T. & Redline, R.W. (1997). Early complete hydatidiform moles contain inner cell mass derivatives. *Am. J. Med. Genet.*, **70**, 273–7.

Zaragoza, M.V., Surti, U., Redline, R.W. *et al.* (2000). Parental origin and phenotype of triploidy in spontaneous abortions: predominance of diandry and association with the partial hydatidiform mole. *Am. J. Hum. Genet.*, **66**, 1807–20.

Zhang, P., McGinniss, M.J., Sawai, S. & Benirschke, K. (2000). Diploid/triploid mosaic placenta with foetus. Towards a better understanding of 'partial moles'. *Early Hum. Dev.*, **60**, 1–11.

DISCUSSION

McLaren   Do you ever see mosaic HM? There are places in the literature (see McLaren 1976) where chimeras are described resulting from double fertilisation of one cell by two sperm at the two-cell stage, but normal fertilisation of the other, or of one sperm fertilising the egg and the other the polar body, and both contributing to the embryo.

R. Fisher   There are cases of mosaicism that involve molar pathology. We recently described a placenta that had large regions that were macroscopically CHM and yet there was a normal live born fetus who continued to develop normally (Makrydimas *et al.* 2002). The regions of the placenta that were molar were genetically complete hydatidiform mole while the regions that were non-molar were genetically normal.

McLaren   I have another question. With dizygotic twins, do you ever get unfortunate women who have an HM pregnancy in the same uterus as a normal fetus?

R. Fisher   Yes, this is not that infrequent. Because of the risk of persistent trophoblastic disease, following a molar pregnancy, the advice used to be to terminate twin pregnancies in which there was an HM. In fact, if these women are allowed to go to term there is approximately a 40% chance of delivering a normal baby with no elevated risk of persistent trophoblastic disease (Sebire *et al.* 2002).

Braude   I think I have another family for you. They were sent to us with the question of whether we could use preimplantation genetic diagnosis (PGD) to try to help them avoid another mole. If these were androgenetic moles then we would have done it in terms of sexing the embryo and replaced male embryos only. However, you raise another possibility and we need to think it through more carefully.

R. Fisher   This is a problem. In vitro fertilisation can be used to prevent an androgenetic CHM or a PHM but is not appropriate for a woman who has familial recurrent HM as the cells will appear genetically normal.

Braude   What advice could you give for this woman? There's probably very little.

R. Fisher   It is difficult to advise these women. We have never seen any normal pregnancies in women with recurrent HM of diploid, biparental origin ourselves. However, there have been occasional normal pregnancies reported in these families by other groups (Helwani *et al.* 1999) so we are unable to say that these women can never have a normal pregnancy. However, having seen women who have had recurrent molar pregnancies and then have had to go through chemotherapy for persistent trophoblastic disease we usually advise that they should consider IVF using oocyte donation rather than risk a probable molar pregnancy. In these circumstances it's clearly important to check whether the recurrent HM are androgenetic or diploid, biparental in origin.

Smith   You said that the familial condition was autosomal recessive.

R. Fisher   We believe so. This is because of the pattern of inheritance and the fact that this disorder often occurs in large consanguineous families.

Smith   Given the fact that the egg is haploid would you not expect the carriers of this condition to have a proportion of affected pregnancies as well?

R. Fisher   No. The defect is only in the oocytes of homozygous women. It is likely to be a defect in the oocyte itself which results in failure to set the maternal imprint. Although the pregnancy is abnormal it is the woman herself who has the inherited defect, not the conceptus.

Ferguson-Smith   Presumably this mutation is present in equal proportions in males and females within the population in the heterozygous state. Do you have any evidence that this problem can be transmitted paternally?

R. Fisher   Presumably the mutated gene can be transmitted paternally. It is not clear what the phenotype of homozygous males is in families with this condition. Very few families have been described, and in those that have there appears to be very few males in the affected generations. Two of the affected families have five and four sisters, respectively, with no male siblings (Kircheisen & Ried 1994, Fisher *et al.* 2002). Mouse models, in which there is a failure to set the maternal imprints (Bourc'his *et al.* 2001), suggest that males that are homozygous for this condition might be sterile.

McLaren   Did you check to see whether the five sisters were XX?

R. Fisher   No, we haven't done this.

Ferguson-Smith   It would be interesting to know whether there is a problem in males in setting paternal methylation marks in the presence of this mutation. I suppose there are probably cultural issues as well with some of these families in terms of male fertility.

R. Fisher   Even in the women there are a lot of cultural issues because of the fact that it is often the Asian community that has these large consanguineous families where the problem occurs.

Jacobs   Is there any clue as to why these CHM have such an enormously different prevalence depending upon ethnic group?

R. Fisher   There clearly is a difference in the incidence of molar pregnancies in different ethnic groups. A large study has recently been completed by the Trophoblastic Screening and Treatment Centre in Sheffield, UK in which they have shown that there is almost twice the risk of having a molar pregnancy in the Asian population than the non-Asian population in their catchment area (Tham *et al.* 2003). Interestingly, in many countries that used to have a very high incidence of molar pregnancy, such as Japan and Korea, the incidence has now reduced to levels comparable with those found in Europe (Kim *et al.* 1998, Matsui *et al.* 2003).

Loke   This is true in Malaysia also. When I was working there 30 years ago we saw HM regularly, but now they can hardly find a case.

Braude   Pat Jacobs, didn't you write an article discussing what happened to Japanese when they moved to Western cultures?

Jacobs   Yes. In Hawaii I looked at all the different racial groups to see what happened with disease prevalences in them. For example, when Japanese women move to Hawaii their breast cancer incidence increases and then when they move to the mainland it is at the same level as in Caucasians. This wasn't the same for moles at all: they kept their own incidence of moles. It is very difficult to equate this with the current observations of a reduction in the rate, which suggests that there is a large environmental component.

Trowsdale   I'd like to ask about the mapping. I was fascinated by the region you identified. We know this region well because the human killer-cell immunoglobulin-like receptor (KIR) genes map to 19q13.4. How was your mapping done?

R. Fisher   The first mapping was done by conventional linkage in Rima Slim's group (Moglabey *et al.* 1999). They identified a common region of homozygosity on chromosome 19q13.3–13.4 in affected individuals. Since then other groups, including ours, have examined affected individuals to see whether they are homozygous for the same region.

Trowsdale   Is that in one family?

R. Fisher   Initially the region was mapped in one family. Subsequently affected members of four families, in which the recurrent hydatidiform moles were shown to be diploid and biparental in origin, were found to be homozygous for this region, which has now been narrowed to approximately 1 Mb on chromosome 19q13.4.

Moffett   The *PEG3* gene is there, isn't it?

R. Fisher   In fact, there is an imprinted domain containing *PEG3* in this region. The first mapping suggested that this was within the region in which the gene, mutated in familial recurrent HM, was located. Now that the region has been refined, the imprinted region is outside the region of interest.

Trowsdale   Do you know which genes are in this region?

R. Fisher   There are approximately 80 genes within the region. A lot of them are not well defined. They are just represented by expressed sequence tags (ESTs) in the databases.

Reik   I have another vague speculation on the different incidence of hydatidiform moles in the human population, and the fact that it may decrease. Imprinting can be polymorphic in the human population. There are reports that the genes can be imprinted in certain populations. This might contribute to that. If imprinting in humans is on the way out there will be fewer and fewer hydatidiform moles! The corollary of this is that you should get androgenetic people walking around.

Braude   There are a number of observations that together lead me to an interesting hypothesis. First, Azim Surani's original studies where he moved pronuclei around and made androgenetic mice and gynogenetic mice. Each had particular outcomes after implantation, namely small but formed fetuses in gynogenetic embryos but vestigial trophoblast; or a tiny or non-existent embryo but normal or large trophoblast in androgenetic embryos (Surani *et al.* 1987). Second, that a CHM was the first tumour that was discovered to be truly androgenetic and existed only in humans. Third, the human teratoma, otherwise known as a dermoid cyst, is of course female. But I have always wondered whether it could be parthenogenetic. In other words, are there certain people who are predisposed to producing parthenogenetically activated eggs? These produce no trophoblastic component. They simply start to make the tissues that they would, should development proceed. Many years ago, when I had to produce my MRCOG case book, I put this up as a hypothesis, but I haven't seen it mentioned since.

Moffett   Complete hydatidiform mole is the human equivalent of what Azim Surani made in mice, but in mice there is a fetus while in humans this is not a normal feature. Can you explain this difference?

Surani   The androgenetic embryos we made in mice are very small, and the ones you see in those pictures are the best ones. Not all of them look like that.

REFERENCES

Bourc'his, D., Xu, G.L., Lin, C.S., Bollman, B. & Bestor, T.H. (2001). Dnmt3L and the establishment of maternal genomic imprints. *Science*, **294**, 2536–9.

Fisher, R.A., Hodges, M.D., Rees, H.C. *et al.* (2002). The maternally transcribed gene p57KIP2 (CDNK1C) is abnormally expressed in both androgenetic and biparental complete hydatidiform moles. *Hum. Mol. Genet.*, **11**, 3267–72.

Helwani, M.N., Seoud, M., Zahed, L. *et al.* (1999). A familial case of recurrent hydatidiform molar pregnancies with biparental genomic contribution. *Hum. Genet.*, **105**, 112–15.

Kim, S.J., Bae, S.N., Kim, J.H. *et al.* (1998). Epidemiology and time trends of gestational trophoblastic disease in Korea. *Int. J. Gynaecol. Obstet.*, **60**(Suppl 1), S33–8.

Kircheisen, R. & Ried, T. (1994). Hydatidiform moles. *Hum. Reprod.*, **9**, 1783–5.

Makrydimas, G., Sebire, N.J., Thornton, S.E. *et al.* (2002). Complete hydatidiform mole and normal live birth: a novel case of confined placental mosaicism: case report. *Hum. Reprod.*, **17**, 2459–63.

Matsui, H., Iitsuka, Y., Yamazawa, K. *et al.* (2003). Changes in the incidence of molar pregnancies. A population-based study in Chiba Prefecture and Japan between 1974 and 2000. *Hum. Reprod.*, **18**, 172–5.

McLaren, A. (1976). *Mammalian Chimeras.* Cambridge: Cambridge University Press.

Moglabey, Y.B., Kircheisen, R., Seoud, M. *et al.* (1999). Genetic mapping of a maternal locus responsible for familial hydatidiform moles. *Hum. Mol. Genet.*, **8**, 667–71.

Sebire, N.J., Foskett, M., Paradinas, F.J. et al. (2002). Twin pregnancies with complete hydatidiform mole and coexistent normal foetus: pregnancy outcome and risk of persistent
trophoblastic disease. *Lancet*, **359**, 2165–6.

Surani, M.A.H., Barton, S.C. & Norris, M.L. (1987). Influence of parental chromosomes on
spatial specificity in androgenetic ↔ parthenogenetic chimaeras in the mouse. *Nature*, **326**,
395–7.

Tham, B.W., Everard, J.E., Tidy, J.A., Drew, D. & Hancock, B.W. (2003). Gestational trophoblastic disease in the Asian population of Northern England and North Wales. *Br. J. Obstet.
Gynaecol.*, **110**, 555–9.

6

Trophoblast and the first trimester environment

Graham J. Burton[1] and Eric Jauniaux[2]

[1] University of Cambridge, UK
[2] Royal Free and University College London, UK

Introduction

Human early placentation is a difficult topic for systematic research due to ethical constraints, the relative inaccessibility of the tissues and the lack of a suitable animal model, yet events taking place lay the foundation for a successful pregnancy. For many years our knowledge had been reliant upon the interpretation of static images of histological material from pregnant hysterectomy or miscarriage samples. The advent of high-resolution ultrasound imaging in the 1980s provided major new impetus, however, for it enabled events to be followed dynamically in vivo with remarkable clarity. Novel findings using this technique prompted a series of physiological investigations that together have led to a radical reappraisal of the environment in which the feto–placental unit develops. Central to this new appreciation is the premise that the human placenta is not fully haemochorial until the start of the second trimester.

The maternal circulation to the human placenta

During the late secretory phase of the menstrual cycle capillaries arising from the distal segments of the spiral arteries form a plexus within the superficial endometrium that connects with the endometrial veins. When the conceptus implants, the invading syncytiotrophoblastic mantle comes into contact with these capillaries, stimulating them to dilate through endothelial proliferation to form sinusoids, before finally breaking into them (Hertig *et al.* 1956, Carter 1997). As a result communications are established with the developing lacunae of the trophoblast mantle, the forerunners of the intervillous space, and maternal erythrocytes can be observed

Biology and Pathology of Trophoblast, eds. Ashley Moffett, Charlie Loke and Anne McLaren.
Published by Cambridge University Press © Cambridge University Press 2005.

in these cavities. Although in the original description it was noted that relatively few maternal erythrocytes are present in normal pregnancies (Hertig *et al.* 1956), accounts in many textbooks of human embryology equate this development with onset of the uteroplacental circulation (Moore & Persaud 1993, Larsen 1997). The suggestion is that such a precocious onset of haemotrophic exchange is an evolutionary advantage of the invasive form of implantation displayed by the human conceptus, and that once established the maternal circulation simply continues to increase gradually in force and volume throughout pregnancy.

This general concept was first challenged by Hustin and Schaaps who presented evidence from a variety of techniques suggesting that maternal blood flow through the placenta is extremely limited during the first trimester (Hustin & Schaaps 1987, Hustin *et al.* 1988, Schaaps & Hustin 1988). Using a transvaginal ultrasound probe, these authors were unable to detect moving echoes indicative of significant fluid movement within the intervillous space prior to 10 weeks of pregnancy. Equally, when they perfused pregnant hysterectomy specimens with radiopaque medium little dye was found to enter the placenta. By contrast, when the same investigations were performed at 12–14 weeks moving echoes could be detected, and contrast medium freely entered the intervillous space. These results suggested that there is a major change in the way the maternal spiral arteries connect with the intervillous space between 10 and 12 weeks. Histological examination revealed the explanation, in that during the early weeks of pregnancy the invading endovascular extravillous trophoblast is so voluminous that it effectively plugs the mouths of the spiral arteries (Hustin *et al.* 1988, Burton *et al.* 1999). Only when these plugs dissipate at the start of the second trimester can it be said that the maternal intraplacental circulation is fully established. Prior to that time the intervillous space is filled with a clear fluid that was initially believed to arise as a plasma filtrate percolating through the intercellular spaces of the trophoblastic plugs or as a transudate from the superficial endometrium (Schaaps & Hustin 1988). Hence, the placenta cannot be considered truly haemochorial during the first trimester.

These initial observations sparked considerable controversy and spirited debate regarding the sensitivity of ultrasound equipment and the precise location of the signals within the placenta and endometrium (Jauniaux *et al.* 1995, Coppens *et al.* 1996, Valentin *et al.* 1996, Jaffe *et al.* 1997, Kurjak & Kupesic 1997, Kurjak *et al.* 1997). However, the demonstration that there are major changes in placental oxygenation at the start of the second trimester provided physiological proof of the new theory, which has now been generally accepted (Rodesch *et al.* 1992, Jauniaux *et al.* 2000, Kliman 2000).

Since then, further investigations have revealed more details concerning onset of the maternal circulation. In normal pregnancies it appears that the circulation starts at the periphery of the placenta at approximately 8 weeks and gradually extends to the central regions by 12 weeks (Jauniaux *et al.* 2003). This pattern correlates with the degree of migration of the extravillous trophoblast cells across the placental bed (Pijnenborg *et al.* 1980, 1981). Invasion is deepest in the central region beneath the original implantation site, and so it might reasonably be assumed that trophoblastic plugging of the arteries is most extensive in this region. By contrast, in abnormal pregnancies ending as missed miscarriages, onset of the maternal circulation is both premature and disorganised throughout the whole placenta (Jaffe & Warsof 1992, Jauniaux *et al.* 1994, 2003, Kurjak & Kupesic 1997, Schwärzler *et al.* 1999). This pattern again correlates with the degree of extravillous trophoblast invasion, for it is particularly shallow in these pregnancies (Khong *et al.* 1987, Hustin *et al.* 1990). Thus, in both normal and abnormal pregnancies there appears to be an association between shallow trophoblast invasion and early onset of the maternal circulation.

Oxygen concentrations and gradients within the early feto–placental unit

One of the principal implications of limited maternal blood flow during the first trimester is that the intraplacental oxygen concentration will be low. Measurements taken in vivo with an oxygen-sensitive probe under ultrasound guidance have confirmed that the concentration within the intervillous space is <20 mmHg prior to 8 weeks of pregnancy, and this is reflected in low expression and activities of the principal antioxidant enzymes within the placental tissues (Rodesch *et al.* 1992, Jauniaux *et al.* 2000). The early development of the villous tree and of the cytotrophoblast cell columns therefore takes place in a low oxygen environment. The oxygen concentration within the underlying decidua is in the region of 60 mmHg prior to 8 weeks, and so when the extravillous trophoblast cells migrate they move into a higher oxygen environment (Rodesch *et al.* 1992, Jauniaux *et al.* 2000). Whether the oxygen concentration changes abruptly at the level of the cytotrophoblastic shell or whether there is a more extensive gradient within the endometrium is not known.

With onset of the full maternal circulation the oxygen concentration within the intervillous space rises to approximately 60 mmHg by 12 weeks (Rodesch *et al.* 1992, Jauniaux *et al.* 2000). Although the concentration in the underlying decidua also rises it does so to a lesser extent, and so the magnitude of the gradient between the placenta and the decidua decreases with gestational age. Onset of the maternal circulation is also associated with the establishment of the lobular arrangement of the villous trees, although whether this configuration is induced by haemodynamic forces or in response to oxygenation is not known (Reynolds 1966). The lobules are sited over the openings of the maternal arteries so that oxygenated blood is delivered into the centre of each lobule and then percolates radially outwards (Freese &

Maciolek 1969, Wigglesworth 1969, Ramsey & Donner 1980). It might be expected therefore that an oxygen gradient will exist across each lobule, and the few measurements that have been performed in the rhesus monkey support this hypothesis (Reynolds *et al.* 1968). More recently, we have demonstrated differences in the expression and activity of antioxidant enzymes across lobules in the human placenta at term that are consistent with the presence of such a gradient (Hempstock *et al.* 2003a).

The influence of oxygen on cell behaviour

Oxygen can exert a powerful influence on cell behaviour through a number of mechanisms, and the consequences range from the physiological responses to pathological changes.

Metabolism

Aerobic respiration is considerably more efficient than anaerobic respiration, for 38 moles of ATP can be generated from 1 mole of glucose in the presence of oxygen compared to 2 moles in its absence. Hence, cellular activities such as protein synthesis and ionic pumping that place heavy demands on ATP supplies may be suppressed when oxygen availability is limited (Carter 2000, Schneider 2000, Hochachka & Lutz 2001). If these adaptations are not sufficient and the ATP concentration falls below the critical threshold, necrosis may ensue (Leist *et al.* 1997).

Redox sensitive transcription factors

A number of redox sensitive transcription factors, such as (nuclear factor-kappaB (NF-κB), activator protein 1 AP-1) and hypoxia-inducible factor 1 (HIF-1), have now been identified that regulate gene expression in response to changes in oxygenation (Arrigo & Kretz-Remy 1998, Semenza 1998, Hensley *et al.* 2000). Hypoxia-inducible factor 1 is a dimeric factor consisting of two subunits, HIF-1α and HIF-1β, that has a wide range of target genes such as those encoding erythropoietin, vascular endothelial growth factor (VEGF), glucose transporters and glycolytic enzymes (Semenza 1998, Lando *et al.* 2003). The activity of HIF-1 is regulated largely at the post-transcriptional level through alterations in the stability of the HIF-1α subunit, for under normoxic conditions this subunit is rapidly degraded. Hydroxylation of a proline residue allows binding by the von Hippel–Lindau protein, marking the complex for ubiquitination and proteasomal degradation. Under hypoxic conditions the reduced oxygen availability becomes rate-limiting, and so the subunit accumulates (Semenza 1998). A second independent regulatory system has recently been described involving hydroxylation of a conserved asparagine residue within a transactivation domain at the C-terminus. Hydroxylation under normoxic conditions prevents binding of transcriptional coactivators, such as cyclic AMP-response element binding protein (CREB)-binding protein (CBP)/p300 and steroid receptor coactivator (SRC-1), that are essential for target gene expression (Lando *et al.* 2002).

Changes in mRNA stability

In addition to regulation by transcription the concentration of mRNA encoding certain genes can be influenced by altering the stability of the mRNA. This is the case for the mRNAs encoding angiopoietin 1, and the mRNA becomes more unstable as the prevailing oxygen concentration falls (Zhang *et al.* 2001). This will shift the balance of angiopoietins 1 and 2 in favour of the latter, promoting new vessel formation.

Reactive oxygen species as signalling molecules

Reactive oxygen species (ROS), free radicals and their non-radical intermediates, are formed as an inevitable by-product of aerobic respiration and other cellular processes (Halliwell & Gutteridge 1999). Once the preserve of chemists, ROS are now increasingly recognised as playing a central role in cellular homeostasis and in the pathogenesis of many disorders (Irani 2000, Droge 2002, Chen *et al.* 2003). The principal intracellular site of formation of free radicals under normal conditions is the mitochondria, where the leakage of electrons from the enzymes of the respiratory chain, in particular Complexes I and III, leads to the formation of the superoxide anion (Raha *et al.* 2000). The rate of formation correlates positively with the prevailing oxygen concentration, but paradoxically is also raised under hypoxia when the decreased availability of oxygen leads to a build-up of electrons on the respiratory chain, increasing the risk of leakage. Another potential source of ROS is the membrane-bound enzyme NAD(P)H oxidase. This enzyme is present on the apical surface of the syncytiotrophoblast, and its activity in generating superoxide is greatest during the first trimester of pregnancy (Matsubara & Tamada 1991, Raijmakers *et al.* 2004).

Many ligand–receptor binding interactions, for example epidermal growth factor with its receptor, are now known to stimulate formation of ROS which act as second messengers. Hence, ROS produced from other cellular processes may mimic these interactions and activate a number of protein kinase cascades, for example the mitogen-activated protein kinases (MAPK), the stress-activated protein kinases (SAPK), and the Janus kinase (JAK)/signal transducer and activator of transcription 3 (STAT) pathway.

Free radicals as toxic agents

Due to their unbalanced electron state, free radicals are highly reactive and can potentially interact with any biological molecule in their immediate vicinity, be it lipid, carbohydrate or nucleic acid. Consequently, a complex system of antioxidant defences has evolved to detoxify them, including the enzymes superoxide dismutase, catalase and glutathione peroxidase. These act in concert with non-enzymatic defences such as vitamins C and E and low molecular weight thiols (Halliwell & Gutteridge 1999). Under normal conditions a homeostatic balance between production and scavenging of ROS exists, but should production exceed the defences then cellular damage can ensue leading to the condition of oxidative stress. For example, peroxidation of lipids may lead to loss of fluidity in the cell membrane and in those of intracellular organelles, and once initiated is a self-propagating reaction. Oxidation of the –SH groups of proteins can result in the formation of additional disulphide bonds, abnormal folding and loss of function. This may stimulate the expression of chaperone heat shock proteins in an attempt to refold or sequester the damaged proteins (Freeman et al. 1999). In the case of mitochondria, oxidation of thiol groups on the inner membrane can trigger opening of the permeability transition pore, causing the release of cytochrome c and other apoptogenic molecules, such as Apaf-1, which activate the caspase pathways leading to apoptosis (Crompton 2000, Kowaltowski et al. 2001). Attacks on the sugar moieties of DNA may cause strand breakages, whereas those on histone proteins can lead to cross-linkages that interfere with chromatin folding, DNA repair and gene transcription. The effects on cell function can therefore be highly varied and difficult to predict.

The influence of oxygen on trophoblast behaviour during the first trimester

Metabolism

Analysis of the fluids within the intervillous space and extraembryonic coelom, which is in free exchange with the placental and fetal tissues, indicates that metabolism is heavily anaerobic during the first trimester (Jauniaux et al. 2001). However, there is no clear evidence that the tissue is hypoxically stressed during this period. We have been unable to detect HIF-1 immunohistochemically in first trimester tissues of <9 weeks' gestational age collected using a chorionic villus sampling (CVS) technique. This is in direct contrast to previously published reports, which described high levels of expression at 5–8 weeks (Caniggia et al. 2000, Rajakumar & Conrad 2000). A possible explanation for the discrepancy is that HIF-1α can be stabilised by other factors, including ROS (Haddad & Land 2001). To test this possibility in placental tissues we exposed our CVS samples to maternal blood in order to mimic conditions during suction curettage, and to other pro-oxidants. In all cases generation of oxidative stress led to increased immunore-activity of HIF-1α in 6-week tissues (Dyson *et al.* 2003). The method used for sample collection may therefore be a confounding factor for the analysis of HIF-1α concentrations. It would also seem unlikely that such a rapidly responsive factor would be up-regulated in placental tissues over a period of weeks when in cells exposed to hypoxia the response is transitory and restored to baseline levels in 4–6 hours (Stroka *et al.* 2001).

Trophoblast behaviour

Since the publication of the first data describing the change in intraplacental oxy-genation with gestational age there has been much interest in the effects of oxygen on trophoblast behaviour. It has long been appreciated that low oxygen concentra-tions stimulate cytotrophoblast proliferation (Fox 1964), and increased numbers of cytotrophoblast cells are seen in the placenta at high altitude (Ali 1997). The explant model system has been used to investigate these effects in vitro, but conflicting data have been reported. In early experiments in which first trimester explants were cultured under 2% or 21% oxygen, it was found that the lower, more physiologi-cal, oxygen concentration favoured cytotrophoblast proliferation and formation of syncytiotrophoblast, whereas under 21% oxygen the cytotrophoblast cells adopted a more invasive phenotype (Genbacev *et al.* 1996). Recent similar experiments comparing the effects of 3% and 21% oxygen produced somewhat different results, for although proliferation was increased under 3% oxygen so too was trophoblast migration from the explants, expression of α5 integrin, synthesis of fibronectin and gelatinase A activity (Caniggia *et al.* 2000). Little outgrowth was observed under 21% oxygen, and these effects appeared to be mediated via HIF-1 and transforming growth factor (TGF)β3. Interpreting these data is difficult because culture under 21% oxygen is clearly unphysiological for placental tissues, particularly at this stage of gestation. It is associated with rapid degeneration of the syncytiotrophoblast layer and this may have a profound effect on the behaviour of the cytotrophoblast cells (Palmer *et al.* 1997). By contrast, differences in cell migration have been demon-strated in an immortalised trophoblast-like cell line maintained under either 1% or 3% oxygen, with low oxygen promoting increased invasiveness through a nitric oxide-mediated pathway (Graham *et al.* 2000). At present, therefore, there seems lit-tle consensus, and further experiments under physiological conditions are required. What must be borne in mind, however, when setting these data in the context of the first trimester environment is the oxygen gradient that exists between the placenta and the decidua. The cytotrophoblast cell columns will be differentiating in the low oxygen environment of the intervillous space, although as mentioned previously the physical extent of the oxygen gradient is not known. It is possible that cells in the distal part of the cell column experience a higher oxygen concentration, but they will only experience that with certainty when they migrate into the endometrium. Extravillous trophoblast invasion occurs from the earliest stages of implantation onwards (Pijnenborg *et al.* 1981), and it is this migration that causes the rise in oxygen concentration within the intervillous space, rather than the other way around as has sometimes been proposed (Caniggia *et al.* 2000).

Other aspects of trophoblast behaviour may also be influenced by oxygen. Thus, reduced fusion of cytotrophoblast cells to form syncytiotrophoblast has been reported under hypoxic conditions (Alsat *et al.* 1996), and this has recently been associated with reduced expression of syncytin, a product encoded by an envelope gene of the human endogenous retrovirus-W (ERV-W) (Mi *et al.* 2000, Kudo *et al.* 2003). Oxygen can also modulate hormonal production by explants in vitro (Esterman *et al.* 1996) and alter cytokine secretion (Benyo *et al.* 1997), but the physiological significance of these effects during the first trimester is not known.

Oxidative stress

Production of ROS within mitochondria is related to the prevailing oxygen concentration (Freeman & Crapo 1981), and so it might be expected that generation will be increased within the placental tissues when the maternal circulation becomes fully established at the start of the second trimester. Evidence that this is the case was provided by the immunohistochemical detection of a transient burst of lipid peroxidation, nitrosylation of proteins and expression of heat shock protein 70 at 9 weeks' gestational age (Jauniaux *et al.* 2000). This was particularly marked in the syncytiotrophoblast, which displays low concentrations of the principal antioxidant enzymes at this stage of development, and was associated with dilatation of the mitochondrial intracristal space indicating involvement of these organelles (Watson *et al.* 1997, 1998a).

Whether this burst of ROS generation plays a physiological role in regulating gene transcription or trophoblast behaviour is not known at present, but if first trimester tissues are exposed to too great an oxidative challenge, for example culture in 21% oxygen, mitochondrial activity is rapidly lost and the syncytiotrophoblast degenerates through what appears to be a necrotic mechanism (Palmer *et al.* 1997, Watson *et al.* 1998b). The cytotrophoblast and stromal cells display higher concentrations of antioxidant enzymes and remain viable; indeed the cytotrophoblast cells differentiate to form a new syncytiotrophoblastic covering. In view of this susceptibility of the syncytium to oxidative stress, we have investigated levels of oxidative stress in normal first trimester placentas on a regional basis. Villi in the peripheral regions where maternal blood flow is first observed, and so where the oxygen concentration is likely to be highest, display significantly greater immunohistochemical and morphological evidence of oxidative stress than their counterparts in the centre (Jauniaux *et al.* 2003). The syncytiotrophoblast is thin with few microvilli on the apical surface, the cytoplasm is highly vacuolated and the mitochondria are distorted with dilated intracristal spaces. The underlying cytotrophoblast cells are characteristically flattened along the basal lamina, a phenotype associated with differentiation and formation of new syncytium. Similar trophoblastic changes are observed in the region of the forming chorion laeve in placenta-*in-situ* specimens, but in addition these villi are avascular (Jauniaux *et al.* 2003). The latter finding is consistent with down-regulation of VEGF expression in response to the elevated oxygen concentration. Since the majority of placental capillaries are not covered with pericytes at this stage of gestation they will be vulnerable to withdrawal of growth factor support in a similar fashion to the vessels of the retina (Benjamin *et al.* 1998, Zhang *et al.* 2002).

In cases of missed miscarriage in which onset of the maternal circulation is both premature and disorganised there is extensive trophoblastic oxidative stress throughout the placenta (Hempstock *et al.* 2003c). The cytotrophoblast cells display an increased rate of apoptosis and decreased proliferation, features that are consistent with exposure to a high oxygen environment. In some cases sheets of degenerate syncytiotrophoblast can be seen sloughing from the villous surface, with a new layer differentiating beneath. This regenerate syncytium fulfils at least some of the functions of the original, for it synthesises human chorionic gonadotrophin (HCG) and consequently serum concentrations of the hormone are maintained (Greenwold *et al.* 2003). If the placenta is retained in utero for some time, regression of the vasculature is observed, and the villi come to resemble closely those seen in the region of the developing chorion laeve.

Hence, a degree of syncytial degeneration induced by oxidative stress appears to be a normal aspect of placental development, particularly in the peripheral regions where villi regress to form the chorion laeve. The balance between degeneration and regeneration may determine the outcome of the pregnancy, and in miscarriage the disorganised onset of the maternal circulation may tip it in favour of degeneration, contributing to pregnancy loss.

The contribution of the endometrial glands to the first trimester environment

If the human placenta is not haemochorial during the first trimester, questions arise as to the origin and nature of the fluid within the intervillous space. In their original descriptions, Hustin and Schaaps proposed that the fluid arises as a filtrate of maternal plasma as it percolates through the labyrinth of intercellular spaces within the trophoblastic plugs (Schaaps & Hustin 1988). Whilst some seepage is likely, we have recently demonstrated that the endometrial glands discharge their secretions through the basal plate into the intervillous space until at least 10 weeks of gestation (Burton *et al.* 2002). Hence, the fluid may have a dual origin, and this raises the possibility that the endometrial glands may provide histiotrophic support to the feto–placental unit during the first trimester. In the earliest specimen available within the Boyd Collection of placenta-*in-situ* specimens, estimated to be 6 weeks' gestational age, the decidua basalis is 5–6mm thick and contains highly active glands. Glandular epithelial cells at 6 weeks of pregnancy contain large aggregations of glycogen and closely resemble those during the late secretory phase of the menstrual cycle (Dockery *et al.* 1988, Burton *et al.* 2002). The thickness of the decidua basalis gradually reduces over the next few weeks, and the glandular epithelium becomes more columnar in form.

We have followed immunohistochemically the discharge of two maternal proteins, glycodelin (PP14) and the mucin MUC-1, into the intervillous space, from where they are taken up by the syncytiotrophoblast and enter into the lysosomal digestive pathway (Burton *et al.* 2002). Breakdown of large glycoproteins will provide the developing placenta with a plentiful supply of carbon and nitrogen for anabolic pathways as well as energy, but the contribution of this route to overall materno–fetal exchange remains to be determined.

The endometrial glands are also a potentially important source of cytokines and growth factors that could modulate placental development. The glandular epithelium is strongly immunoreactive for VEGF, leukaemia inhibitory factor (LIF), epidermal growth factor (EGF) and TGFβ_3 during the first trimester (Hempstock *et al.* 2003b), and receptors for these factors are present on the trophoblast and villous endothelial cells (Ladines-Llave *et al.* 1991, Mühlhauser *et al.* 1993, Cooper *et al.* 1995, Sharkey *et al.* 1999). Epidermal growth factor appears to have a dual action on trophoblast dependent on gestational age, for in the samples of 4–5 weeks of age it stimulates cytotrophoblastic proliferation whereas at 6–8 weeks it promotes syncytiotrophoblastic differentiation and secretion of HCG (Maruo *et al.* 1992). Vascular endothelial growth factor and LIF may both be involved in regulation of angiogenesis, and LIF may also modulate HCG production (Kojima *et al.* 1995).

Another category of proteins expressed by the glands is that of transport carriers. Of particular importance may be tocopherol transfer protein, which is highly expressed and may facilitate the transport of vitamin E to the fetus, boosting antioxidant defences (Jauniaux *et al.* 2004).

The endometrial glands therefore potentially play more diverse roles in early pregnancy than previously anticipated. Attempts to match endometrial function with pregnancy outcome have met with mixed success. Whilst reduced concentrations of MUC-1, LIF and glycodelin in uterine flushings have been reported in women suffering recurrent miscarriages (Dalton *et al.* 1998, Mikolajczyk *et al.* 2003), expression of these markers within the endometrium shows no significant association (Tuckerman *et al.* 2004).

A comparative perspective

It is now apparent that early development of the human feto–placental unit takes place in a low oxygen environment, supported not by a precocious onset of the maternal circulation as previously thought but by a plasma filtrate supplemented by secretions from the endometrial glands. This brings the human into line with most other mammalian species. The initial support for the mammalian conceptus is provided by the cells of the oviduct, followed when it enters the uterus by the endometrial glands. The endometrial secretions contain high quantities of lipid, giving them a white opaque appearance, and so they have been referred to variously as uterine milk or histiotroph (Amoroso 1952, Wooding & Flint 1994). In the human it has always been considered that this phase of histiotrophic nutrition is brief due to the invasive form of implantation, but in many species, particularly those displaying non-invasive implantation, there is often a considerable period before placental attachment and development takes place (Mossman 1987, Wooding & Flint 1994). During this period growth factors such as EGF secreted by the endometrial glands play a key role in promoting proliferation and growth of the extraembryonic membranes (Lennard *et al.* 1998, Gray *et al.* 2000).

Besides providing the conceptus with a rich and complex array of growth factors there are other potential benefits to a reliance on histiotrophic nutrition during early pregnancy. The exclusion of significant quantities of maternal blood from the intervillous space during the first trimester ensures that the oxygen concentration is kept low within the feto–placental unit during the critical phase of embryogenesis. Metabolism in most mammalian embryos is heavily anaerobic during this phase of development (New 1978), and this may protect the developing fetus from the damaging effects of ROS (Burton *et al.* 2003). Disruption of signalling pathways or damage to DNA could lead to aberrant gene expression and teratogenesis. Once organogenesis is complete at approximately 10 weeks, the oxygen concentration can safely rise, and onset of the maternal circulation permits the rapid growth of the fetus seen during the second and third trimesters.

Conclusion

The invasive implantation and the haemochorial form of placentation displayed by the human conceptus appears to present a paradox. Whilst the extensive and intimate apposition of the maternal and fetal circulations it creates is ideally suited for supporting rapid growth of the fetus in later pregnancy, it may pose a risk to the differentiating embryo through free radical-mediated damage during the first trimester. Plugging of the spiral arteries and reliance more on histiotrophic nutrition from the endometrial glands may be a solution to this problem. However, the transition from histiotrophic to haemotrophic nutrition is a vulnerable phase, and must be carefully coordinated to prevent the pregnancy ending in failure.

ACKNOWLEDGEMENTS

The authors are grateful to the Medical Research Council, the Wellcome Trust, Tommy's the Baby Charity, WellBeing and the Special Trustees of University College London who have supported the work described here.

REFERENCES

Ali, K. Z. M. (1997). Stereological study of the effect of altitude on the trophoblast cell populations of human term placental villi. *Placenta*, **18**, 447–50.

Alsat, E., Wyplosz, P. & Malassiné, A. (1996). Hypoxia impairs cell fusion and differentiation process in human cytotrophoblast cells, *in vitro*. *J. Cell. Physiol.*, **168**, 346–53.

Amoroso, E. C. (1952). Placentation. In A. S. Parkes, ed., *Marshall's Physiology of Reproduction*. London: Longmans, Green and Co, pp. 127–311.

Arrigo, A.-P. & Kretz-Remy, C. (1998). Regulation of mammalian gene expression by free radicals. In O. I. Aruoma & B. Halliwell, eds., *Molecular Biology of Free Radicals in Human Diseases*. Saint Lucia: OICA International, pp. 183–223.

Benjamin, L. E., Hemo, I. & Keshet, E. (1998). A plasticity window for blood vessel remodelling is defined by pericyte coverage of the preformed endothelial network and is regulated by PDGF-B and VEGF. *Development*, **125**, 1591–8.

Benyo, D. F., Miles, T. M. & Conrad, K. P. (1997). Hypoxia stimulates cytokine production by villous explants from the human placenta. *J. Clin. Endocrinol. Metab.*, **82**, 1582–8.

Burton, G. J., Jauniaux, E. & Watson, A. L. (1999). Maternal arterial connections to the placental intervillous space during the first trimester of human pregnancy; the Boyd Collection revisited. *Am. J. Obstet. Gynecol.*, **181**, 718–24.

Burton, G. J., Watson, A. L., Hempstock, J., Skepper, J. N. & Jauniaux, E. (2002). Uterine glands provide histiotrophic nutrition for the human foetus during the first trimester of pregnancy. *J. Clin. Endocrinol. Metab.*, **87**, 2954–9.

Burton, G. J., Hempstock, J. & Jauniaux, E. (2003). Oxygen, early embryonic metabolism and free radical-mediated embryopathies. *Reprod. Bio. Med. Online.*, **6**, 84–96.

Caniggia, I., Mostachfi, H., Winter, J. *et al.* (2000). Hypoxia-inducible factor-1 mediates the biological effects of oxygen on human trophoblast differentiation through $TGF\beta_3$. *J. Clin. Invest.*, **105**, 577–87.

Carter, A. M. (1997). When is the maternal placental circulation established in man? *Placenta*, **18**, 83–7.

(2000). Placental oxygen consumption. Part I: *in vivo* studies – a review. *Placenta*, **21** (Suppl A), S31–7.

Chen, K., Thomas, S.R. & Keaney, J.F. (2003). Beyond LDL oxidation: ROS in vascular signal transduction. *Free Radic. Biol. Med.*, **35**, 117–32.

Cooper, J.C., Sharkey, A.M., McLaren, J., Charnock Jones, D.S. & Smith, S.K. (1995). Localization of vascular endothelial growth factor and its receptor, flt, in human placenta and decidua by immunohistochemistry. *J. Reprod. Fertil.*, **105**, 205–13.

Coppens, M., Loquet, P., Kollen, F., De Neubourg, F. & Buytaert, P. (1996). Longitudinal evaluation of uteroplacental and umbilical blood flow changes in normal early pregnancy. *Ultrasound Obstet. Gynecol.*, **7**, 114–21.

Crompton, M. (2000). Mitochondrial intermembrane junctional complexes and their role in cell death. *J. Physiol.*, **529**, 11–21.

Dalton, C.F., Laird, S.M., Estdale, S.E., Saravelos, H.G. & Li, T.C. (1998). Endometrial protein PP14 and CA-125 in recurrent miscarriage patients; correlation with pregnancy outcome. *Hum. Reprod.*, **13**, 3197–202.

Dockery, P., Li, T.C., Rogers, A.W., Cooke, I.D. & Lenton, E.A. (1988). The ultrastructure of the glandular epithelium in the timed endometrial biopsy. *Hum. Reprod.*, **3**, 826–34.

Droge, W. (2002). Free radicals in the physiological control of cell function. *Physiol. Rev.*, **82**, 47–95.

Dyson, C.A.J., Hempstock, J., Jauniaux, E., Charnock-Jones, D.S. & Burton, G.J. (2003). Regulation of the level of immunoreactive HIF-1α by oxidative stress in the early human placenta. *Placenta*, **24**, A6.

Esterman, A., Finlay, T.H. & Dancis, J. (1996). The effect of hypoxia on term trophoblast: hormone synthesis and release. *Placenta*, **17**, 217–22.

Fox, H. (1964). The villous cytotrophoblast as an index of placental ischaemia. *J. Obstet. Gynaecol. Br. Commw.*, **71**, 885–93.

Freeman, B.A. & Crapo, J.D. (1981). Hyperoxia increases oxygen radical production in rat lungs and lung mitochondria. *J. Biol. Chem.*, **256**, 10986–92.

Freeman, M.L., Borrelli, M.J., Meredith, M.J. & Lepock, J.R. (1999). On the path to the heat shock response: destabilization and formation of partially folded protein intermediates, a consequence of protein thiol modification. *Free Radic. Biol. Med.*, **26**, 737–45.

Freese, U.E. & Maciolek, B.J. (1969). Plastoid injection studies of the uteroplacental vascular relationship in the human. *Obstet. Gynecol.*, **33**, 8–16.

Genbacev, O., Joslin, R., Damsky, C.H., Polliotti, B.M. & Fisher, S.J. (1996). Hypoxia alters early gestation human cytotrophoblast differentiation/invasion in vitro and models the placental defects that occur in preeclampsia. *J. Clin. Invest.*, **97**, 540–50.

Graham, C.H., Postovit, L.M., Park, H., Canning, M.T. & Fitzpatrick, T.E. (2000). Adriana and Luisa Castellucci Award Lecture 1999: role of oxygen in the regulation of trophoblast gene expression and invasion. *Placenta*, **21**, 443–50.

Gray, C.A., Bartol, F.F., Taylor, K.M. *et al.* (2000). Ovine uterine gland knock-out model: effects of gland ablation on the estrous cycle. *Biol. Reprod.*, **62**, 448–56.

Greenwold, N., Jauniaux, E., Gulbis, B. *et al.* (2003). Relationships between maternal serum endocrinology, placental karyotype and intervillous circulation in early pregnancy failure. *Fertil. Steril.*, **79**, 1373–9.

Haddad, J.J. & Land, S.C. (2001). A non-hypoxic, ROS-sensitive pathway mediates TNF-α-dependent regulation of HIF-1. *FEBS Lett.*, **505**, 269–74.

Halliwell, B. & Gutteridge, J.M.C. (1999). *Free Radicals in Biology and Medicine.* Oxford: Oxford Science Publications.

Hempstock, J., Bao, Y.-P., Bar-Issac, M. *et al.* (2003a). Intralobular differences in antioxidant enzyme expression and activity reflect oxygen gradients within the human placenta. *Placenta*, **24**, 517–23.

Hempstock, J., Jauniaux, E. & Burton, G.J. (2003b). Secretory activity of the endometrial glands is maintained throughout the first trimester of human pregnancy. *Placenta*, **24**, A19.

Hempstock, J., Jauniaux, E., Greenwold, N. & Burton, G.J. (2003c). The contribution of placental oxidative stress to early pregnancy failure. *Hum. Pathol.*, **34**, 1265–75.

Hensley, K., Robinson, K.A., Gabbita, S.P., Salsman, S. & Floyd, R.A. (2000). Reactive oxygen species, cell signaling, and cell injury. *Free Radic. Biol. Med.*, **28**, 1456–62.

Hertig, A.T., Rock, J. & Adams, E.C. (1956). A description of 34 human ova within the first 17 days of development. *Am. J. Anat.*, **98**, 435–94.

Hochachka, P.W. & Lutz, P.L. (2001). Mechanism, origin, and evolution of anoxia tolerance in animals. *Comp. Biochem. Physiol. B Biochem. Mol. Biol.*, **130**, 435–59.

Hustin, J. & Schaaps, J.P. (1987). Echographic and anatomic studies of the maternotrophoblastic border during the first trimester of pregnancy. *Am. J. Obstet. Gynecol.*, **157**, 162–8.

Hustin, J., Schaaps, J.P. & Lambotte, R. (1988). Anatomical studies of the utero-placental vascularisation in the first trimester of pregnancy. *Troph. Res.*, **3**, 49–60.

Hustin, J., Jauniaux, E. & Schaaps, J.P. (1990). Histological study of the materno-embryonic interface in spontaneous abortion. *Placenta*, **11**, 477–86.

Irani, K. (2000). Oxidant signaling in vascular cell growth, death, and survival. A review of the roles of reactive oxygen species in smooth muscle and endothelial cell mitogenic and apoptotic signaling. *Circ. Res.*, **87**, 179–83.

Jaffe, R. & Warsof, S.L. (1992). Color Doppler imaging in the assessment of uteroplacental blood flow in abnormal first trimester intrauterine pregnancies: an attempt to define the etiologic mechanisms. *J. Ultrasound Med.*, **11**, 41–4.

Jaffe, R., Jauniaux, E. & Hustin, J. (1997). Maternal circulation in the first-trimester human placenta – myth or reality? *Am. J. Obstet. Gynecol.*, **176**, 695–705.

Jauniaux, E., Zaidi, J., Jurkovic, D., Campbell, S. & Hustin, J. (1994). Comparison of colour Doppler features and pathologic findings in complicated early pregnancy. *Hum. Reprod.*, **9**, 243–7.

Jauniaux, E., Jurkovic, D. & Campbell, S. (1995). Current topic: *In vivo* investigation of the placental circulations by Doppler echography. *Placenta*, **16**, 323–31.

Jauniaux, E., Watson, A.L., & Hempstock, J. *et al.* (2000). Onset of maternal arterial bloodflow and placental oxidative stress; a possible factor in human early pregnancy failure. *Am. J. Pathol.*, **157**, 2111–22.

Jauniaux, E., Watson, A.L. & Burton, G.J. (2001). Evaluation of respiratory gases and acid-base gradients in fetal fluids and uteroplacental tissue between 7 and 16 weeks. *Am. J. Obstet. Gynecol.*, **184**, 998–1003.

Jauniaux, E., Hempstock, J., Greenwold, N. & Burton, G.J. (2003). Trophoblastic oxidative stress in relation to temporal and regional differences in maternal placental blood flow in normal and abnormal early pregnancies. *Am. J. Pathol.*, **162**, 115–25.

Jauniaux, E., Cindrova-Davies, T. & Johns, J. (2004). Distribution and transfer pathways of antioxidant molecules inside the first trimester human gestational sac. *J. Clin. Endocrinol. Metab.*, **89**, 1452–8.

Khong, T.Y., Liddell, H.S. & Robertson, W.B. (1987). Defective haemochorial placentation as a cause of miscarriage. A preliminary study. *Br. J. Obstet. Gynaecol.*, **94**, 649–55.

Kliman, H.J. (2000). Uteroplacental blood flow. The story of decidualisation, menstruation and trophoblast invasion. *Am. J. Pathol.*, **157**, 1759–68.

Kojima, K., Kanzaki, H., Iwai, M. *et al.* (1995). Expression of leukaemia inhibitory factor (LIR) receptor in human placenta: a possible role for LIF in the growth and differentiation of trophoblasts. *Hum. Reprod.*, **10**, 1907–11.

Kowaltowski, A.J., Castilho, R.F. & Vercesi, A.E. (2001). Mitochondrial permeability transition and oxidative stress. *FEBS Lett.*, **495**, 12–15.

Kudo, Y., Boyd, C.A., Sargent, I.L. & Redman, C.W. (2003). Hypoxia alters expression and function of syncytin and its receptor during trophoblast cell fusion of human placental BeWo cells: implications for impaired trophoblast syncytialization in preeclampsia. *Biochim. Biophys. Acta*, **1638**, 63–71.

Kurjak, A. & Kupesic, S. (1997). Doppler assessment of the intervillous blood flow in normal and abnormal early pregnancy. *Obstet. Gynecol.*, **89**, 252–6.

Kurjak, A., Kupesic, S., Hafner, T. *et al.* (1997). Conflicting data on intervillous circulation in early pregnancy. *J. Perinat. Med.*, **25**, 225–36. ·

Ladines-Llave, C.A., Maruo, T., Manalo, A.S. & Mochizuki, M. (1991). Cytologic localization of epidermal growth factor and its receptor in developing human placenta varies over the course of pregnancy. *Am. J. Obstet. Gynecol.*, **165**, 1377–82.

Lando, D., Peet, D.D., Whelan, D.D., Gorman, J.J. & Whitelaw, M.L. (2002). Asparagine hydroxylation of the HIF transactivation domain: a hypoxic switch. *Science*, **295**, 858–61.

Lando, D., Gorman, J.J., Whitelaw, M.L. & Peet, D.D. (2003). Oxygen-dependent regulation of hypoxia-inducible factors by prolyl and asparaginyl hydroxylation. *Eur. J. Biochem.*, **270**, 781–90.

Larsen, W.J. (1997). *Human Embryology*. New York: Churchill Livingstone.

Leist, M., Single, B., Castoldi, A.F., Kühnle, S. & Nicotera, P. (1997). Intracellular adenosine triphosphate (ATP) concentration: a switch in the decision between apoptosis and necrosis. *J. Exp. Med.*, **185**, 1481–6.

Lennard, S.N., Gerstenberg, C., Allen, W.R. & Stewart, F. (1998). Expression of epidermal growth factor and its receptor in equine placental tissues. *J. Reprod. Fertil.*, **112**, 49–57.

Maruo, T., Matsuo, H., Murata, K. & Mochizuki, M. (1992). Gestational age-dependent dual action of epidermal growth factor on human placenta early in gestation. *J. Clin. Endocrinol. Metab.*, **75**, 1362–7.

Matsubara, S. & Tamada, T. (1991). Ultracytochemical localization of NAD(P)H oxidase activity in the human placenta. *Acta Obstet. Gynaecol. Jap.*, **43**, 117–21.

Mi, S., Lee, X., Li, X. *et al.* (2000). Syncytin is a captive retroviral envelope protein involved in human placental morphogenesis. *Nature*, **403**, 785–9.

Mikolajczyk, M., Skrzypczak, J., Szymanowski, K. & Wirstlein, P. (2003). The assessment of LIF in uterine flushing – a possible new diagnostic tool in states of impaired infertility. *Reprod. Biol.*, **3**, 259–70.

Moore, K. L. & Persaud, T. V. N. (1993). *The Developing Human: Clinically Orientated Embryology.* Philadelphia: W. B. Saunders.

Mossman, H. W. (1987). *Vertebrate Fetal Membranes: Comparative Ontogeny and Morphology; Evolution; Phylogenetic Significance; Basic Functions; Research Opportunities.* London: Macmillan.

Mühlhauser, J., Crescimanno, C., Kaufmann, P. *et al.* (1993). Differentiation and proliferation patterns in human trophoblast revealed by c-erbB-2 oncogene product and EGF-R. *J. Histochem. Cytochem.*, **41**, 165–73.

New, D. A. T. (1978). Whole-embryo culture and the study of mammalian embryos during organogenesis. *Biol. Rev.*, **53**, 81–122.

Palmer, M. E., Watson, A. L. & Burton, G. J. (1997). Morphological analysis of degeneration and regeneration of syncytiotrophoblast in first trimester villi during organ culture. *Hum. Reprod.*, **12**, 379–82.

Pijnenborg, R., Dixon, G., Robertson, W. B. & Brosens, I. (1980). Trophoblastic invasion of human decidua from 8 to 18 weeks of pregnancy. *Placenta*, **1**, 3–19.

Pijnenborg, R., Bland, J. M., Robertson, W. B., Dixon, G. & Brosens, I. (1981). The pattern of interstitial trophoblastic invasion of the myometrium in early human pregnancy. *Placenta*, **2**, 303–16.

Raha, S., McEachern, G. E., Myint, A. T. & Robinson, B. H. (2000). Superoxides from mitochondrial complex III: the role of manganese superoxide dismutase. *Free Radic. Biol. Med.*, **29**, 170–80.

Raijmakers, M. T. M., Burton, G. J., Jauniaux, E., Seed, P. T. & Poston, L. (2004). Increased placental NAD(P)H oxidase mediated superoxide generation in early pregnancy. *J. Physiol.*, **555P**, C104.

Rajakumar, A. & Conrad, K. P. (2000). Expression, ontogeny, and regulation of hypoxia-inducible transcription factors in the human placenta. *Biol. Reprod.*, **63**, 559–69.

Ramsey, E. M. & Donner, M. W. (1980). *Placental Vasculature and Circulation: Anatomy, Physiology, Radiology, Clinical Aspects, Atlas and Textbook.* Stuttgart: Georg Thieme.

Reynolds, S. R. M. (1966). Formation of fetal cotyledons in the hemochorial placenta. A theoretical consideration of the functional implications of such an arrangement. *Am. J. Obstet. Gynecol.*, **94**, 425–39.

Reynolds, S. R. M., Freese, U. E., Bieniarz, J. *et al.* (1968). Multiple simultaneous intervillous space pressures recorded in several regions of the hemochorial placenta in relation to functional anatomy of the fetal cotyledon. *Am. J. Obstet. Gynecol.*, **102**, 1128–34.

Rodesch, F., Simon, P., Donner, C. & Jauniaux, E. (1992). Oxygen measurements in endometrial and trophoblastic tissues during early pregnancy. *Obstet. Gynecol.*, **80**, 283–5.

Schaaps, J. P. & Hustin, J. (1988). *In vivo* aspect of the maternal–trophoblastic border during the first trimester of gestation. *Troph. Res.*, **3**, 39–48.

Schneider, H. (2000). Placental oxygen consumption. Part II: *in vitro* studies – a review. *Placenta*, 21 (Suppl A), S38–44.

Schwärzler, P., Holden, D., Nielsen, S. *et al.* (1999). The conservative management of first trimester miscarriages and the use of colour Doppler sonography for patient selection. *Hum. Reprod.*, 14, 1341–5.

Semenza, G.L. (1998). Hypoxia-inducible factor 1: master regulator of O_2 homeostasis. *Curr. Opin. Genet. Dev.*, 8, 588–94.

Sharkey, A.M., King, A., Clark, D.E. *et al.* (1999). Localization of leukaemia inhibitory factor and its receptor in human placenta throughout pregnancy. *Biol. Reprod.*, 60, 355–64.

Stroka, D.M., Burkhardt, T., Desbaillets, I. *et al.* (2001). HIF-1 is expressed in normoxic tissue and displays an organ-specific regulation under systemic hypoxia. *FASEB J.*, 15, 2445–53.

Tuckerman, E., Laird, S.M., Stewart, R., Wells, M. & Li, T.C. (2004). Markers of endometrial function in women with unexplained recurrent pregnancy loss: a comparison between morphologically normal and retarded endometrium. *Hum. Reprod.*, 19, 196–205.

Valentin, L., Sladkevicius, P., Laurini, R., Söderberg, H. & Marsal, K. (1996). Uteroplacental and luteal circulation in normal first-trimester pregnancies: Doppler ultrasonographic and morphologic study. *Am. J. Obstet. Gynecol.*, 174, 768–75.

Watson, A.L., Palmer, M.E., Jauniaux, E. & Burton, G.J. (1997). Variations in expression of copper/zinc superoxide dismutase in villous trophoblast of the human placenta with gestational age. *Placenta*, 18, 295–9.

Watson, A.L., Skepper, J.N., Jauniaux, E. & Burton, G.J. (1998a). Changes in the concentration, localization and activity of catalase within the human placenta during early gestation. *Placenta*, 19, 27–34.

(1998b). Susceptibility of human placental syncytiotrophoblastic mitochondria to oxygen-mediated damage in relation to gestational age. *J. Clin. Endocrinol. Metab.*, 83, 1697–1705.

Wigglesworth, J.S. (1969). Vascular anatomy of the human placenta and its significance for placental pathology. *J. Obstet. Gynaecol. Br. Commw.*, 76, 979–89.

Wooding, F.B.P. & Flint, A.P.F. (1994). Placentation. In G.E. Lamming, ed., *Marshall's Physiology of Reproduction*. London: Chapman & Hall, pp. 233–460.

Zhang, E.G., Smith, S.K., Baker, P.N. & Charnock-Jones, D.S. (2001). The regulation and localization of angiopoietin-1, -2, and their receptor Tie2 in normal and pathologic human placentae. *Mol. Med.*, 7, 624–35.

Zhang, E.C., Burton, G.J., Smith, S.K. & Charnock-Jones, D.S. (2002). Placental vessel adaptation during gestation and to high altitude: changes in diameter and perivascular cell coverage. *Placenta*, 23, 751–62.

DISCUSSION

Pijnenborg During normal early development of the placenta, Eric Jauniaux did measurements of the flow up to 13 weeks, didn't he?

Burton Yes.

Pijnenborg So at 13 weeks you still have more flow in the periphery than in the centre.

Burton   It becomes more balanced as you move towards 12 weeks.

Pijnenborg I was trying to link this up with the observations I made when I tried to map out the degree of trophoblast invasion through the whole placental bed area. Between 8 and 12 weeks, almost all the invasion is in the central part, but later on it goes to the periphery: there is a sort of ring-like distribution throughout the placental bed. Can you persuade Eric to do these measurements in the 14–18 week interval, to see whether he can see plugging in the peripheral vessels and shutting down the flow in that area?

Burton   The latest ones were about 14 weeks.

Pijnenborg You have the plugs in the endings of the spiral arteries. More than 20 years ago De Wolf *et al.* (1980) made electron microscopic observations of what the plugs look like. There are plenty of desmosomes that join the trophoblastic cells together. There must be a mechanism of de-plugging. Have you any idea about this?

Burton   I agree. There must be. I would very much like to link this to regression of the glands but have no evidence to do so as yet. What is unique about the human placenta is that the same structure is perfused in a very different way from the first trimester to the second. You would expect that as the glands regress, and one form of nutrition gives way to the other, that there should be some sort of dialogue between the two.

Pijnenborg Also, you then have all the different growth factors and cytokines which might redirect differentiation processes in the trophoblast.

Burton   It may be that the nature of the glandular secretions changes, allowing those cells to migrate more. There are changes of glycosylation of glycodelin, for example, in pregnancy. This is an area to explore.

Pijnenborg Many years ago there were a lot of challenges to the new concept of low-to-high flow. One of the arguments made by Anthony Carter (1997) was that some flow is needed to explain the crown-like arrangements of the villi which develop during the first few months. He thought these crown-like arrangements were related to the spiral artery outlets. In his opinion some flow was needed to explain this phenomenon.

Burton   In 1966 Reynolds published a paper (Reynolds 1966) in which he commented that lobules aren't seen until 14 weeks of pregnancy. He felt that the haemodynamics were responsible for forming the lobules. These are not seen early on.

Kunath   I want to ask about the oxygen tension experiments. What happens to the cytotrophoblast if you let these experiments go on for longer?

Burton   If you leave them they will fuse to form a new syncytiotrophoblast layer.

Kunath   Is there a proliferative effect with high and low oxygen tension on cytotrophoblast, or do they all eventually become a syncytium?

Burton   On those villous explants there is such a lot of syncytial degeneration going on that the cytotrophoblast cells are kicked into a differentiation pathway. Colin Sibley has seen the same with the term placenta.

Sibley	Yes, but there is evidence that oxygen affects proliferation of the cytotrophoblast cells. Some of the interpretations of your high-altitude work suggest that.
Burton	Is it increased proliferation or is it decreased fusion? The proliferation studies that have been done have been comparing 2% oxygen with 21% oxygen. What we really need to be looking at is the difference between 2% and 5%, because 21% is clearly non-physiological. For example, Charles Graham reckons that it is necessary to get down to about 1% oxygen to show a difference in invasiveness in his model system.
Kunath	In our mouse work we use 20% oxygen and the trophoblast stem cells grow fine. They do change at low oxygen though.
Burton	Cells will adapt. At high oxygen they will up-regulate their antioxidant defences. The syncytiotrophoblast is not capable of adapting, for some reason.
S. Fisher	We have looked at this issue of early gestation, with isolated cytotrophoblast or explanted villi. We have done 1% and 2% intervals up to 20% oxygen. Anywhere between 2% and 8% we get proliferation and decreased differentiation. We have thought for a long time that oxygen tension is a very important variable in regulating human trophoblast differentiation.
Sibley	On this same topic, in explants we have cultured first trimester and term villous placenta. Contrary to what we predicted, the term placental tissue is much more sensitive to oxygen in terms of HCG production. The first trimester tissue looks fairly happy whatever oxygen concentration we put it in.
Cross	Sensitive meaning high was bad, or low was bad?
Sibley	I'm not sure you can say good or bad. One of the interpretations of our data is that oxygen might be the switch that people have searched for, for why HCG goes down after the end of the first trimester.
Cross	Let me rephrase: does high oxygen suppress HCG?
Sibley	Yes. I want to return to the nutrition of the fetus in the first trimester. Graham and I have had this discussion before, but I feel the need to repeat it. You can see secretion of MUC-1 and glycoproteins into the intervillous space, but what you state is that you have a plasma filtrate: I can't see why this filtrate does not have the same concentrations of amino acids, glucose and ions that the fetus needs. This is a time when the fetus hasn't started growing yet, and the filtrate will have all the same sorts of nutrients needed. I am yet to be convinced that the fact you see more glycoprotein there really makes a difference to the sorts of nutrient processes taking place. In addition, when we look at transport, we hypothesise that in the trophoblast if there was a switch in the sorts of nutrition before and after turning on blood flow and oxygen, then you might see a change in the pattern of transporter expression. Having bought a new quantitative (Q)-PCR machine, we have been working it to death and have looked at large numbers of samples from before 10 weeks, after 10 weeks and at term. The major difference is between first

trimester and term, but not between before 10 weeks and after 10 weeks. Although it makes a bit of difference, it doesn't bother me whether you call it histiotrophic or haemotrophic – I'm not sure it makes that much difference to what the fetus really sees.

Burton   You wouldn't want a major change in protein composition, because that would provide a huge shock to the placenta. We only looked at MUC-1 and glycodelin because they are unique to the glands and so we could use them to trace the glandular secretions. I have perhaps emphasised in the past nutrition more than growth factors, but Twink Allen's group has shown a spatiotemporal correlation in the horse between EGF activity in the glands and cellular proliferation in the chorion immediately above it. Factors such as EGF or LIF coming out of the endometrial glands could have an important local effect on the trophoblast.

Sibley   Our Q-PCR machine tells us that IGF2 is very high in first trimester compared with term.

Keverne   To me it sounds counterintuitive that the fetus should be deprived of oxygen during its development. Is this to slow development down? We know that there are some developmental genes that are sensitive to hypoxia. Is it concerning the switching on of these particular genes?

Burton   I can't say. If you look across the mammalian species, organogenesis takes place in a low oxygen environment. Our view is that in all species you want a low oxygen environment during organogenesis to prevent free radical-mediated damage. In the human, the way to achieve this is to stop the maternal blood flow. Once organogenesis is complete at the end of the first trimester, you need growth and thus oxygen. It is this unique transition in the human that might contribute to the higher rates of miscarriage and pre-eclampsia that are peculiar to our species.

Braude   The discussion here reminds those of us who are embryologists that this is what has been happening with in vitro culture of embryos for years. The only reason a high oxygen (20%) environment is used in IVF incubators is because it is more convenient to use air rather than a special gas mixture. There is lots of evidence suggesting that the fallopian tube is a low oxygen environment. A better way to culture cells and early embryos is in a low oxygen (5%) environment. It may be that when you have such systems in place, it is easier for the embryo to deal with any extra free radicals than the vast amount produced in a higher oxygen environment.

Burton   If you take diabetic rats and increase expression of superoxide dismutase, you can knock down the rate of congenital malformations to normal. Reactive oxygen species are teratogenic molecules.

REFERENCES

Carter, A. M. (1997). When is the maternal placental circulation established in man? *Placenta*, **18**, 83–7.

De Wolf, F., De Wolf-Peeters. C., Brosens, I. & Robertson, W. B. (1980). The human placental bed: electron microscopic study of trophoblast invasion of spiral arteries. *Am. J. Obstet. Gynecol.*, **137**, 58–70.

Reynolds, S. R. M. (1966). Formation of fetal cotyledons in the hemochorial placenta. A theoretical consideration of the functional implications of such an arrangement. *Am. J. Obstet. Gynecol.*, **94**, 425–9.

7

Implantation is a sticky situation

Olga Genbacev[1], Akraporn Prakobphol[2], Russell A. Foulk[3] and
Susan J. Fisher[4]

[1] University of California San Francisco, USA
[2] University of California San Francisco, USA
[3] The Nevada Center for Reproductive Medicine, USA
[4] University of California San Francisco, USA

Abstract. For many reasons the implantation process has been extraordinarily difficult to study. The molecules that orchestrate this highly specialised event are likely localised to the interacting surfaces of only a few embryonic and maternal cells. Additionally, their expression, which is precisely timed, may also be transient. Therefore, much of what we know about this process at a molecular level, such as the importance of leukaemia inhibitory factor (LIF), is a by-product of studying mutant mice that were generated for other purposes. In other cases, the 'candidate molecule' approach has been fruitful, as exemplified by recently published evidence that L-selectin and its carbohydrate ligands are involved in the initial stages of implantation. In this review we discuss the current body of knowledge regarding L-selectin functions, which prompted experiments to examine expression of this receptor and its specialised carbohydrate ligands during implantation and the early stages of placentation. The results highlight the amazing plasticity of trophoblast cells that have co-opted portions of vascular and leukocyte differentiation programmes. The challenge now is to use our knowledge of the trophoblast L-selectin adhesion system to benefit women who fail to conceive due to defects in the implantation process.

Introduction

After fertilization, the next major hurdle for human reproduction is trophoblast differentiation, which is required for implantation, followed in lockstep by rapid assembly of these embryonic cells into a functional placenta. Thus, by the time implantation occurs, the trophoblast layer of the blastocyst has acquired the repertoire of embryonic molecules necessary to initiate adhesion to the uterine

Biology and Pathology of Trophoblast, eds. Ashley Moffett, Charlie Loke and Anne McLaren.
Published by Cambridge University Press © Cambridge University Press 2005.

wall. New data suggest that the cells' expression of L-selectin, which interacts with specialised carbohydrate ligands that are presented at the luminal surfaces of receptive uterine epithelial cells, is an important part of this specialised set of molecules. As discussed below, a great deal is known about how L-selectin and its carbohydrate receptors function in the blood–vascular system. We now have evidence that some of these functions are also critical components of implantation and the early stages of placentation. Taken together, this discovery and the results of studies we published previously suggest that a subset of trophoblast functions that are vital to reproduction are accomplished by molecules whose expression, in the adult, is largely restricted to blood and vascular cells. These new insights suggest novel strategies for increasing implantation rates in women who are having difficulty becoming pregnant, as well as ways to prevent early pregnancy loss.

L-selectin and its carbohydrate ligands in the blood and vascular systems

In the 1950s and 1960s, James Gowans at the Sir William Dunn School of Pathology, Oxford University, discovered that lymphocytes move from the blood into lymphoid organs, a process he termed 'homing', after which they return to the circulation (Gowans & Knight 1964). Specifically, the lymphocytes enter the nodes through high endothelial venules (HEV), and the cells composing them are called high endothelial cells (HEC). Gowans & Knight (1964) noted that the walls of HEV contain many small lymphocytes in various stages of extravasation. The restriction of infiltrating cells to this class of leukocyte led to their prediction of a 'special affinity' between the endothelium and the small lymphocytes. These landmark studies provided the first evidence of a role for lymphocyte recirculation in immune surveillance; namely, this process enables small numbers of specialised lymphocytes to come in contact with antigens in regional lymphoid organs. As a result, homing underlies primary sensitisation of naive lymphocytes and restimulation of memory cells (Butcher & Picker 1996, Salmi & Jalkanen 1997, von Andrian & Mackay 2000).

In 1976, through the development of an in vitro adhesion assay for lymphocyte–HEV binding, it became possible to approach the molecular basis of homing. By overlaying viable lymphocytes onto cryostat-cut sections of lymph node, Stamper & Woodruff (1976) observed highly specific adherence of exogenous lymphocytes to HEV. Using function-perturbing monoclonal antibodies to decipher the molecular basis of this interaction, Gallatin *et al.* (1983) discovered that a cell surface antigen on lymphocytes (gp90 MEL-14) was the target of the MEL-14 antibody. The cloning of this molecule led to the identification of L-selectin (CD62L), a type I membrane protein with a C-type lectin domain at the N-terminus (Lasky 1995). The structure of the molecule validated earlier cell-biological work, showing that gp90 MEL-14 functions as a calcium-dependent lectin-like receptor that recognises specific carbohydrate-based ligands on lymph node HEV (Stoolman & Rosen 1983, Rosen *et al.* 1985, Yednock *et al.* 1987). A definitive role for L-selectin in lymphocyte homing to lymph nodes was subsequently established by gene targeting (Arbones *et al.* 1994).

L-selectin is now recognised as essential for homing of naive lymphocytes to all HEV-bearing secondary lymphoid organs (Butcher & Picker 1996). Homing to secondary lymphoid organs occurs through a cascade of events that involve the stepwise action of adhesion and signalling receptors. The most fully elucidated adhesion cascade is for homing of naive lymphocytes to mouse peripheral lymph nodes (von Andrian & Mackay 2000). For naive lymphocytes and some memory cells, L-selectin serves as a primary adhesion receptor. First, L-selectin mediates the tethering and rolling of lymphocytes along the apical aspects of HEV. Second, HEV-associated chemokines such as CC chemokine ligand 21(CCL21) (secondary lymphoid chemokine; SLC) engage specific G-protein-coupled receptors on lymphocytes (CC chemokine receptor CCR7 in the case of SLC), which leads to the activation of LFA-1 (integrin $\alpha L\beta 2$) on the lymphocytes. Firm arrest of the lymphocytes occurs when LFA-1 interacts with intercellular adhesion molecule-1 (ICAMs) on the HEV. Finally, the lymphocytes transmigrate into the lymph node parenchyma. Generalised aspects of this model also account for the exquisite spatiotemporal specificity of inflammatory leukocyte trafficking by which leukocyte populations are selectively targeted with precise timing to particular vascular beds (Springer 1994, Butcher & Picker 1996).

As might be expected, the carbohydrate ligands with which L-selectin interacts are composed of highly specialised structures. Gesner & Ginsburg (1964) were the first to suggest that cell surface carbohydrates serve as recognition determinants in lymphocyte homing. The key finding was that sialidase treatment of lymph node sections completely abrogates the binding of lymphocytes to HEV. Another important finding was that HEV avidly incorporate $^{35}SO_4$ into macromolecules, suggesting an important function for sulphated moieties in the process of lymphocyte homing (Andrews *et al.* 1980). These early observations have now been rationalised by structural analysis of actual ligands.

The first HEV-expressed ligands to be identified were glycosylation-dependent cell adhesion molecule-1 (GlyCAM-1), CD34 and podocalyxin (Imai *et al.* 1991, Lasky 1995, Puri *et al.* 1995, Sassetti *et al.* 1998). Notably, all are sialomucins. Mucins are glycoproteins with multiple O-linked (via Ser or Thr) glycans. Whereas CD34 and podocalyxin are type I membrane proteins, GlyCAM-1 is a secreted molecule that is found at high levels in plasma. Podocalyxin and CD34 are broadly expressed on the vascular endothelium, as well as on haematopoietic precursor cells (McNagny *et al.* 1997, Renkonen *et al.* 2002). Another L-selectin sialomucin, endoglycan, differs from the other two by having an acidic amino region that contains two tyrosine sulphates. In addition, endoglycan is modified with chondroitin sulphate glycosaminoglycan chains.

Production of the MECA-79 monoclonal antibody provided a powerful tool for the identification of L-selectin ligands (Streeter *et al.* 1988). This antibody strongly stains lymph node HEV in mouse, blocks lymphocyte attachment to HEV in the Stamper-Woodruff in vitro adherence assay and inhibits lymphocyte homing to lymph nodes. As revealed by intravital microscopy, MECA-79 effectively blocks the tethering and rolling of lymphocytes along HEV, thus preventing the initiation of the homing cascade (von Andrian 1996). Additionally, null mice have been generated for GlyCAM-1 (Rosen 1999) and CD34 (Suzuki *et al.* 1996) with no obvious abnormality in homing to lymph nodes. It is strongly suspected that the HEV-expressed sialomucins are functionally redundant such that the loss of one member is compensated by the activity of the others. In contrast, significant deficiencies in homing are seen when specific post-translational modifications shared by these ligands are eliminated by gene targeting (Maly *et al.* 1996).

Thus, there is a not a strict requirement for a particular core protein; rather, a set of specific post-translational modifications are necessary. For example, all three selectins recognise sialyl-Lewis x, sLe^x ($Sia\alpha2\rightarrow3Gal\beta1\rightarrow4(Fuc\alpha1\rightarrow3)GlcNAc$) but with relatively low affinity (Varki 1997, Lowe 2002). The 6-sulphation of sLe^x enhances its interaction with L-selectin in cell-free assays (Scudder *et al.* 1994, Rosen 1999). Also, changing sLe^x to 6-sulpho sLe^x on the surface of transfected cells increases binding by L-selectin (Bistrup *et al.* 1999, Kimura *et al.* 1999, Kanamori *et al.* 2002). In fact, structural investigation of mouse GlyCAM-1 found sulphation at C-6 of GlcNAc (i.e. $GlcNAc$-6-SO_4) (Hemmerich *et al.* 1995). In the simplest *O*-glycans carried by this molecule, 6-sulpho sLe^x ($Sia\alpha2\rightarrow3(SO_3\rightarrow6)$ $Gal\beta1\rightarrow4(Fuc\alpha1\rightarrow3)GlcNAc$) occurs as a capping group on one of the oligosaccharide branches. Taken together, these findings qualify 6-sulpho sLe^x as a minimal recognition determinant for L-selectin.

The structural elucidation of the MECA-79 epitope has provided further insights into the structure of L-selectin ligands (Yeh *et al.* 2001). The critical structure is 6-sulphated *N*-acetyl-lactosamine (6-sulpho LacNAc) on an extended core 1 *O*-glycan. This oligosaccharide is found in the *O*-glycans of both native and recombinant GlyCAM-1. In its fully substituted form, the structure is modified with $\alpha2\rightarrow3$ sialylation on galactose and $\alpha1\rightarrow3$ fucosylation on GlcNAc, thus providing the 6-sulpho sLe^x determinant as a capping group. Interestingly, sialylation and fucosylation are dispensable for the MECA-79 epitope, whereas they are required for optimal binding by L-selectin. Native GlyCAM-1 from murine lymph nodes exhibits biantennary *O*-glycans, both of which are capped by 6-sulpho sLe^x. The lower arm is the extended core 1 glycan containing the MECA-79 epitope, and the upper arm is the core 2 branch. Mass spectrometry analysis of human tonsillar

CD34 is consistent with the existence of the sulphated extended core 1 structure (Satomaa *et al.* 2002).

The special nature of these molecules foreshadows unique functions. For most eukaryotic cells, changes in cell adhesion to other cells or extracellular matrix takes minutes to hours. In contrast, leukocytes, whose functions depend on rapid deployment over large distances, develop adhesive interactions quickly, and the interactions are usually readily reversible. An extreme example of rapid kinetics is the rolling interaction of blood-borne leukocytes on the vascular endothelium. Here, within seconds of contact, the leukocyte is converted from a free-moving cell to a rolling cell propelled by the blood flow (Butcher & Picker 1996). The rolling interaction with the endothelium involves the rapid formation of bonds at the leading edge of the leukocyte and rapid bond dissociation at the trailing edge: rolling increases and then decreases (Finger *et al.* 1996). Rolling via L-selectin is also very stable: rolling velocity plateaus with increasing wall shear stress (Chen & Springer 1999). This property minimises variation in the velocity of rolling leukocytes with fluctuations in wall shear stress and provides sufficient time for the leukocytes to be exposed to activating stimuli present on the vessel wall.

L-selectin and its carbohydrate ligands in human implantation and placentation

At a morphological level, analogies can be drawn between key steps in leukocyte emigration from blood and trophoblast attachment to the uterine wall. Implantation begins with apposition: the trophectoderm of the originally free-floating embryo lies adjacent to the uterine epithelium, but the blastocyst is easily dislodged (Carson *et al.* 2000). Soon thereafter, blastocyst adhesion to the uterine wall is stabilised, and trophoblasts transmigrate across the uterine epithelium, a process that in humans buries the entire embryo beneath the uterine surface. Subsequent development depends on the ability of trophoblasts to adhere under conditions of shear stress created when these fetal cells breach uterine vessels; this process diverts maternal blood flow to the placenta. At a molecular level, trophoblast adhesion from implantation onward is an integrin-dependent process that takes place in a chemokine- and cytokine-rich milieu analogous to the blood–vascular interface (Guleria & Pollard 2000, Drake *et al.* 2001). Together, these findings raised the possibility that implantation and placentation utilise other components of the leukocyte emigration system, such as selectins and their ligands.

To determine whether selectin ligands are present at appropriate times and locations to function in blastocyst adhesion to the uterus, we studied their expression at the maternal–fetal interface with antibodies that bind sulphated oligosaccharides that interact with L-selectin. We found that tissue sections of uterine

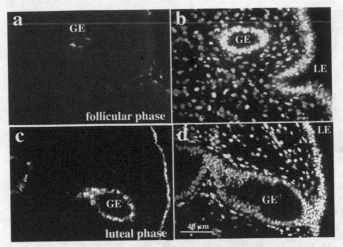

Figure 7.1   Receptive human uterine epithelial cells up-regulate the expression of sulphated selectin oligosaccharide ligands *in situ*. (a and c) Staining of human uterine epithelial cells with MECA-79 was weak and patchy during the follicular phase and intense and uniform during the luteal phase. (b and d) Cell nuclei were visualised by staining with Hoechst. LE, luminal epithelium; GE glandular epithelium.

biopsy samples obtained from patients during the follicular phase of the menstrual cycle reacted with the MECA-79 antibody, which recognises carbohydrate epitopes on all L-selectin ligands (particularly $SO_3 \rightarrow 6$ GlcNAc). In all cases, MECA-79 reactivity localised to the surface of glandular and luminal epithelia. When the uterus was not receptive, staining was patchy and weaker (Fig. 7.1a) than the more intense immunoreactivity observed when the uterus was receptive (Fig. 7.1c). We also stained the same samples with the HECA-452 antibody, which reacts with sLe^x and related sulphated structures, including 6-sulpho sLe^x, with essentially the same results (data not shown). Analyses of samples later in gestation showed that staining with these antibodies was lost during the second trimester, a situation that persisted until birth. Immunoblot analyses with MECA-79 confirmed up-regulation of selectin oligosaccharide ligands as the window of human receptivity opens. Together, these results suggest that uterine expression of specialised carbohydrate structures that support selectin-mediated adherence is dramatically up-regulated as the uterus becomes receptive.

These findings prompted us to ask whether the trophectoderm of implantation-competent human embryos expresses L-selectin. Accordingly, we stained blastocysts, without permeabilisation, using fluorescein isothiocyanate (FITC) conjugated anti-L-selectin. After hatching, strong staining was observed in association with the trophectoderm over the entire embryo surface (Fig. 7.2b). In additional experiments, we asked whether placental trophoblasts retain L-selectin

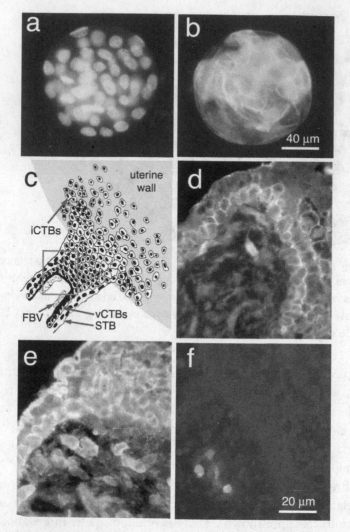

Figure 7.2   Human trophoblasts express L-selectin. (a) After hatching, a human blastocyst was stained with Hoechst to visualise the nuclei. (b) The trophoblast covering of the same embryo stained brightly for L-selectin expression. (c) Scheme of the human materno–fetal interface showing a placental anchoring villus attaching to the uterus through invasive cytotrophoblasts (iCTBs). (d) Before 16 weeks of gestation, villous cytotrophoblast progenitors (vCTBs), column cytotrophoblasts and invasive cytotrophoblasts within the uterine wall stained with anti-human L-selectin, as did macrophages and syncytiotrophoblasts. After 17 weeks of gestation, this staining pattern changed dramatically. (e) The general cellular arrangement of cytotrophoblasts in the villi did not change, as demonstrated by staining for cytokeratin. (f) However, the trophoblast populations no longer reacted with anti-L-selectin, although macrophages did. FBV, fetal blood vessel; STB, syncytiotrophoblast.

expression later in gestation. To answer this question, we analysed L-selectin expression in tissue sections of the human materno–fetal interface. Between 6 and 16 weeks of gestation, cytotrophoblast progenitors, cytotrophoblasts in cell columns and invasive cytotrophoblasts strongly reacted with an antibody that recognises the extracellular domain of L-selectin (Fig. 7.2d). The pattern of reactivity was indicative of antibody binding to cell surface L-selectin. Overlying syncytiotrophoblasts also stained, as did macrophages in the villus stromal cores. To establish that trophoblast L-selectin staining was not due to adsorption of shed L-selectin from blood, antibodies that recognised the C-terminus of the molecule were also used in immunolocalisation experiments. The same populations of cells stained with both antibodies (data not shown). However, from 17 weeks of gestation to term, there was reduced or no staining, although macrophages continued to react strongly (Fig. 7.2f). Because the selectins have overlapping functions in mediating leukocyte rolling adhesion, we examined human trophoblast expression of P- and E-selectin. Anti-P-selectin inconsistently demonstrated weak staining of first- and second-trimester syncytiotrophoblasts, and anti-E-selectin did not react with any of the samples (data not shown).

To support our *in situ* observations, we characterised human trophoblast L-selectin expression in vitro by using two culture systems that model cytotrophoblast differentiation along the pathway that leads to uterine attachment and invasion. In an organ culture model, explanted anchoring villi are cultured on Matrigel-coated wells; villi attach to the extracellular matrix via the remnants of severed cytotrophoblast columns that subsequently give rise to invasive cytotrophoblasts (Genbacev *et al.* 1992). Sections of explants cultured for 72h were stained with anti-L-selectin. The pattern of antibody reactivity was very similar to that observed *in situ*: cytotrophoblast stem cells within the villi and column cytotrophoblasts that invaded the Matrigel stained, as did the syncytial surface (data not shown). At higher magnification, the pattern of cytotrophoblast staining was indistinguishable from that of Jurkat cells that express L-selectin. In a second in vitro model, purified cytotrophoblast stem cells plated on Matrigel differentiate to invasive cells over 48 to 72h. After 48h these cells also reacted with anti-L-selectin (data not shown). To confirm antigen identity, lysates prepared from isolated cytotrophoblasts and the columns dissected from explants were analysed by immunoblotting samples that were separated on 10% polyacrylamide gels. These samples contained a broad ~75–90kDa band. Jurkat and neutrophil lysates contained the same bands. Together, these data indicate that trophoblast up-regulation of L-selectin expression occurs concomitantly with the opening of the window of blastocyst attachment to the uterine epithelium, and cytotrophoblast invasion of the underlying parenchyma.

Next we assessed the functional state of trophoblast L-selectin in vitro (data not shown). Under shear stress, beads coated with 6-sulpho sLe^x bound to explants of the human chorionic villus tree. They associated with cytotrophoblast column remnants of anchoring villi and with the syncytiotrophoblasts at the surfaces of the villi, i.e. the cells that express L-selectin *in situ* and in vitro. Beads that displayed sLe^x also bound to villous explants, but in fewer numbers. Very few control (uncoated) phosphatidylcholine-conjugated beads bound to cytotrophoblast cell columns or syncytiotrophoblasts. Likewise, uncoated beads did not bind. Beads that displayed 6-sulpho sLe^x did not adhere to explants preincubated with an antibody that blocks L-selectin function, suggesting that the binding was specific.

We also compared cytotrophoblast and Jurkat adhesion to tissue sections cut from uterine biopsies – a variation of the aforementioned method that allows visualisation of leukocyte adhesion through L-selectin to lymph node HEV (data not shown). Under shear stress, cytotrophoblasts, as single cells and clusters, primarily bound to the epithelial portion of the receptive (luteal phase) uterus, including the lumen. Adherent cells stained for L-selectin. Cytotrophoblasts also bound to glands and their contents. Adherence to both luminal (data not shown) and glandular epithelium was inhibited by adding anti-L-selectin. Adherence was also inhibited when the tissue sections were preincubated with MECA-79. Many fewer cytotrophoblasts bound to tissue sections of non-receptive (follicular phase) biopsies; epithelial adhesion was nearly absent. As a positive control, Jurkat binding to tissue sections of luteal phase uterine biopsies was tested. The cells preferentially adhered to epithelia, and binding was inhibited by adding anti-L-selectin or MECA-79. Like cytotrophoblasts, the cells often adhered to glands that contained MECA-79-reactive secretions.

Our finding of L-selectin function outside the blood–vascular system has several important implications for implantation and placentation. Shear stress, required for L-selectin-mediated adhesion through its specialised oligosaccharide ligands, is likely to be an important component of both processes. During implantation, apposition may be analogous to leukocyte transient tethering and rolling. Although the magnitude of shear stress at the surface of the receptive uterus is unknown, distractive forces are likely derived from several sources, including fluid secretions and uterine contractions. During the early stages of placentation, cytotrophoblasts that invade and line maternal vessels experience the same shear stress as the resident vascular cells. Given the many and varied causes of infertility and early pregnancy loss, it seems likely that defects in the shear-stress-activated selectin adhesion system at the materno-fetal interface account for some unexplained reproductive failures.

In conclusion, our data offer further insights into the highly unusual nature of trophoblasts. Previously, we showed that invasive cytotrophoblasts of ectodermal origin undergo a novel differentiation process, taking on characteristics of vascular cells. Our finding that the same cells also share leukocyte adhesion mechanisms raises the possibility that trophoblasts have characteristics of the haemangioblast stem cell population that gives rise to both blood cells and blood vessels.

Future directions

The results of recent experiments suggest that the adhesion cascade that leads to embryo implantation may be analogous at a molecular level to the stepwise process whereby leukocytes home to regional lymph nodes or, in other locations, extravasate from blood into the tissues. This novel concept suggests many new testable hypotheses for explaining enigmatic aspects of the complex process that ultimately buries the embryo in the decidualised uterine stroma. In this regard, research into the upstream regulatory mechanisms will benefit from the large body of ongoing work regarding L-selectin interactions with its ligands in the blood and vascular systems. For example, it will be interesting to identify the uterine protein scaffolds that carry the bioactive carbohydrate ligands that interact with trophoblast L-selectin. Could they include any of the known selectin ligands? Additionally, we expect that the activities of the glycosyl- and sulphotransferases that build these unique sugar structures will be responsive, either directly or indirectly, to the same hormones that render the uterus receptive. Recent data in support of this concept come from studies showing that L-selectin-dependent lymphocyte–endothelial interactions in secondary lymph nodes and the uterus are coordinated by pregnancy-associated hormones (Chantakru *et al.* 2003). Whether or not these hormonal influences extend to the blastocyst, additional evidence of the cross-talk that is thought to play an important role in implantation (Paria *et al.* 2002) remains to be determined.

The discovery of extravascular functions for the L-selectin adhesion system during implantation and the early stages of placentation has many possible clinical applications, at both conceptual and practical levels. For example, gene expression profiling of endometrium suggests that GlcNAc 6-sulphotransferase-1, one of the enzymes that can provide the sulphation modification recognised by the MECA-79 monoclonal antibody, is up-regulated during the window of implantation (Kao *et al.* 2002). Accordingly, MECA-79 could be a useful tool, in conjunction with other markers, for assessing uterine receptivity. This possibility is strengthened by the fact that GlcNAc 6-sulphotransferase-1 expression, as determined by gene expression profiling, is diminished in women with endometriosis (Kao *et al.* 2003). Whether this finding is related to infertility in this and other patient populations remains to be determined. For example, uterine inflammation secondary to infections could trigger premature shedding of L-selectin, which we predict could decrease the likelihood of implantation.

Is there a downside to involving molecules with powerful immune functions in implantation? It will take years to answer this question, but based on our current evidence the possibility exists. If the expression of selectin ligands outside the uterus is hormonally regulated, as suggested by data in the mouse (Chantakru *et al.* 2003) and human (Prakobphol, Ma, Genbacev and Fisher, unpublished observations), then in cycling women leukocyte extravasation and exposure to tissue antigens may occur to varying degrees on a monthly basis, peaking approximately six days after ovulation, i.e. at the time of maximal uterine receptivity. We are very interested in exploring this concept in the context of the long-standing observation that women have a far greater risk than men of developing most of the common auto-immune disorders.

ACKNOWLEDGEMENTS

This work was supported by grants from the UC Discovery Program and the National Institutes of Health (DE 07244, HL 64597, U01 HD 42283 (part of the Cooperative Program on Trophoblast–Maternal Tissue Interactions) and HD 30367.

REFERENCES

Andrews, P., Ford, W. L. & Stoddart, R. W. (1980). Metabolic studies of high-walled endothelium of postcapillary venules in rat lymph nodes. *Ciba Found. Symp.*, **71**, 211–30.

Arbones, M. L., Ord, D. C., Ley, K. *et al.* (1994). Lymphocyte homing and leukocyte rolling and migration are impaired in L-selectin-deficient mice. *Immunity*, **1**, 247–60.

Bistrup, A., Bhakta, S., Lee, J. K. *et al.* (1999). Sulfotransferases of two specificities function in the reconstitution of high endothelial cell ligands for L-selectin. *J. Cell Biol.*, **145**, 899–910.

Butcher, E. C. & Picker, L. J. (1996). Lymphocyte homing and homeostasis. *Science*, **272**, 60–6.

Carson, D. D., Bagchi, I., Dey, S. K. *et al.* (2000). Embryo implantation. *Dev. Biol.*, **223**, 217–37.

Chantakru, S., Wang, W. C., Van Den Heuvel, M. *et al.* (2003). Coordinate regulation of lymphocyte-endothelial interactions by pregnancy-associated hormones. *J. Immunol.*, **171**, 4011–19.

Chen, S. & Springer, T. A. (1999). An automatic braking system that stabilizes leukocyte rolling by an increase in selectin bond number with shear. *J. Cell Biol.*, **144**, 185–200.

Drake, P. M., Gunn, M. D., Charo, I. F. *et al.* (2001). Human placental cytotrophoblasts attract monocytes and CD56 (bright) natural killer cells via the actions of monocyte inflammatory protein 1alpha. *J. Exp. Med.* **193**, 1199–212.

Finger, E. B., Puri, K. D., Alon, R. *et al.* (1996). Adhesion through L-selectin requires a threshold hydrodynamic shear. *Nature*, **379**, 266–9.

Gallatin, W. M., Weissman, I. L. & Butcher, E. C. (1983). A cell-surface molecule involved in organ-specific homing of lymphocytes. *Nature*, **304**, 30–4.

Genbacev, O., Schubach, S. A. & Miller, R. K. (1992). Villous culture of first trimester human placenta – model to study extravillous trophoblast (EVT) differentiation. *Placenta*, **13**, 439–61.

Gesner, B.M. & Ginsburg, V. (1964). Effect of glycosidases on the fate of transfused lymphocytes. *Proc. Natl. Acad. Sci. U.S.A.*, **52**, 750–5.

Gowans, J.L. & Knight, E.J. (1964). The route of re-circulation of lymphocytes in the rat. *Proc. R. Soc. Lond. B. Biol. Sci.*, **159**, 257–82.

Guleria, I. & Pollard, J.W. (2000). The trophoblast is a component of the innate immune system during pregnancy. *Nat. Med.*, **6**, 589–93.

Hemmerich, S., Leffler, H. & Rosen, S.D. (1995). Structure of the O-glycans in GlyCAM-1, an endothelial-derived ligand for L-selectin. *J. Biol. Chem.*, **270**, 12035–47.

Imai, Y., Singer, M.S., Fennie, C., Lasky, L.A. & Rosen, S.D. (1991). Identification of a carbohydrate-based endothelial ligand for a lymphocyte homing receptor. *J. Cell Biol.*, **113**, 1213–21.

Kanamori, A., Kojima, N., Uchimura, K. *et al.* (2002). Distinct sulfation requirements of selectins disclosed using cells that support rolling mediated by all three selectins under shear flow. L-selectin prefers carbohydrate 6-sulphation to tyrosine sulphation, whereas P-selectin does not. *J. Biol. Chem.*, **277**, 32578–86.

Kao, L.C., Tulac, S., Lobo, S. *et al.* (2002). Global gene profiling in human endometrium during the window of implantation. *Endocrinology*, **143**, 2119–38.

Kao, L.C., Germeyer, A., Tulac, S. *et al.* (2003). Expression profiling of endometrium from women with endometriosis reveals candidate genes for disease-based implantation failure and infertility. *Endocrinology*, **144**, 2870–81.

Kimura, N., Mitsuoka, C., Kanamori, A. *et al.* (1999). Reconstitution of functional L-selectin ligands on a cultured human endothelial cell line by cotransfection of alpha1→3 fucosyl-transferase VII and newly cloned GlcNAcbeta:6-sulfotransferase cDNA. *Proc. Natl. Acad. Sci. U.S.A.*, **96**, 4530–5.

Lasky, L.A. (1995). Selectin–carbohydrate interactions and the initiation of the inflammatory response. *Annu. Rev. Biochem.*, **64**, 113–39.

Lowe, J.B. (2002). Glycosylation in the control of selectin counter-receptor structure and function. *Immunol. Rev.*, **186**, 19–36.

Maly, P., Thall, A., Petryniak, B. *et al.* (1996). The alpha(1,3)fucosyltransferase Fuc-TVII controls leukocyte trafficking through an essential role in L-, E-, and P-selectin ligand biosynthesis. *Cell*, **86**, 643–53.

McNagny, K.M., Pettersson, I., Rossi, F. *et al.* (1997). Thrombomucin, a novel cell surface protein that defines thrombocytes and multipotent hematopoietic progenitors. *J. Cell Biol.*, **138**, 1395–407.

Paria, B.C., Reese, J., Das, S.K. & Dey, S.K. (2002). Deciphering the crosstalk of implantation: advances and challenges. *Science*, **296**, 2185–8.

Puri, K.D., Finger, E.B., Gaudernack, G. & Springer, T.A. (1995). Sialomucin CD34 is the major L-selectin ligand in human tonsil high endothelial venules. *J. Cell Biol.*, **131**, 261–70.

Renkonen, J., Tynninen, O., Hayry, P., Paavonen, T. & Renkonen, R. (2002). Glycosylation might provide endothelial zip codes for organ-specific leukocyte traffic into inflammatory sites. *Am. J. Pathol.*, **161**, 543–50.

Rosen, S.D. (1999). Endothelial ligands for L-selectin: from lymphocyte recirculation to allograft rejection. *Am. J. Pathol.*, **155**, 1013–20.

Rosen, S. D., Singer, M. S., Yednock, T. A. & Stoolman, L. M. (1985). Involvement of sialic acid on endothelial cells in organ-specific lymphocyte recirculation. *Science*, **228**, 1005–7.

Salmi, M. & Jalkanen, S. (1997). How do lymphocytes know where to go: current concepts and enigmas of lymphocyte homing. *Adv. Immunol.*, **64**, 139–218.

Sassetti, C., Tangemann, K., Singer, M. S., Kershaw, D. B. & Rosen, S. D. (1998). Identification of podocalyxin-like protein as a high endothelial venule ligand for L-selectin: parallels to CD34. *J. Exp. Med.*, **187**, 1965–75.

Satomaa, T., Renkonen, O., Helin, J. *et al.* (2002). O-glycans on human high endothelial CD34 putatively participating in L-selectin recognition. *Blood*, **99**, 2609–11.

Scudder, P. R., Shailubhai, K., Duffin, K. L., Streeter, P. R. & Jacob, G. S. (1994). Enzymatic synthesis of a 6'-sulfated sialyl-Lewis x which is an inhibitor of L-selectin binding to peripheral addressin. *Glycobiology*, **4**, 929–32.

Springer, T. A. (1994). Traffic signals for lymphocyte recirculation and leukocyte emigration: the multistep paradigm. *Cell*, **76**, 301–14.

Stamper, H. B. Jr & Woodruff, J. J. (1976). Lymphocyte homing into lymph nodes: in vitro demonstration of the selective affinity of recirculating lymphocytes for high-endothelial venules. *J. Exp. Med.*, **144**, 828–33.

Stoolman, L. M. & Rosen, S. D. (1983). Possible role for cell-surface carbohydrate-binding molecules in lymphocyte recirculation. *J. Cell Biol.*, **96**, 722–9.

Streeter, P. R., Rouse, B. T. & Butcher, E. C. (1988). Immunohistologic and functional characterization of a vascular addressin involved in lymphocyte homing into peripheral lymph nodes. *J. Cell Biol.*, **107**, 1853–62.

Suzuki, A., Andrew, D. P., Gonzalo, J. A. *et al.* (1996). CD34-deficient mice have reduced eosinophil accumulation after allergen exposure and show a novel crossreactive 90-kD protein. *Blood*, **87**, 3550–62.

Varki, A. (1997). Selectin ligands: will the real ones please stand up? *J. Clin. Invest.*, **100**, S31–5.

von Andrian, U. H. (1996). Intravital microscopy of the peripheral lymph node microcirculation in mice. *Microcirculation*, **3**, 287–300.

von Andrian, U. H. & Mackay, C. R. (2000). T-cell function and migration. Two sides of the same coin. *New Engl. J. Med.*, **343**, 1020–34.

Yednock, T. A., Butcher, E. C., Stoolman, L. M. & Rosen, S. D. (1987). Receptors involved in lymphocyte homing: relationship between a carbohydrate-binding receptor and the MEL-14 antigen. *J. Cell Biol.*, **104**, 725–31.

Yeh, J. C., Hiraoka, N., Petryniak, B. *et al.* (2001). Novel sulfated lymphocyte homing receptors and their control by a Core 1 extension beta 1,3-N-acetylglucosaminyltransferase. *Cell*, **105**, 957–69.

DISCUSSION

Cross   Have you been able to localise L-selectin in the blastocyst? In particular, if there is preferential localisation in the blastocyst, does it correlate with how a human blastocyst implants as opposed to a mouse one?

S. Fisher	We are trying to do this now. It is very hard to stain human blastocysts because they collapse. In the USA we can't work on human embryos, so this is all done off campus, which has slowed us down.
McLaren	This links up with a question I was going to ask. You showed a picture of cytotrophoblast with all those cytokine receptors listed, but they were not identified on the trophectoderm of the implanted blastocyst.
S. Fisher	We have not done this yet. Because we have so little access to human embryos we do a lot of our work first in early gestation, and then we take it back to the embryo.
Braude	It is interesting that when it comes to a field where there is money to be made, medicine often proceeds far ahead of the scientific information. At the moment you can buy embryo 'glue'. This is basically hyaluronic acid, which you can coat embryos with prior to transfer and it is alleged to improve implantation rate. There are no reliable data to prove or disprove this effect.
Loke	You drew the analogy with binding of leukocytes in inflamed blood vessels. The final event here is extravasation of these leukocytes. Do you envisage this is what happens with endovascular trophoblast, that it also gets out of the blood vessel into the surroundings?
S. Fisher	No. We think this extravasation event is when the cells go through the uterine epithelium. The endovascular trophoblast doesn't make much L-selectin. You wouldn't expect it to, because by then it is the equivalent of the endothelium. One of the things we are looking at is whether it now switches and makes the ligands.
Loke	The controversy is whether the trophoblast in the wall of blood vessels is derived from the endovascular trophoblast migrating from inside the vessel or from the trophoblast invading from outside.
Pijnenborg	This debate is ongoing.
Loke	If it is inside-to-out, then Susan Fisher's mechanism can provide an explanation.
Pijnenborg	Susan Fisher, you mentioned the endovascular trophoblast lining the inner side of the spiral arteries. This is a temporary stage. It is seen in the first and early part of the second trimester, but not at the end of pregnancy. All the trophoblast is incorporated into the wall and is covered by fresh endothelium. I'm sure that your comparison with the extravasation event is a valid one. I think that most of the trophoblast getting into the wall is originally derived from the endovascular trophoblast. Part of the controversy concerns how much of the interstitial trophoblast contributes to this. I am not sure that there is none there at all. Other investigators are still working on this.
McLaren	Does this link up with what pathologists sometimes describe as 'trophoblastic rests'? They claim to be able to identify trophoblast cells hanging around in women who have been pregnant.

S. Fisher   There is good evidence that there are fetal cells hanging around, but their identity is quite inscrutable. I don't think we have the right markers. People here may have other ideas.

Sharkey   I wanted to discuss this extravasation issue. In other species there is quite a lot of evidence that this is more like apoptosis induction in the epithelial cells underneath the uterus: this is the dogma. In other species such as big cats there is more of an actual extravasation event. There seems to be quite a lot of heterogeneity in how this actually happens. What is currently known about the situation in the human? This is almost impossible to look at, but what do people think is going on?

S. Fisher   In humans, from the few sections we have to go on in the Carnegie collection, it looks like the trophoblast very quickly goes in without doing much harm to the uterine epithelium. Then it heals over very quickly. This is one of the reasons why human embryos have been so hard to find because they bury themselves in the uterus so quickly.

Sharkey   People have done in vitro work putting embryos onto polarised epithelial cells.

S. Fisher   From our experience in culture, I think it is rather hard to do these cultures in the right way. The conclusions from the Carnegie collection are pretty clear. There aren't many samples, though.

Pijnenborg   With regard to culturing blastocysts on polarised epithelia, there is one publication by Lindenberg *et al.* (1989) who compared the 'implantation' of human, mouse and bovine blastocysts on a uterine monolayer. What we see in the implanting human blastocyst is very similar to what has been described in Rhesus monkeys, with an insertion of multinucleated trophoblastic cells in between epithelial cells.

Burton   The trophoblast that seems to be invading is a multinucleated syncytial mass. Does anyone know at what point the first syncytium is formed in the human? Is it cytotrophoblast cells that are doing the invasion or syncytium?

S. Fisher   The electron microscopy shows that both cytotrophoblasts and syncytiotrophoblasts are there. So it could be either one. I am not convinced that it is totally syncytial.

McLaren   Are we talking about invasion of the stroma once it is through the epithelium, which is syncytial, or are we talking about invasion actually through the uterine epithelium?

S. Fisher   Both. We see both cell types from the beginning, at least from the blastocyst stage.

Moffett   Do you know where the L-selectin ligand is expressed temporally and spatially in the uterus? Is there a window of expression?

S. Fisher   We know temporally. With the window of implantation this ligand goes from being almost undetectable to being highly expressed. It is at the right place at the right time. What we don't know is the spatial expression pattern with regard to different areas of the uterine wall such as fundus versus the lower segment.

Pijnenborg I would also be very interested in looking at the interaction between trophoblastic cells and the deeper myometrial cells, not just the decidual cells. When there is pre-eclampsia or other defects in implantation or placentation, that is where the problems are.

S. Fisher We are getting those experiments going.

McLaren I wanted to mention the work of David Kirby, a very talented mammalian embryologist killed in a tragic car accident 35 years ago when he was in his late 30s. Kirby & Cowell (1968) described in the mouse the difference between putting a blastocyst into a properly hormonally primed uterus, in which case you get a decidual response to the trophoblast – it invades but doesn't invade too far – and the consequences of putting a mouse trophoblast into a mouse uterus that is not hormonally primed, when the trophoblast not only gets through the endothelium but also is much more aggressive and destroys the entire uterus. Would you say that human trophoblast is even more aggressive than mouse?

S. Fisher Yes, the human trophoblast is very aggressive. It is known from ectopic pregnancies that the pregnancy can go to term as long the placenta gets a good blood supply without initiating bleeding. I assume it would be quite invasive in any tissue.

REFERENCES

Kirby, D.R.S. & Cowell, T.P. (1968). Trophoblast–host interaction. In R. Fleischmajer and R.E. Billingham, eds., *Epithelial–Mesenchymal Interactions*. Baltimore: Williams & Wilkins, pp. 64–77.

Lindenberg, S., Hyttel, P., Sjogren, A. & Geve, T. (1989). A comparative study of attachment of human, bovine and mouse blastocysts to uterine epithelial monolayer. *Hum. Reprod.*, **4**, 446–56.

8

Trophoblast regulation of maternal endocrine function and behaviour

E. B. Keverne

University of Cambridge, UK

Trophoblast cell lineage exerts considerable influence on maternal endocrine function. Progesterone is the steroid hormone that dominates pregnancy and is necessary to sustain pregnancy. The sustained production of progesterone beyond the normal duration of the oestrous cycle is common to all mammals and is referred to as the maternal recognition of pregnancy. However, the means of producing high levels of progesterone in maternal circulation varies according to species and the stage of pregnancy, and involves different cell types of the trophectoderm lineage. There are three important mechanisms for progesterone regulation by trophoblast cells (a) by direct synthesis, (b) indirectly by production of hormones that sustain the maternal corpus luteum (prolactin in rodents; chorionic gonadotrophins in primates and horses), and (c) indirectly by paracrine factors (antiluteolysins) that prevent uterine production of prostaglandins and luteal regression (sheep and cows trophoblast produce interferon).

The effects of progesterone on maternal tissues are mediated through its interaction with specific intracellular receptors that are members of the nuclear receptor superfamily of transcription factors (Tsai & O'Malley 1994). Progesterone receptor binding induces conformational changes in receptor structure leading to dimerisation, post-translational modification by recruitment of coactivator proteins and binding to specific enhancer DNA elements in promoters that initiate gene transcription. Progesterone has a broad spectrum of effects by acting on many maternal target tissues (Fig. 8.1).

Progesterone function in pregnancy

Implantation

A null mutation of the progesterone receptor in mice prevents decidualisation and pregnancy. Moreover, two key enzymes, cytochrome P450 and 3β-hydroxysteroid

Biology and Pathology of Trophoblast, eds. Ashley Moffett, Charlie Loke and Anne McLaren.
Published by Cambridge University Press © Cambridge University Press 2005.

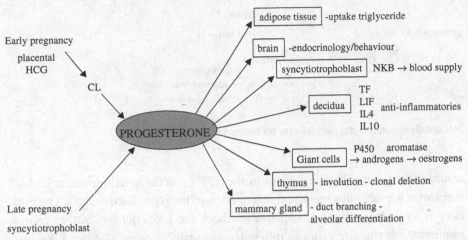

Figure 8.1   Placental progesterone production and maternal target tissues. CL, corpus luteum, HCG, human chorionic gonadotrophin, IL, interleukin, LIF, leukaemia inhibitory factor, NKB, neurokinin B, TF, tissue factor.

dehydrogenase, that are essential for progesterone production, are induced by implantation (Arensburg *et al.* 1999). This takes place in the decidual cells at the antimesometrial side of the uterine wall, but these same transcripts also become highly abundant in the giant trophoblast cells that surround the embryonic cavity by days 8.5–11 of mouse gestation.

The question arises as to what might be the function of local progesterone production at the implantation site in the face of high maternal circulation of progesterone originating from the corpus luteum? It has been suggested that progesterone produced during the first trimester by trophoblast cells acts in a paracrine manner on the decidua serving an immunological role, reducing the production of leukaemia inhibitory factor (LIF), interleukin (IL)4 and IL10 by decidual T cells (Arensburg *et al.* 1999). Progesterone is also known to regulate the expression of the cell adhesion molecule cadherin II in the decidua.

Behaviour

As pregnancy is established the proliferation of trophoblasts results in high levels of progesterone production (300 mg per day in humans), which acts as a hormone on maternal target tissues. Notable among these are the brain, the mammary gland and the thymus. In the hypothalamic region of the brain, high levels of progesterone exert a negative feedback on the pulsatile release of gonadotrophin-releasing hormone (GnRH). The GnRH neurons are not themselves steroid receptive cells but it is thought that negative feedback inhibition occurs via γ-aminobutyric acid (GABA)-ergic interneurons (Everitt & Keverne 1986). Gonadotrophin releasing hormone

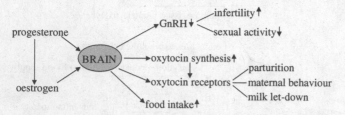

Figure 8.2   Placentally regulated steroids: effects on maternity.

results in the release of luteinising hormone (LH) from the anterior pituitary, which
is essential for folliculogenesis and reactivation of the reproductive cycle. The pituitary is an additional site of negative feedback for progesterone, but its relative
importance at this site varies in different mammalian species (Everitt & Keverne
1986). In most mammalian species, progesterone negative feedback inhibits folliculogenesis and hence oestrogen production resulting in a complete suppression
of female fertility and sexual receptivity. In large-brained primates, where sexual
receptivity has become substantially emancipated from endocrine determinants,
high levels of progesterone in pregnancy reduce sexual activity as a consequence
of peripheral actions on the reproductive tract and sexual skin swellings (Keverne
1984).

Not only is placental progesterone important in suppressing pregnant female
sexual behaviour, but it is also important for priming the brain for promotion
of maternal behaviour. Other hormones of importance in the context of maternal behaviour are prolactin and oestrogen. In the late stages of pregnancy, prior
to parturition and the onset of maternal behaviour, notable changes occur in the
circulating levels of hormones in the female, which have much in common across
most mammalian species studied. These changes involve a fall in progesterone levels and an increase in oestrogen and prolactin, maternal endocrine changes that
are dependent on the placenta. Prolactin-like hormones produced by trophoblasts
become the primary luteotrophins in the latter half of rodent pregnancy and peak
in the maternal circulation at parturition (Grattan 2002). Oestrogen levels, which
increase towards the end of pregnancy are also indirectly dependent on the placenta. Placental trophoblasts are the major site for conversion of progestins into
androgen, which then serves as the precursor for aromatisation to oestrogen by the
maternal ovary. In the female rodent brain, placental lactogens (PL-I and PL-II)
have been shown to promote maternal behaviour by priming the brain possibly by
an action on dopamine neurons (Mann & Bridges 2001). Progesterone and oestrogen are steroids that readily enter the brain and both have effects on oxytocinergic
neurons (Fig. 8.2). Oxytocin is produced in the brain's parvocellular neurons to
activate maternal behaviour, while the magnocellular production of oxytocin is

important for parturition and milk let-down. High levels of progesterone promote oxytocin synthesis but inhibit neural firing and hence oxytocin release (Kendrick & Keverne 1992). Around the time of parturition, the falling levels of progesterone and increasing levels of oestrogen promote the synthesis of oxytocin receptors in the brain, uterus and mammary gland (Johnson *et al.* 1989, Broad *et al.* 1999). Hence the conceptus, via the hormones of the extraembryonic trophectoderm, capitalises on the maternal neuroendocrine system to ensure the synchronisation of birth with milk let-down and maternal care. In order to ensure fetal control over parturition, the placental trophoblast cell lineage silences maternal oxytocinergic neurons by producing or inducing high levels of progesterone, and any oxytocin leakage from the pituitary is taken care of by a proteolytic enzyme (oxytocinase) produced by the placenta, rendering this oxytocin biologically inactive.

Mammary glands

Progesterone, acting on receptor B (PR-B), has an important role in the normal proliferative responses of the mammary gland, aided by placental lactogens (Ismail *et al.* 2003, Bailey *et al.* 2004). These proliferative changes include pregnancy-associated lateral duct branching and lobular alveolar differentiation. Lactogenesis does not occur until the end of pregnancy, or following parturition because of the inhibitory effects of progesterone on prolactin action. Leptin is also produced by the placenta (cytotrophoblasts of labyrinthine layer and giant cells) and is high in maternal circulation from week 36 to term in women (Domali & Messinis 2002). This peptide has also been suggested to affect milk production by inhibition of prolactin response.

Thymus

Progesterone acts on the maternal thymus to reduce lymphocyte development and produce thymic involution, reducing the output of mature T cells (Tibbetts *et al.* 1999). The mechanism by which progesterone regulation of T cell development protects the conceptus is not clear. However, it has been shown that T cells capable of recognising paternal antigens undergo clonal deletion or anergy during pregnancy. Pregnancy studies of thymectomised wild-type mice with replacement thymic transplants taken from the null progesterone receptor mutant mice, show a significant reduction of implantation sites and increases in embryo resorption (Conneely *et al.* 2001).

Feeding and metabolism

In rodents, food intake, fat storage and overall body mass increase during pregnancy. In the early stages of pregnancy this is thought to be due to progesterone alone. In

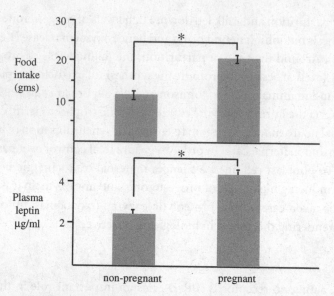

Figure 8.3   Food intake versus plasma leptin, constructed from data in Seeber *et al.* (2002).

the later stages of pregnancy both oestrogen and progesterone are at high levels in maternal circulation, and act on adipose tissue to affect lipoprotein lipase (LPL), which mediates the uptake of triglycerides. Progesterone activates LPL activity and oestrogen is required to induce production of progesterone receptors. Pregnancy also increases food intake in many mammalian species as well as fat storage. A failure to obtain sufficient food intake by the mother during pregnancy results in elevated levels of placental corticotrophin-releasing hormone (CRH) and preterm delivery (Smith & Waddell 2003).

Maternal food intake alone in the last trimester of pregnancy is not sufficient to sustain the enhanced growth of the feto–placental unit stimulated by the increased release of insulin-like growth factors (IGFs). Therefore, increased food intake stimulated by progesterone in the early stages of pregnancy serves as an energy store in the form of increased adiposity. Theoretically, this increase in fat together with the high levels of maternal insulin should result in reduced maternal food intake. Fat produces leptin, a peptide which serves as an adiposity signal to the brain (inhibits neuropeptide γ (NPY) and stimulates pro-opiomelanocortin (POMC)-derived melanocyte-stimulating hormone (MSH)), which responds by reducing food intake to restore adipose tissue to normal level (Elmquist *et al.* 1999). However, high calorie intake is sustained throughout pregnancy despite high fat stores and the pregnant female develops leptin resistance (Fig. 8.3) and insulin resistance (gestational diabetes and increased glucose tolerance) (Sagawa *et al.* 2002). Precisely how this is brought about is complex and dependent on placental neuropeptides. Leptin is produced by the cytotrophoblasts and by the giant cells in the junctional zone at the maternal interface. The placental release of leptin into the fetal circulation is very low while the release into maternal circulation is very high (Jakimuik *et al.* 2003). Likewise, high levels of placental IGFs are released into maternal circulation and act on the insulin receptor. It is well known that sustained high levels of leptin and IGF will result in down-regulation of the receptors, which, in turn, could account for the maternal resistance to leptin and insulin during pregnancy. Precisely how this receptor down-regulation allows increased food intake, increased adiposity and susceptibility to diabetes is a topical issue in obesity research. It is known that leptin resistance in the arcuate nucleus of the hypothalamus allows the neuropeptides that influence feeding (NPY and MSH) to be regulated without the negative feedback from increased adiposity (Rahmouni & Haynes 2001). However, it is interesting to note that both insulin and IGF1 act on the insulin receptor that activates the IRS2 (insulin receptor substrate 2) signalling pathway, and IRS2-deficient mice have high blood sugar, increase food intake and develop obesity (Burks *et al.* 2000). Resistin, a polypeptide known to increase insulin resistance, has recently been shown to be produced in chorionic placental tissue and increases throughout pregnancy (Yura *et al.* 2003).

Fertility requires the integration of reproductive and metabolic signals. Deletion of the IRS2 receptor also causes female infertility by an action on both the ovary and the pituitary. Hence, high levels of the cytokine (IGF1) produced by the placenta enhances transfer of nutrients to the fetus while ensuring high food intake and reduced fertility in the pregnant mother by uncoupling the insulin receptor from the IRS2 signalling cascade. Down-regulation of the insulin receptor IRS2 signalling pathway in the placenta therefore ensures that the increased calorie intake is directed into maternal fat stores and not fetal growth, while growth of the fetus is ensured by coupling the IGF1 signalling cascade to another member of the insulin receptor substrate family, IRS1. It is also important that the placenta receives an adequate blood flow. Neurokinin B, a tachykinin produced by the syncytiotrophoblast is a potent vasoconstrictor that acts on NK3 receptors in the portal vein and mesenteric veins of the mother and increases heart rate. Hence, during pregnancy these vasoconstrictive actions would reduce the large blood flow through the liver to satisfy the needs of the placenta where, paradoxically, neurokinin B causes concentration-dependent relaxation of the placental vessels (Laliberte *et al.* 2004). This is brought about as a consequence of another placental peptide of the prolactin family, proliferin, which is produced by the giant cells in mice (Linzer & Fisher 1999). Production of proliferin enables these migratory trophoblasts to displace the vascular endothelial cells (Hemberger *et al.* 2003, Weimers *et al.* 2003a) resulting in vessels entirely lined by trophoblast cells. Proliferin stimulates endothelial cell migration and neovascularisation of placental vessels by binding to the IGF2R (Volpert *et al.* 1996).

Growth

Insulin-like growth factors (IGF1 and IGF2) are produced by the placenta and are important for growth of extraembryonic membranes, the fetus and regulation of extracellular fluid volume (Accili *et al.* 1999, Evain-Brion & Malassine 2003). Autocrine effects of trophoblast-derived IGF2 have been shown to enhance growth of the cytotrophoblast and to control placental supply of nutrients (Constancia *et al.* 2002). The *Igf2* gene is expressed in fetal tissue at the fetal–maternal interface of invading trophoblast and later in pregnancy *Igf2* production increases in the syncytiotrophoblast. It has an autocrine action on placental growth via the IGF receptor and stimulates endothelial migration via the IGF2/M6P (mannose-6-phosphate) receptor (Volpert *et al.* 1996). In mice, but not human, placental growth is affected only by manipulation of the *Igf2* gene (Han & Carter 2000), while the *Igf1* gene regulates fetal growth in relation to nutrient supply. Insulin-like growth factors are normally buffered in maternal circulation by binding to a protein (IGFBP), which is formed in the liver and avidly binds IGF1 and IGF2 (Fowden 2003). Although during pregnancy phosphorylated isoforms of IGFBP are found in placental circulation, placental alkaline phosphatase is able to dephosphorylate IGFBPs at the syncytial interface. Insulin-like growth factor binding protein 1 occurs in abundance in the decidua and is thought to have an important role in interactions between the decidua and invading trophoblast (Guidice *et al.* 1998). It is thought to act as a local modulator of IGF action at the interface between the decidua and the placenta (Pekonen *et al.* 1988).

Placental growth hormone (PGH) is the product of the *GH-V* gene specifically expressed in the syncytiotrophoblast layer of the human placenta. It differs from pituitary GH by 13 amino acids and has high somatogenic and low lactogenic activities. Assays of PGH by specific monoclonal antibodies reveal that in human maternal circulation from 15–20 weeks prior to term, PGH gradually replaces pituitary GH, which becomes undetectable. Placental GH is secreted by the placenta in a non-pulsatile manner, which is important in the control of maternal IGF1 levels. Placental GH does not appear to have a direct effect on fetal growth, as this hormone is not detectable in the fetal circulation. The physiological role of PGH does, however, promote placental development via an autocrine or paracrine mechanism as suggested by the presence of specific GH receptors in this tissue.

Placental lactogens

In rodents, a variety of prolactin-like hormones influence wide aspects of maternal physiology throughout pregnancy (Weimers *et al.* 2003b). From the earliest stages of implantation, local autocrine/paracrine signalling at the deciduo–trophectoderm interface is crucial to the establishment of pregnancy (Jabbour & Critchley 2001).

Prolactin is secreted by the decidualised endometrium at the time of conception and local expression persists until parturition (Soares *et al.* 1998). There are two distinct placental lactogens (I and II), the former (I) being produced at the time of implantation until mid-gestation when placental lactogen II takes over. These two hormones bind to the same receptor. A third placental hormone in mice, which also binds to the prolactin receptor, proliferin, is specifically produced by the trophoblast giant cells. Proliferin is functionally related to placental angiogenesis by stimulation of endothelial cell migration and is produced by trophoblast giant cells (Lee *et al.* 1988). A second placental specific hormone, proliferin-related protein (PRP), also acts on endothelial cells of uterine blood vessels. It has the opposite effect to proliferin and inhibits endothelial cell migrations (Linzer & Fisher, 1999). Proliferin-related peptide is expressed in giant cells and spongiotrophoblast and may act as a 'brake' that slows down vessel growth in response to proliferin and other angiogenic factors. It may also act as a barrier to prevent maternal blood vessels extending from the uterus or fetus into the placenta.

In humans two other related hormones, prolactin-like protein A (PLPA) binds to natural killer (NK) cells reducing their cytotoxicity whereas PLPE binds to megakaryocytes, stimulating their differentiation, i.e. they regulate the maternal blood system. In rodents, two additional prolactin genes (PLP-L and PLP-M) are highly expressed in invasive trophoblast cells lining the central placental vessel and are produced in the latter half of rodent pregnancy (days 11–20). Prolactin-like hormones produced by the trophoblasts become the primary luteotrophins in the latter half of pregnancy.

Genomic imprinting and trophoblast function

The placental trophoblast is an extraordinary tissue capable of producing a vast range of endocrine secretions, which enable the fetus to regulate its own destiny. Most of these placental hormones function by acting on maternal receptors, an interaction that has required genomic coadaptation between mother and fetus. Hence, the functioning of two genomes (maternal and fetal) as part of a single phenotype (pregnant mother) provide a template for coadaptive selection pressures to operate. Early mortality often accounts for the majority of variance in viability fitness in many species (Wolf 2000), providing a substantial opportunity for selection on traits that are expressed early in life.

One possible way in which such coadaptation could be organised would be through genomic imprinting especially if the maternal oocyte is able to regulate allelic exclusion and, hence, gene dosage. Imprints are reset in the germ line with a maternal imprint resulting in the expression of the paternal allele (Kafri *et al.* 1992). This exclusivity for expression of the paternal allele is therefore dependent on methylation being maintained on the maternal allele following the genome-wide demethylation that occurs after fertilisation (Monk *et al.* 1987). The paternal allele acquires its expression by an active process of demethylation, which occurs in the egg (Mayer *et al.* 2000). Hence, which maternal alleles are suppressed and which paternal alleles are expressed is dependent on events that occur in the fertilised egg. The importance of the environment within the egg is seen with interspecific hybrids (*Peromyscus maniculatus* × *Peromyscus polionotus*) where disruption of imprinting occurs due to nuclear–cytoplasmic incompatibility (Vrana *et al.*, 1998). The oocyte cytoplasm contains proteins (Oct4 and polycomb proteins) that are known to play critical roles in epigenetic inheritance (Ferguson-Smith & Surani 2001). Hence, for a paternally expressed gene, passage through oogenesis is essential to repress the maternal allele.

Paternally expressed gene 3 (*Peg3*) and feto–maternal coadaptation

The conflict theory of genomic imprinting predicts that paternal expression of imprinted genes in embryos should demand more from a mother than maternally expressed genes in the same pregnancy (Haig & Graham 1991). The outcome of paternally expressed genes should therefore tend to increase offspring size and survival. This has been tested in mice by studying the mutant offspring of a wild-type mother that have a null mutation in the *Peg3* gene they have inherited from their father (Li *et al.* 1999, Keverne 2001, Curley *et al.* 2004). These offspring are smaller (Fig. 8.4) and exhibit impaired infant suckling, poor weight gain and growth. Litter size is reduced in primiparous females suggesting prenatal mortality is high, and this trend continues into the post-partum period when significant pup loss continues. The placental size of mutant embryos is reduced by 25%, which has a major impact on birth weight. This is especially notable in mixed mutant/wild-type litters where mutant pups are smaller than in litters that are all mutant, and wild-type offspring are larger than in litters that are all wild-type. Hence, when there is intrauterine competition for maternal resources the smaller placenta of the *Peg3* mutant pup results in them being more severely growth impaired and wild-type pups of the same litter are more advantaged. Also, when the mutation is in the fetus, their mothers eat less and fail to increase their food intake in the last trimester of pregnancy, suggesting an impairment of placental endocrine signals that are, in part, responsible for regulating maternal food intake. Moreover, *Peg3*$^{+/-}$ mutant pups are also slower to regulate thermogenesis and maintain homeothermy, and are later to commence puberty onset. Although crucial to infant survival these features do not fit comfortably with the conflict hypothesis.

The *Peg3*$^{+/-}$ mutation in the mother produces a complementarity of dysfunctions, which can be studied independently of the mutation in pups. Mutant females

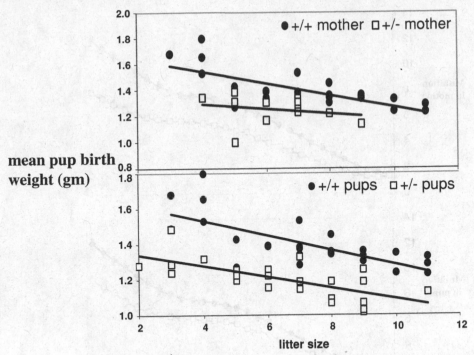

Figure 8.4   Pup weights and litter sizes in *Peg3* mutant mice compared with wild-type mice from mutant mothers. White squares denote mutation of *Peg3*. (Modified after Curley *et al.* 2004.).

fail to increase their food intake in the early stages of pregnancy, eat less throughout pregnancy and carry over less bodyweight reserve into the post-partum period. Milk let-down is impaired in the mutant females during the post-partum period and their pups lose weight on day 1 following birth. Wild-type pups born to *Peg3* mutant mothers remain significantly weight reduced throughout the post-partum period (Fig. 8.5), and this also delays the onset of puberty (Fig. 8.6). Regardless of whether the *Peg3* mutation is expressed in the mother or in the pup the dysfunctional outcome is remarkably similar (Figs 8.4–8.6). The *Peg3* gene mutation influences suckling in the pup and food intake in the mother; postnatal growth in the pups and the time the mother takes to achieve weaning weight of her pups. Finally, provision of warmth by maternal crouching and nest building, and the early onset of thermogenesis by pups are also complementary aspects of maintaining body temperature, and both are impaired by mutation of the *Peg3* gene. While independently producing a complementarity of dysfunctions when mutations are either in mother or pups, the outcome is lethal with only 6% of pups surviving beyond day 1 when the *Peg3* gene is simultaneously mutated in mother and infant.

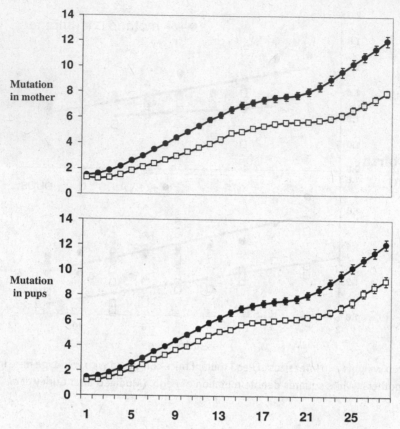

Figure 8.5   Post-partum growth in mice with *Peg3* mutations compared with wild-type mice from mothers with *Peg3* mutations. White squares denote mutation of *Peg3*. (Modified after Curley *et al.* 2004.)

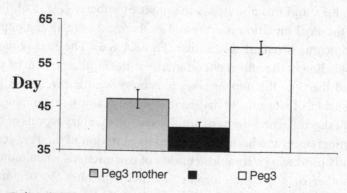

Figure 8.6   Delayed puberty in *Peg3* mutant pups (white column) and wild-type (WT) pups from a *Peg3* mutant mother (grey column) and wild-type pups from wild-type mother (black column).

Although consequences of this mutation in mother versus offspring are functionally complementary, the mechanisms whereby the effects are brought about are quite different. In the case of the mother, *Peg3* is expressed strongly in the developing and adult hypothalamus and is known to affect size and structure of the paraventricular nucleus, especially involving oxytocinergic neurons (Li *et al.* 1999). The paraventricular nucleus of the hypothalamus regulates milk let-down, maternal care and nest building, food intake and body temperature (Russell *et al.* 2001), all of which are impaired in the adult female carrying a *Peg3* mutation. Hence, these hypothalamic dysfunctions could account for all of the phenotypic impairments seen in the adult, while the delayed postnatal growth and late weaning of infants born to mutant mothers are probably secondary to the failure of the mother's hypothalamus to respond to placental hormone signals and postnatal suckling signals. In the fetus, prenatal effects that reduce birth weight are probably secondary to *Peg3* action in the placenta. Impaired suckling by the infant also delays postnatal growth and weaning, and defects in the onset of infant thermogenesis are probably consequences of hypothalamic dysfunction (Smith *et al.* 1998).

The advantages of evolving imprinting for *Peg3* gene regulation is probably in terms of its actions in the placenta and hypothalamus, tissues that interact with each other while the development and functioning of each structure is regulated by different genotypes. All of the maternal consequences of the mutation have been shown in other studies to be produced by lesions of the hypothalamus (food intake, maternal behaviour, body temperature, milk production). Moreover, all of these hypothalamic phenotypes are influenced by hormones produced by the placenta (food intake, maternal behaviour, milk let-down) or by postnatal pup development (prenatal thermogenesis and maternal body temperature) and behaviour of pups (suckling: milk production and milk let-down). These interactions between the two genotypes, involving the hypothalamus and placenta, provide the template for coadaptive selection pressures to operate. Moreover, since early infant mortality accounts for the major part of the variance in viability fitness, this provides a substantial opportunity for selection on traits that are expressed early in life (Mousseau & Fox 1998). The evolutionary outcome of this linked coadaptation is that offspring that have extracted 'good' maternal nurturing would themselves be both well provisioned for and genetically predisposed towards good mothering when adult, thereby enhancing the spread of this gene in the population.

Concluding remarks

The placenta is not only an endocrine organ in its own right producing hormones that act in an autocrine/paracrine manner to regulate implantation, placental growth and development, but many of these hormones enter the maternal circulation to influence maternal physiology, metabolism and behaviour. Therefore impairments in placental growth and development not only perturb transfer of nutrients to the offspring, but may also disturb many endocrine aspects of maternity. Hence an efficient placenta can be seen as one which not only optimises prenatal transfer of maternal resources and ensures provision of these resources by regulating maternal feeding behaviour and metabolism, but also prepares for postnatal events by priming the brain for maternal behaviour and priming the mammary gland for milk production.

The placental trophectoderm is a very special tissue in that it interfaces with maternal circulation. I have emphasised those aspects of this interface that impinge on the mother, but equally important is the growth and development of the fetus for which the energetic requirements need to be synchronised with the transfer capacity of the placenta. Fetal growth is a complex process with some tissues, such as the brain, being more energetically demanding than others. Brain growth occurs late in development and not surprisingly most of mammalian brain growth is postponed to the postnatal period. Fetal growth and form require tight regulation of gene dosage involving homeobox genes, growth factors and their receptors, helix-loop-helix (HLH) transcription factors and cell cycle regulators. Many of these genes are imprinted (expressed according to parent of origin in a haploid condition) and many of the imprinted genes so far investigated are expressed in the placenta. One way to ensure tight regulation of synchronised fetal growth with the growth and provisioning capacity of the placenta is by the coordinated expression of these regulatory genes in mother and placenta. Genomic imprinting has undoubtedly been instrumental in achieving such regulatory coordination (a) by ensuring that gene expression in the fetus and placenta occurs from the same allele, thereby circumventing polymorphic irregularities, (b) by expressing maternal and paternal alleles that are in conflict and hence regulate each other according to supply and demand, and (c) by expressing the same growth promoting genes postnatally, the regulation of which is also balanced between supply and demand. For all of these reasons, the evolution of the placenta has been pivotal in the evolution of mammalian form and speciation.

REFERENCES

Accili, D., Nakae, J., Kim, J. J., Park, B. C. & Rother, K. I. (1999). Targeted gene mutations define the roles of insulin and IGF-1 receptors in mouse embryonic development. *J. Pediatr. Endocrinol. Metab.*, **12**, 475–85.

Arensburg, J., Payne, A. H. & Orly, J. (1999). Expression of steroidogenic genes in maternal and extra-embryonic cells during early pregnancy in mice. *Endocrinology*, **140**, 5220–31.

Bailey, J.P., Neiport, K., Herbst, M.P. *et al.* (2004). Prolactin and transforming growth factor-(beta) signaling exert opposing effects on mammary gland morphogenesis, involution, and the Akt-forkhead pathway. *Mol. Endocrinol.*, **18**, 1171–84.

Broad, K.D., Levy, F., Evans, G. *et al.* (1999). Previous maternal experience potentiates the effect of parturition on oxytocin receptor MRNA in the paraventricular nucleus. *Eur. J. Neurosci.*, **11**, 3725–37.

Burks, D.J., Font de Mora, J., Schubert, M. *et al.* (2000). IRS-2 pathways integrate female reproduction and energy homeostasis. *Nature*, **407**, 377–82.

Conneely, O.M., Mulac-Jericevic, B., Lydon, J.P. & De Mayo, F.J. (2001). Reproductive junctions of the progesterone receptor isoforms: lessons from knock-out mice. *Mol. Cell. Endocrinol.*, **179**, 97–103.

Constancia, M., Hemberger, M., Hughes, J. *et al.* (2002). Placental-specific IGF-II is a major modulator of placental and fetal growth. *Nature*, **417**, 945–8.

Curley, J.P., Barton, S.C., Surani, A.M. & Keverne, E.B. (2004). Co-adaptation in mother and infant regulated by a paternally expressed imprinted gene. *Proc R. Soc. Lond. B Biol. Sci.*, **271**, 1303–9.

Domali, E. & Messinis, I.E. (2002). Leptin in pregnancy. *J. Matern. Fetal Neonatal Med.*, **12**, 222–30.

Elmquist, J.K., Elias, C.F. & Saper, C.B. (1999). From lesions to leptin: hypothalamic control of food intake and body weight. *Neuron*, **22**, 221–32.

Evain-Brion, D. & Malassine, A. (2003). Human placenta as an endocrine organ. *Growth Horm. IGF Res.*, **13**, S34–7.

Everitt, B.J. & Keverne, E.B. (1986). Reproduction. In S.L. Lightman and B.J. Everitt, eds., *Neuroendocrinology*. Oxford: Blackwell Scientific Publications, pp. 472–537.

Ferguson-Smith, A.C. & Surani, M.A. (2001). Imprinting and the epigenetic asymmetry between parental genomes. *Science*, **293**, 1086–9.

Fowden, A.L. (2003). The insulin-like growth factors and feto-placental growth. *Placenta*, **24**, 803–12.

Grattan, D.R. (2002). Behavioural significance of prolactin signaling in the central nervous system during pregnancy and lactation. *Reproduction*, **123**, 497–506.

Guidice, L.C., Mark, S.P. & Irwin, J.C. (1998). Paracrine actions of insulin-like growth factors and IGF binding protein-1 in non-pregnant human endometrium and at the decidual–trophoblast interface. *J. Reprod. Immunol.*, **39**, 133–48.

Haig, D. & Graham, C. (1991). Genomic imprinting and the strange case of the insulin-like growth factor II receptor. *Cell*, **64**, 1045–6.

Han, V.K. & Carter, A.M. (2000). Spatial and temporal patterns of expression of messenger RNA for insulin-like growth factors and their binding proteins in the placenta of man and laboratory animals. *Placenta*, **4**, 289–305.

Hemberger, M., Nozaki, T., Masutani, M. & Cross, J.C. (2003). Differential expression of angiogenic and vasodilatory factors by invasive trophoblast giant cells depending on depth of invasion. *Dev. Dyn.*, **227**, 185–91.

Ismail, P.M., Amato, P., Soyal, S.M. *et al.* (2003). Progesterone involvement in breast development and tumorigenesis – as revealed by progesterone receptor 'knockout' and 'knockin' mouse models. *Steroids*, **68**, 779–87.

Jabbour, H.N. & Critchley, H.O.D. (2001). Potential roles of decidual prolactin in early pregnancy. *Reproduction*, **121**, 197–205.

Jakimuik, A.J., Skalba, P., Huterski, D. *et al.* (2003). Leptin messenger ribonucleic acid (mRNA) content in the human placenta at term: relationship to levels of leptin in cord blood and placental weight. *Gynecol. Endocrinol.*, **17**, 311–16.

Johnson, A.E., Ball, G.F., Coirini, H. *et al.* (1989). Time course of the estradiol-dependent induction of oxytocin receptor binding in the ventromedial hypothalamic nucleus of the rat. *Endocrinology*, **125**, 1414–19.

Kafri, T., Ariel, M., Brandeis, M. *et al.* (1992). Developmental pattern of gene-specific DNA methylation in the mouse embryo and germ line. *Genes Dev.*, **6**, 705–14.

Kendrick, K.M. & Keverne, E.B. (1992). Control of synthesis and release of oxytocin in the sheep brain. In C.A. Pederson, J.D. Caldwell, G.F. Jirikowski & T.R. Insel, eds., Annals of the New York Academy of Sciences Volume 652: *Oxytocin in Maternal, Sexual, and Social Behaviors.* New York: New York Academy of Sciences, pp. 102–21.

Keverne, E.B. (1984). Reproductive behaviour. In C.R. Austin and R.V. Short, eds., *Reproduction in Mammals. Book 4, Reproductive Fitness.* Cambridge: Cambridge University Press, pp. 133–75.

Keverne, E.B. (2001). Genomic imprinting, maternal care, and brain evolution. *Horm. Behav.*, **40**, 146–55.

Laliberte, C., DiMarzo, L., Morrish, D.W. & Kaufman, S. (2004). Neurokinin B causes concentration-dependent relaxation of isolated human placental resistance vessels. *Regul. Pept.*, **117**, 123–6.

Lee, S.J., Talamantes, F., Wilder, E., Linzer, D.I.H. & Nathans, D. (1988). Trophoblastic giant cells of the mouse placenta as the site of proliferin synthesis. *Endocrinology*, **122**, 1761–8.

Li, L.L., Keverne, E.B., Aparicio, S. *et al.* (1999). Regulation of maternal behavior and offspring growth by paternally expressed *Peg3. Science*, **294**, 330–3.

Linzer, D.I. & Fisher, S.J. (1999). The placenta and the prolactin family of hormones: regulation of the physiology of pregnancy. *Mol. Endocrinol.*, **13**, 837–40.

Mann, P.E. & Bridges, R.S. (2001). Lactogenic hormone regulation of maternal behavior. *Prog. Brain Res.*, **133**, 251–62.

Mayer, W., Niveleau, A., Walter, J., Fundele, R. & Haaf, T. (2000). Demethylation of the zygotic paternal genome. *Nature*, **203**, 501–2.

Monk, M., Boubelik, M. & Lehnert, S. (1987). Temporal and regional changes in DNA methylation in the embryonic, extra-embryonic and germ cell lineages during mouse embryo development. *Development*, **99**, 371–82.

Mousseau, T.S. & Fox, C. (1998). The adaptive significance of maternal effects. *Trends Ecol. Evol.*, **13**, 403–7.

Pekonen, F., Suikkari, A.M., Makinen, T. & Rutanen, E.M. (1988). Different insulin-like growth factor binding species in human placenta and decidua. *J. Clin. Endocrinol. Metab.*, **67**, 1250–7.

Rahmouni, K. & Haynes, W.G. (2001). Leptin signaling pathways in the central nervous system: interactions between neuropeptide Y and melanocortins. *BioEssays*, **23**, 1095–9.

Russell, J.A., Douglas, A.J. & Ingram, C.D. (2001). Brain preparations for maternity – adaptive changes in behavioural and neuroendocrine systems during pregnancy and lactation. An overview. *Prog. Brain Res.*, **133**, 1–38.

Sagawa, N., Yura, S., Itoh, H. *et al.* (2002). Possible role of placental leptin in pregnancy: a review. *Endocrine*, **19**, 65–71.

Seeber, R.M., Smith, J.T. & Waddell, B.J. (2002). Plasma leptin binding activity and hypothalamic leptin receptor expression during pregnancy and lactation in the rat. *Biol. Reprod.*, **66**, 1762–7.

Smith, J.T. & Waddell, B.J. (2003). Leptin distribution and metabolism in the pregnant rat: transplacental leptin passage increases in late gestation but is reduced by excess glucocorticoids. *Endocrinology*, **144**, 3024–30.

Smith, J.E., Jansen, A.S.P., Gilbey, M.P. & Loewy, A.D. (1998). CNS cell groups projecting to sympathetic outflow of tail artery: neural circuits involved in heat loss in the rat. *Brain Res.*, **786**, 153–64.

Soares, M.J., Muller, H., Orwig, K.E., Peters, T.J. & Dai, G. (1998). The uteroplacental prolactin family and pregnancy. *Biol. Reprod.*, **58**, 273–84.

Tibbetts, T.A., DeMayo, F., Rich, S., Conneely, O.M. & O'Malley, B.W. (1999). Progesterone receptors in the thymus are required for thymic involution during pregnancy and for normal fertility. *Proc. Natl. Acad. Sci. U.S.A.*, **96**, 12021–6.

Tsai, M.J. & O'Malley, B.W. (1994). Molecular mechanisms of action of steroid. Thyroid receptor superfamily members. *Annu. Rev. Biochem.*, **63**, 451–86.

Volpert, O., Jackson, D., Bouck, N. & Linzer, D.I. (1996). The insulin-like growth factor II/mannose 6-phosphate receptor is required for proliferin-induced angiogenesis. *Endocrinology*, **137**, 3871–6.

Vrana, P.B., Guan, X.-J., Ingram, S. & Tilghman, S.M. (1998). Genomic imprinting is disrupted in interspecific *Peromyscus* hybrids. *Nat. Genet.*, **20**, 362–5.

Weimers, D.O., Ain, R., Ohboshi, S. & Soares, M.J. (2003a). Migratory trophoblast cells express a newly identified member of the prolactin gene family. *J. Endocrinol.*, **179**, 335–46.

Weimers, D.O., Shao, L.J., Ain, R., Dai, G. & Soares, M.J. (2003b). The mouse prolactin gene family locus. *Endocrinology*, **144**, 313–25.

Wolf, J.B. (2000). Gene interactions from maternal effects. *Evolution*, **54**, 1882–98.

Yura, S., Sagawa, N., Itoh, H. *et al.* (2003). Resistin is expressed in the human placenta. *J. Clin. Endocrinol. Metab.*, **88**, 1394–7.

DISCUSSION

McLaren   You mentioned all these different neuropeptides and trophic factors, but it wasn't clear to me whether it was different trophoblast cell lineages that produced different factors, or the same lineage producing them one after the other.

Keverne   It is all of those things. For example, the giant cells are important in producing proliferin. Resistin is produced by the choroid, and neurokinin is produced by the syncytiotrophoblast as is IGF2 and PGH. Proliferin-related protein is produced by the spongiotrophoblast. There is also the timing aspect. Leptin is initially produced by the cytotrophoblast and then by the giant cells. I didn't have time to go into the details, but I wanted to illustrate the vast range of factors that are being produced. I have already heard that some of these actions are controversial and depend on the species. For example, someone already mentioned the role of migration of the endothelial cells from the spiral arteries and their replacement with trophoblast, which occurs in mouse but not human.

Cross If we look across species, it is very hard to make a generalised story about production of these hormones. For example, Dan Linzer assures me that there is not a human homologue of proliferin. The genome simply doesn't have it. In another case, the mouse has an aromatase gene but it is not expressed in the placenta, and therefore the mouse placenta does not make oestrogen.

Keverne The mouse placenta produces the androgen, which is then aromatised to oestrogen in the ovary. The outcome is the same although the method may be different in mouse and human. If the human doesn't produce proliferin, a peptide of the prolactin family, then what I have said probably doesn't apply, but there is still migration of the endothelial cells from the spiral arteries. It could be that one other of the many prolactin family members has taken over this role in humans.

Evain-Brion I have the same comment. The endocrine functions of the placenta are very different from one species to another. One of the things you showed was a drop of progesterone at the end of pregnancy, which doesn't occur in humans. Progesterone is also not produced by the mouse placenta. It is very difficult to take a general view across species.

Keverne I agree, but I didn't say that the mouse placenta produces progesterone. In the mouse it is coming from the corpus luteum, but the human placenta produces progesterone. All my experimental data were taken from the mouse, and where I could complement these with human data I did. I am not attempting to provide the detailed comparative endocrinology of the placenta. The point I am trying to illustrate is that although the mechanisms may differ, the fact remains that the placenta is acting as an endocrine organ in its own right and it is actually capitalising on receptors that are present in the mother in order to influence metabolism, feeding and behaviour of the mother.

Evain-Brion I agree that the placenta produces hormones that adapt the maternal metabolism to pregnancy.

Sibley There is another thing about the placenta as an endocrine organ. Hormones go both ways, not just into the maternal circulation but also into the fetal circulation where they could have quite different effects.

Keverne Some of the peptide hormones, such as leptin, don't. Leptin is produced by the placenta but only released into maternal circulation.

Sibley   Neurokinin B certainly gets into the fetal circulation, where it is a vasodilator, not a vasoconstrictor.

Keverne   It acts on NK3 in the maternal portal system and mesenteric veins, where it is a vasoconstrictor and reduces the large blood flow through the liver in order to satisfy the increased needs of the placenta, where, paradoxically, neurokinin B causes concentration-dependent relaxation of the placental vessels.

Sibley   There is also redundancy in the endocrine function of the placenta. The standard redundancy quoted is human placental lactogen (HPL). You can have a trophoblast that makes grand quantities of HPL at the end of pregnancy and yet you can have normal pregnancies that make no HPL at all. It is a complex system.

Keverne   I was quite surprised to hear that proliferin, a member of the prolactin family, acts on the M6P receptor. This was news to me because I always thought this receptor was exclusively for IGF2.

Lever   Quite a number of the endogenous retroviruses (HERVs) that are known to be expressed in the placenta have hormone-responsive elements in their promoter regions. It is probably no coincidence that they are highly expressed in the placenta.

Keverne   What are they doing?

Lever   I don't think anyone really knows. They are implicated in syncytiotrophoblast formation by expression of HERV-W envelope. There they may have various other functions. For example, they express immunosuppressive peptides.

McLaren   So do they play any part in methylation? Andrew Sharkey, you were speculating earlier about retroviruses and methylation.

Sharkey   I was under the impression that the placenta is the only place where these endogenous retroviruses are expressed in humans, even though they are exposed to progesterone all the time.

Lever   They are expressed in a number of tissues, but they are most highly expressed in the placenta. Interestingly, they are expressed in the placenta but not the fetus. I was speculating earlier how this might relate to the different methylation systems which control gene expression in the placenta versus the fetus.

Evain-Brion It is important to notice that the trophoblast cells are the placental cells where the retroviral envelope proteins are expressed. What seems to be specific for the trophoblast is that the envelope protein is expressed and is directly involved in placental morphogenesis such as, for example, human trophoblast fusion. Then there are also retroviral sequences located near the promoters of some genes, which could explain the specific expression of some hormones in the trophoblast.

Ferguson-Smith   We have looked at a family of non-long terminal repeats (LTR)-containing retrotransposons. It is a small family with six X-linked and four autosomal transposons. Two of the autosomal ones are imprinted. The one we work on is expressed in the fetus and in the placenta. We don't know the tissue distribution at the moment, but we are working on this. The expression levels are higher in the fetus.

Moffett   I think Danielle Evain-Brion is right: the fact that the envelope protein is there means that we should think of trophoblast as infected in some rather primitive way. There is viral protein expressed. The interest for us is whether or not the maternal immune system sees it as being an infected cell. Could these proteins act as target ligands?

Braude   I wanted to pick up on Barry Keverne's comments about the sexually deprived and lactating feeding mouse. There was a paper by Roger Short in 1976 in the *Proceedings of the Royal Society* entitled 'The evolution of human reproduction' (Short 1976). In this he cites reproductive habits in three different tribes: the Kung bushwomen, the Hutterites of North America and the women in Western societies. What he noted was that the Bushwomen were lactating or pregnant for the majority of their lives. Many of the children died and they would have four or five well-spaced pregnancies in order to reproduce themselves. I annoy my students when I suggest that the natural state of women is pregnant or lactating, which is quite true but not very PC. We have a very artificial society now where because contraception is widespread, women menstruate much more frequently and breasts are exposed for many more years to cyclic hormone environments.

Renfree   Roger would say that menstruation is an iatrogenic disease.

Keverne   One of the things that is different about humans is the independence of maternal behaviour on hormones of pregnancy. That is, women don't have to have gone through pregnancy or parturition to be maternal, which isn't true for any non-primate mammal. Once the brain has evolved a vast neocortex, maternal or parental care may continue long beyond weaning. It needs to. One of the important evolutionary developments has been the postponement of most of our brain development to the postnatal period. Such extended postnatal brain development is only possible through extended parental or alloparental care. This is extended even for decades in humans, but also occurs to a lesser extent in large-brained primates. Our brains grow in size until about age 7, and cortical areas are remodelled when we go through puberty. The prefrontal and temporal cortex are still differentiating at the age of 22. Part of our being able to grow a big brain has required this emancipation of the maternal care from the determining influence of the hormones. I agree with what you said about our ancestors. They used to come into menarchy later, die younger, lactate for longer and continuously produce babies. Even so, this is very different from the female mouse, since although the hormones of pregnancy and lactation act as nature's contraceptive in women, they do not inhibit or restrict sexual activity to only the fertile period.

Renfree   Our ancestors would have had only five or six babies in their lifetime. They would have a long lactation that lasted four years.

Keverne	Even four years of hormonal exposure would not be time enough to sustain human reproductive success. Children are not developmentally independent at four.
Reik	I'd like to switch gears a little to the *Peg3* story. The *Peg3* mothers will have undergone growth restriction themselves in utero, as well as not having the *Peg3* product in their brains. So do they do what they do because they have been treated badly as embryos themselves, and therefore they treat their offspring badly, or is it because of the brain?
Keverne	We can't rule out the fact that mutant offspring from normal mothers have experienced these growth problems in utero and postnatally, and have also come into puberty later. But the fact remains that where we see the impairment in maternal behaviour, this is a result of deleted *Peg3* expression in the hypothalamus. Littermates that do not carry the mutation are normal in their maternal behaviour.
Reik	Do you attribute the phenotype to the brain disruption of the gene expression?
Keverne	Yes. The thing about 129 and C57 BL/6 mouse strains is that they can be spontaneously maternal anyway. What we are seeing here is not so much an all-or-none effect. Mice will show spontaneous maternal care, provided they have been exposed to infants for some time. We are, undoubtedly, getting a real impairment with the *Peg3* mutation compared with the controls but we don't think that it is the impaired growth and development of the fetus that has produced these kinds of effects on maternal behaviour.
Redman	Have you swapped the fetuses to wild-type mothers?
Keverne	There is no need, you can have a wild-type mother with the infants carrying the mutation and compare this with a mutant mother carrying wild-type pups. Both are impaired in early postnatal growth and have later puberty onset, but only those females carrying the mutation are behaviourally impaired.
Reik	You really need a conditional knockout.
Keverne	Ideally yes, otherwise we can't separate the effects of early growth impairment. However, if you get at the mechanism, both neural and placental, and show the gene is independently affecting the brain, then this gets you part of the way there.
Cross	You have talked about the fate of wild-type pups that are reared by a mutant female. Why can't you just breed these and see whether they give rise to smaller young or abuse their pups?
Keverne	They don't. However, they do come into puberty later and their lifetime's reproductive success is impaired in comparison to wild-type pups reared by wild-type mothers.
Cross	Is their maternal behaviour normal?
Keverne	Yes. We are in the process of studying this in detail, but the breeding records would suggest they are not abnormal

Fowden   Considering this is potentially a hypothalamic disorder, is gestational length altered? Some of the other maturational effects operate through the hypothalamus.

Keverne   We found in the knockout that some of the pregnancies actually extend for longer, and primiparous mutant females do experience problems in giving birth.

Fowden   So you don't know whether it is the oxytocin or the fetal trigger to the onset of labour that has been changed.

Keverne   I would put it down to oxytocin, because we know there are fewer oxytocinergic neurons in the hypothalamus of mutants.

REFERENCE

Short, R. V. (1976). The evolution of human reproduction. *Proc. R. Soc. Lond. B Biol. Sci.*, **195**, 3–24.

General discussion II

McLaren	I'd like to go back to Rosemary Fisher and her work on hydatidiform moles. I am not sure that we really settled the question of why they are so much more common in Southeast Asia. Second, in time, rather than space, why are they so much less common now than they used to be?
R. Fisher	I don't have any explanation for this.
Jacobs	I have been thinking about this. Not only were they commoner in Southeast Asia, they were also much more common among the lower socioeconomic classes. If this has something to do with it, it could explain why there are more of them among rural communities than city communities. If they are suddenly all disappearing it could be because populations are now much better off socioeconomically. Of course, this doesn't address the mechanism.
Braude	Unless some dietary factor changes with better nutrition or a change in type of diet with more international influences.
Jacobs	In communities where they were very common they are now unusual.
Trowsdale	If there is socioeconomic clustering, we might be talking about malnutrition or infection.
Renfree	I was wondering whether it had something to do with a frequency of twinning. Roger Short has recently been looking at frequency rates of both dizygotic (DZ) and monozygotic (MZ) twinning in various populations, particularly in Asian populations where there is a much lower incidence of DZ twinning under the control of particular genes that induce multiple ovulation (Tong *et al.* 1997). These are possibly related to the X-linked and genomically imprinted genes of sheep that induce multiple ovulation (Montgomery *et al.* 2001). You were saying that you had 'empty eggs'.
R. Fisher	That was just how we described them. The cytoplasm in the eggs seems to be intact and the mitochondrial DNA is normal.

Biology and Pathology of Trophoblast, eds. Ashley Moffett, Charlie Loke and Anne McLaren.
Published by Cambridge University Press © Cambridge University Press 2005.

169

Renfree   If you have multiple ovulations, could there be a correlation between the twinning rate and the rate of moles?

Braude   I am worried about the term 'empty egg', as I don't understand how it occurs unless it is proposed that the egg has lost all its chromosomes into the polar body, or they have all fragmented in some strange way. I understand that for a complete mole there is only one set of chromosomes that are paternal, but the simple explanation of an empty egg is not that plausible as a common phenomenon in certain racial groups or species.

McLaren   To me an empty egg is what cloners use, where they have removed all the nuclear genetic material.

Jacobs   The effect is exactly that. What is wrong with the polar body?

Braude   It is a very odd business to have everything in the polar body.

Jacobs   But triploidy can occur: something similar is happening but the other way round – all the chromosomes then remain in the egg.

Braude   I can understand that, where there is non-extrusion of the polar body. But I find it odd that all the chromosomes suddenly disappear into the polar body.

McLaren   Also extrusion of the second polar body doesn't occur until the sperm has entered.

Surani   Has anyone seen an empty egg?

McLaren   There are reports of one pronucleus, two pronuclei and three pronuclei, but never zero pronuclei.

Braude   It is possible to see a single pronucleus after the injection of a sperm at ICSI, which is quite interesting. Where is the female pronucleus?

S. Fisher   Are any of the genes in this deleted area involved in the formation of the centrosome, where you could imagine that there is unequal partitioning of the chromosomes?

R. Fisher   We don't see unequal partitioning of the chromosomes.

S. Fisher   If you have divisions with failure of the centrosome, you will end up with unequal partitioning. We are talking about how you might get an empty egg. In *Drosophila*, with some of the centrosome defects you do end up with cells that have almost no chromosomes or cells that have very few.

Sharkey   This has all been worked out in yeast. Everyone has worked out all the things that during meiosis cause spindle defects.

S. Fisher   That would get you to the point where there are very few or non-functional chromosomes in the egg.

Reik   This can't be related to Rosemary's genetic locus because they are biparental.

R. Fisher   The androgenetic moles involve the empty egg but the biparental ones don't.

Braude   It is presumed that all diandric eggs – the ones that are going to make moles – contain one sperm that has duplicated. Is that correct?

R. Fisher   About 25% of them involve two sperm.

Braude   Why couldn't it be two sperm that have entered the egg?

Jacobs   Because of the genetics. The highest proportion are completely homozygous. It is one sperm that has gone in to the 'empty egg' and has duplicated.

Braude   It could be a 46,XX sperm.

Jacobs   No, because then it would be entirely paternal but it would be heterozygous.

Loke   What happens if there is reduplication of a YY sperm?

Jacobs   It is lethal.

Surani   What proportion are XY?

R. Fisher   Probably about 10%. About 75% are homozygous for XX. The remaining 25% are heterozygous, but these could be XX or XY.

Ferguson-Smith   Presumably the identification and recognition of the phenomenon of a biparental complete mole is a relatively recent one.

Jacobs   They have been in the literature for a long time. There are extraordinary families who have nine consecutive moles, which is unusual even in a population where moles are relatively common. The elucidation of this condition is very recent, though.

Ferguson-Smith   It may be that they have been reduced in frequency because of reduced incidence of cosanguinity.

Jacobs   The ones that are reduced in frequency are the ordinary moles, not these rare biparental moles.

Loke   What about teratomas: are they all XX?

R. Fisher   Teratomas are all XX.

Cross   Are teratomas that occur in the testis XX?

R. Fisher   They are quite different to ovarian teratomas.

Braude   If they are parthenotes, they would have to be haploid or reduplicated diploids. Is that correct? If they are in the female they will be 23,X or 46,XX. In the male they would be 23,X or 23,Y if they were haploid, 46,XX or 46,YY if they were diploid.

McLaren   Are you talking about testicular teratomas? They could never be parthenotes. One thing mentioned earlier intrigued me. This goes back to the question of trophoblast invasion and its aggressiveness. Someone mentioned that Anne Croy has natural killer (NK)-deficient mice with giant trophoblast cells that invaded further. We know it is the decidual response in the mouse that prevents invasion, but is this also the case in humans?

S. Fisher   One of the things we see with trophoblast invasion is that it is timed. At any time we take cytotrophoblasts out of the human placenta, they are always declining in the ability to invade. The earliest we can isolate them is 5–6 weeks. They are dramatically less invasive at 6 weeks than 5. There is some sort of temporal programme that they carry in their heads, so to speak. We have looked at several ectopic sites. In the ectopic pregnancy it is obviously very ragged, so I think the uterus does play a big role in organising invasion.

McLaren   Humans do have a decidual response. It is just not induced by the embryo.

Pijnenborg   We could also refer to those rare cases of placenta accreta, where there is no decidua at all. In this case we have a deeper invasion than normal. Normally trophoblast invasion takes place over the whole length of the spiral arteries up to the point where they are sprouting from the radial arteries. In cases of placenta accreta, trophoblast goes deeper and invades the radial arteries as well. This supports the idea that decidual tissue may act as a brake to trophoblast invasion.

Moffett   If we look at human ectopic pregnancies and intrauterine pregnancies that have implanted where there is no decidua, the difference is very noticeable. It is remarkable that when the trophoblast invades there is no destruction. There is no necrosis like that found with tumour invasion, apart from the necrosis of the arterial media (the middle layer of the arterial wall). If trophoblast invades without going through decidua, then there is destruction of smooth muscle. In the wall of the uterus, fibrinoid change in the myometrium occurs. This indicates that trophoblast may be making something that is specifically damaging to smooth muscle. It needs to go through the decidua to be modified.

McLaren   Does it seem like a signalling molecule?

Moffett   This is based on histology, which doesn't tell us what the mechanism is. The arterial media is entirely destroyed and replaced by fibrinoid accretions. The rest of the decidua is fine.

REFERENCES

Montgomery, G. W., Galloway, S. M., Davis, G. H. & McNatty, K. (2001). Genes controlling ovulation rate in sheep. *Reproduction*, **121**, 843–52.

Tong, S., Caddy, D. & Short, R. V. (1997). Use of dizygotic to monozygotic twinning ratio as a measure of fertility. *Lancet*, **349**, 843–5.

9

Molecular signalling in embryo–uterine interactions during implantation

S. K. Dey and Susanne Tranguch

Vanderbilt University Medical Center, USA

The process of implantation involves complex interactions between embryonic and uterine cells. The major events of this process include synchronised development of the preimplantation embryo into an implantation-competent blastocyst and establishment of the uterus to the receptive state (Psychoyos 1973a), escape of the semiallogenic embryo from the maternal immunological response (Beer & Billingham 1978), increased capillary permeability and blood flow at the site of blastocyst apposition (Psychoyos 1973a), post-attachment localised stromal decidualisation (De Feo 1967, Psychoyos 1973a) and controlled uterine invasion by embryonic trophoblasts (Kirby & Cowell 1968). Uterine receptivity is defined as a restricted period when the uterus supports blastocyst attachment (Psychoyos 1973b). Therefore, successful implantation of an embryo is contingent upon the initiation of these critical events during this 'window' of receptivity, and failure to initiate these events results in early pregnancy failure.

Preimplantation embryo development, which culminates in the formation of a blastocyst, requires the activation of the embryonic genome. Upon activation of the embryonic genome, the embryo grows rapidly to form a blastocyst. At the blastocyst stage, embryos mature and escape from their zona pellucidae to gain implantation competency. The differentiated and expanded blastocyst is composed of three cell types: the outer polarised epithelial trophectoderm, the primitive endoderm and the pluripotent inner cell mass (ICM). The ICM provides the future cell lineages for the embryo proper (McLaren 1990, Hogan *et al.* 1994), while the trophectoderm, the very first epithelial cell type in the developmental process, makes the initial physical and physiological connection with the uterine luminal epithelium. The formation of the trophectoderm and its subsequent development into trophoblast tissue are crucial steps for the initiation of implantation and establishment of pregnancy. Trophoblast cells produce a variety of growth factors, cytokines and hormones that

Biology and Pathology of Trophoblast, eds. Ashley Moffett, Charlie Loke and Anne McLaren.
Published by Cambridge University Press © Cambridge University Press 2005.

influence the conceptus and maternal physiology in an autocrine, paracrine and/or juxtacrine manner (Petraglia *et al.* 1998, Roberts *et al.* 1999).

The ability of blastocysts to remain dormant for a prolonged period of time creates a unique physiological condition of delayed implantation (Mead 1993). While the blastocysts become dormant, the uterus remains in a quiescent state. Ovariectomy prior to the oestrogen secretion on the morning of day 4 of pregnancy results in the failure of implantation and initiates blastocyst dormancy in mice and rats (Yoshinaga & Adams 1966, Psychoyos 1973a). This delayed implantation can be maintained for many days by continuous treatment with progesterone. Implantation can be initiated by a single injection of oestrogen in the progesterone-primed uterus (Yoshinaga & Adams 1966, Psychoyos 1973a). Because coordinated interactions of progesterone and oestrogen make the uterus receptive and the blastocyst activated, the delayed implantation model can be exploited to understand better the molecular signalling that occurs during the embryo–uterine dialogue.

On the first day of pregnancy (vaginal plug) in mice, uterine epithelial cells undergo proliferation under the influence of preovulatory oestrogen secretion. Rising levels of progesterone secreted from freshly formed corpora lutea initiate stromal proliferation from day 3 onward. This stromal cell proliferation is further stimulated by a small amount of ovarian oestrogen secreted on the morning of day 4. These coordinated effects of progesterone and oestrogen result in uterine epithelial cell differentiation (Huet *et al.* 1989). During normal pregnancy, the presence of an implantation-competent blastocyst in the uterus is the stimulus for the implantation reaction. After the attachment reaction is initiated around midnight on day 4, stromal cells surrounding the implanting blastocyst begin to proliferate extensively and differentiate into decidual cells, forming an area called the primary decidual zone (PDZ) (Dey 1996). The cells within the PDZ subsequently apoptose; however, cells adjacent to the PDZ continue to proliferate and differentiate, forming the secondary decidual zone (SDZ) (Tan *et al.* 2002). Eventually the SDZ also undergoes apoptosis, enlarging the implantation chamber to accommodate the growing embryo. A defect in any of these events affects pregnancy outcome; therefore, close examination of the signalling pathways involved in the embryo–uterine dialogue is essential for the development of strategies to correct implantation failures and pregnancy losses.

In the mouse, while the uterus is fully receptive on day 4, it is considered pre-receptive on days 1–3 of pregnancy or pseudopregnancy. Evidence suggests that the uterus is most receptive to implantation on day 4 (Paria *et al.* 1993) and the efficiency of implantation then decreases with time (Song *et al.* 2002). By day 6, the uterus becomes completely refractory to blastocyst implantation. Recent evidence suggests that the concentration of oestrogen within a very narrow range determines the duration of this 'window' of receptivity; uterine receptivity remains open for an extended period at lower oestrogen levels, but rapidly closes at higher levels. Uterine non-receptivity induced at higher oestrogen levels is accompanied by aberrant uterine expression of implantation-related genes (Ma *et al.* 2003).

Recent evidence also suggests that even a short delay in the attachment reaction can produce an adverse ripple effect throughout pregnancy, causing defective development of the feto–placental unit (Song *et al.* 2002). This concept of timing being such a crucial component of normal feto–placental development and determinant of pregnancy outcome comprises a novel theme whereby early embryo–uterine interaction directs the developmental programming for the remainder of gestation.

Numerous cytokines, growth factors, vasoactive factors and other signalling proteins are implicated in implantation (Salamonsen *et al.* 1986, Lim *et al.* 2002, Paria *et al.* 2002). This review focuses on the genetically altered mouse models and gene expression studies on the following compounds: heparin-binding epidermal growth factor (EGF)-like growth factor (HB-EGF), leukaemia inhibitory factor (LIF), cyclooxygenase (COX)-2 derived prostaglandins, bone morphogenetic proteins (BMPs), Wnt signalling and Hoxa-10/Hoxa-11. Because each of these signalling pathways plays a critical role in the embryo–uterine cross-talk during implantation, any alteration of these signalling pathways can dramatically alter the implantation process and, therefore, decrease the probability of a successful pregnancy. While this review consists of data generated primarily from mouse models, it is with the assumption that many of the findings will be relevant to the process in humans.

Heparin-binding EGF-like growth factor is the earliest known marker of implantation in mice that is expressed in the uterine luminal epithelium surrounding the blastocyst 6–7 hours before the initial attachment of the blastocyst to the uterus (Lim *et al.* 2002). It is not induced at the site of the blastocyst during delayed implantation, but is rapidly induced by the termination of delay by oestrogen. This induction is followed by the expression of betacellulin, epiregulin, neuregulin-1 and COX-2 around the time of the attachment reaction (Chakraborty *et al.* 1996, Das *et al.* 1997, Lim *et al.* 1998). In contrast, amphiregulin is expressed throughout the uterine epithelium on the morning of day 4 of pregnancy and is a progesterone-responsive gene in the uterus (Das *et al.* 1995). While these results suggest that amphiregulin has a role in implantation, amphiregulin-deficient mice or compound knockout mice for *EGF/transforming growth factor (TGF)α/amphiregulin* do not exhibit implantation defects (Luetteke *et al.* 1993, 1999). Since HB-EGF, betacellulin, epiregulin, neuregulin and amphiregulin all show overlapping uterine expression patterns around the implanting blastocyst at the time of attachment (Das *et al.* 1997, Carson *et al.* 2000), it is assumed that a compensatory mechanism rescues implantation in the absence of one or more members of the EGF family.

Uterine HB-EGF has been shown to interact with ErbBs expressed on the blastocyst cell surface in a paracrine and/or juxtacrine manner during implantation (Das *et al.* 1994a, b, Lim *et al.* 1998). However, the evidence for absolute necessity of HB-EGF in implantation requires genetic evidence. A recent report shows that most HB-EGF mutant mice die early in postnatal life due to cardiac defects, precluding critical examination of the implantation phenotype (Iwamoto *et al.* 2003). Heparin-binding EGF-like growth factor also appears to play a role in implantation and embryonic development in humans. Its expression is maximal during the late secretory phase (cycle days 20–24) when the endometrium is receptive for implantation (Yoo *et al.* 1997, Leach *et al.* 1999), and cells expressing the transmembrane form of HB-EGF adhere to human blastocysts displaying cell surface ErbB4 (Chobotova *et al.* 2002). Furthermore, HB-EGF was shown to be one of the most potent growth factors for enhancing the development of human IVF-derived embryos to blastocysts and subsequent zona-hatching (Martin *et al.* 1998). The importance of the EGF family is emphasised by the expression of multiple ligands and multiple receptors during implantation, perhaps ensuring the efficacy and success of embryo development and implantation. Collectively, these studies suggest that HB-EGF plays a significant role in preimplantation embryo development and implantation.

Spatial and transient expression of cytokines and their receptors in the uterus and embryo during early pregnancy suggests their roles in various aspects of implantation (Chard 1995, Stewart & Cullinan 1997, Sharkey 1998, Carson *et al.* 2000). However, gene-targeting studies show that mice lacking tumour necrosis factor (TNF)α, interleukin 1β (IL1β), IL1 receptor antagonist (IL1ra), IL1 receptor type 1, IL6 or granulocyte/macrophage-colony stimulating factor (GM-CSF) apparently do not manifest overt reproductive defects (Stewart & Cullinan 1997). These observations suggest that either these molecules have only minor roles in implantation, or the loss of one cytokine is compensated by other cytokines with overlapping functions. In contrast, some cytokines are crucial to implantation (Pollard *et al.* 1991, Stewart *et al.* 1992, Robb *et al.* 1998). For example, mice with a null mutation of the *Lif* gene show complete failure of implantation, and blastocysts in these mutant mice undergo dormancy (Stewart *et al.* 1992, Escary *et al.* 1993). Studies using *Il11rα* mutant mice have shown that IL11 is crucial to decidualisation, but not for the attachment reaction (Robb *et al.* 1998). Both LIF and IL11 are members of the IL6 family, which includes IL6 itself, oncostatin M, ciliary neurotrophic factor and cardiotrophin (Kishimoto *et al.* 1994). Leukaemia inhibitory factor and IL11 bind to ligand-specific receptors, LIFR and IL11R, respectively, and share gp130 as a signal transduction partner (Kishimoto *et al.* 1994), suggesting that gp130 signalling is critically involved in implantation. Leukaemia inhibitory factor is transiently expressed in uterine glands on day 4 of pregnancy in mice, suggesting its role in uterine preparation for implantation (Bhatt *et al.* 1991). However, our recent studies show that uterine LIF expression is biphasic on day 4. Not only is LIF expressed in the glands on day 4 morning, it is also expressed in stromal cells surrounding the blastocyst at the time of attachment (Song *et al.* 2000). This suggests that LIF has dual roles: first in preparation of the uterus and later in the attachment reaction. However, the molecular mechanism by which LIF executes its effects on implantation is not yet known. A recent report, however, does show that inactivation of gp130 by deletion of all signal transducer and activator of transcription (STAT) binding sites results in implantation failure (Ernst *et al.* 2001), reinforcing the importance of LIF signalling in implantation. The uterine environment in *Lif* mutant mice fails to support implantation irrespective of the blastocyst genotype, suggesting that maternal LIF is crucial to implantation (Stewart *et al.* 1992, Escary *et al.* 1993). Expression of LIF in the uterus is maximal around the time of implantation in most species examined, although the steroid hormonal requirements for the preparation for uterine receptivity and implantation differ according to species. In humans, LIF is expressed at higher levels in the glandular epithelium of the secretory endometrium. Furthermore, LIF deficiency has been associated with unexplained recurrent abortions and infertility in women (Hambartsoumian 1998).

One hallmark of implantation is increased vascular permeability and angiogenesis at the site of the blastocyst. Because of their roles in angiogenesis, cell proliferation and differentiation in various systems, prostaglandins (PGs) are likely to participate in uterine vascular permeability and angiogenesis during implantation and decidualisation. Prostaglandins are synthesised by the liberation of arachidonic acid by phospholipase A_2 (PLA_2) followed by participation of cyclooxygenases. The mammalian PLA_2 superfamily consists of four major subfamilies that include cytosolic ($cPLA_2$), secretory ($sPLA_2$), Ca^{2+}-independent ($iPLA_2$), and platelet-activating factor (PAF) acetylhydrolase. Cyclooxygenase is the rate-limiting enzyme in PG synthesis and exists in two isoforms, COX-1 and COX-2 (Lim *et al.* 1997). Whereas the expression of COX-1 is considered constitutive, that of COX-2 is inducible (Smith *et al.* 1996). Cytosolic $PLA_2\alpha$ is known to couple functionally to COX-2 in specific cell types (Reddy & Herschman 1997, Takano *et al.* 2000).

Cyclooxygenase genes exhibit spatiotemporal expression patterns in the uterus during the peri-implantation period. Cyclooxygenase-1 is expressed in the epithelium throughout the uterus on day 4 of pregnancy prior to the time of implantation, while COX-2 is expressed in the luminal epithelium and stroma surrounding the blastocyst at the time of attachment. This restriction of COX-2 expression to the implantation site occurs in most species studied, including primates (Lim *et al.* 1997, 2002). While mice deficient in *Cox-1* are fertile with limited parturition defects, *Cox-2$^{-/-}$* mice have defective implantation and decidualisation, independent of faulty ovulation and fertilisation (Dinchuk *et al.* 1995, Langenbach *et al.*

1995, Lim *et al.* 1997), proving that COX-2-derived PGs are essential for successful implantation and decidualisation.

Cytosolic Pla$_2\alpha^{-/-}$ mice have small litters with presumed parturition defects and often show pregnancy failures (Bonventre *et al.* 1997, Uozumi *et al.* 1997). Recent evidence shows that in *cPla$_2\alpha^{-/-}$* females, a significant number of blastocysts implant beyond the normal 'window' of implantation when the uterus can no longer optimally support a normal pregnancy. Interestingly, the decidualisation process still occurs, raising the idea that the on-time initial attachment reaction governs the subsequent embryonic developmental processes (Song *et al.* 2002). Mice lacking *cPla$_2\alpha$*, along with showing a delay in the attachment of the blastocyst to the uterus, show aberrant expression of genes encoding HB-EGF and LIF at the site of blastocysts. This suggests that *cPla$_2\alpha^{-/-}$*-derived arachidonic acids and/or eicosanoids coordinate these signalling pathways for implantation. There is also overlap between the *cPLA$_2\alpha$* and COX pathways. The ability of cPLA$_2\alpha$ to couple functionally with COX-2, and the obvious defects in both *Cox-2$^{-/-}$* and *cPla$_2\alpha^{-/-}$* mice contribute to the idea that the initiation of implantation and subsequent progression of pregnancy are the result of the integration of various signals between the embryo and uterus.

Cyclooxygenase is present in both the endoplasmic reticulum membrane and the nuclear envelope (Spencer *et al.* 1998), suggesting that PGs can exert their effects via different classes of receptors. Prostaglandins synthesised in the endoplasmic reticulum can exit cells and function via G-protein-coupled surface receptors. In the mouse, cell surface receptors for PGE$_2$, PGF$_{2\alpha}$, PGD$_2$ and prostacyclin (PGI$_2$) are EP$_1$–EP$_4$, FP, DP and IP, respectively (Negishi *et al.* 1995). Although PGE synthase is expressed at the implantation sites with the presence of PGE$_2$ and EP receptors (Yang *et al.* 1997, Ni *et al.* 2002, 2003), and although PGE$_2$ has been shown to be associated with implantation and decidualisation (Kennedy 1985), gene-targeting experiments show that three of the four EP receptor subtypes (EP$_1$–EP$_3$) are not critical for implantation. Deficiency in EP$_4$ mostly results in perinatal lethality and thus its role in implantation has yet to be determined (Lim & Dey 2000). Mice deficient in FP or IP show normal implantation.

Prostaglandins produced via nuclear COX can also exert their effects directly on the nucleus by activating peroxisome proliferator-activated receptors (PPARs), members of the nuclear hormone receptor superfamily (Mangelsdorf & Evans 1995). The PPAR family members include PPARα, PPARγ and PPARδ(β) (Kliewer *et al.* 1994). Peroxisome proliferator-activated receptor must form heterodimers with a member of the retinoid X receptor (RXR) subfamily (Kliewer *et al.* 1992, Lim *et al.* 1999a) to be functional.

Among various PGs, the levels of PGI$_2$ are highest at implantation sites of wild-type mice, and implantation defects are partially restored in *Cox-2$^{-/-}$* mice by administration of a more stable PGI_2 agonist, carbaprostacyclin (Lim *et al.* 1999a). Consistent with the finding that COX-2-driven uterine PG production is crucial to implantation, *Cox-2* and *prostacyclin synthase* (*Pgis*) are co-expressed at the implantation site, suggesting the availability of PGI_2 directly to uterine cells. In searching for a receptor for PGI_2 in the uterus, *PPARδ* was co-localised at similar regions of the implantation sites with *Cox-2* and *Pgis*. In contrast, the expression of *IP*, *PPARα* and *PPARγ* was low to undetectable. Three independent groups have reported diverse phenotypes of *PPARδ* knockout mice (Peters *et al.* 2000, Michalik *et al.* 2001, Barak *et al.* 2002). However, because of severe early developmental defects of *PPARδ* mutant embryos, it is difficult to utilise this model to address whether the absence of maternal PPARδ affects implantation as in *Cox-2*-deficient mice. Therefore, the conditional knockout mouse model with uterine-specific deletion of *PPARδ* is necessary to address this issue. Nonetheless, it is apparent that COX-2–PGI_2–PPARδ signalling is important for successful implantation.

Genetic mutation of various components of the PG synthetic and signalling pathways in mice has provided important information on distinct and overlapping functions of various PGs in female reproduction, providing the consensus that lipid mediators are essential for successful pregnancy (Langenbach *et al.* 1995, Lim *et al.* 1997, 1999a). Recently, it has been shown that, depending on the genetic background, there is also a shift in the normal 'window' of implantation in *Cox-2*-deficient females, leading to developmental anomalies and small litter sizes (Wang *et al.* 2003). This similarity between $cPla_2\alpha^{-/-}$ and $Cox-2^{-/-}$ mice demonstrates the significance of the concept that a short delay in the initial attachment reaction can propagate detrimental effects throughout the remaining pregnancy, and also provides evidence for a $cPLA_2\alpha$–COX-2 axis as an essential determinant for on-time implantation. This is of clinical relevance since it has been shown in humans that implantation beyond the normal 'window' of receptivity leads to an increase in pregnancy loss (Wilcox *et al.* 1999).

The intricate dialogue between the blastocyst and the uterus required for successful implantation has several features of the reciprocal epithelial–mesenchymal interactions during embryogenesis that involve evolutionary conserved pathways. Of central importance are the hedgehog (HH), fibroblast growth factor (FGF), BMP, and the Wnt family of proteins, as well as their agonists, receptors and components of intracellular signalling pathways (Hogan 1996, Ingham 1998, Massague & Chen 2000). The uterine expression of many members of these important gene families is just now being investigated during early implantation.

The BMPs are a group of growth and differentiating factors that belong to the TGFβ family (Kingsley 1994). To date, at least 15 members of the group have been identified, termed BMP-2 through BMP-15 (Onagbesan *et al.* 2003). Bone morphogenetic proteins are disulphide-linked dimeric proteins, with each monomer normally containing seven cysteine residues. Heterodimers can form between BMP-2 or BMP-4 and BMP-7, and these heterodimers are much more potent in their activation than their corresponding homodimers (Aono *et al.* 1995, Israel *et al.* 1996). The BMPs bind to serine/threonine kinase type I and II receptors, designated BMPR-IA, BMPR-IB and BMPR-II (Kawabata *et al.* 1998). Bone morphogenetic proteins, specifically BMP-2 and BMP-4, have important roles in early development. Null mutation of the *Bmp-4* gene results in defects in extraembryonic and posterior/ventral formation with embryonic death occurring between day 6.5 and 9.5 (Winnier *et al.* 1995), while BMP-2-deficient mice die between embryonic day 7.5 and 9.0 (Zhang & Bradley 1996). Whether BMPs are crucial to implantation is not known. Recently, it has been shown that the uterus expresses BMP-2 in the stroma around the site of the implanting blastocyst. After implantation, BMP-2 transcripts were also detected in the decidua but by day 7, BMP-2 expression was absent in cells of the PDZ but present in the SDZ (Paria *et al.* 2001). Bone morphogenetic protein-4 transcripts, however, are detected in the luminal epithelium on day 1 of pregnancy, while on day 4, expression shifts to the stroma. Neither BMP-4, -5, -6 or -7 shows the same highly localised expression as BMP-2, indicating a perhaps unique role for BMP-2 in embryo implantation.

In many developing systems, antagonists of growth factors, including those of BMPs and Wnts, are key components of intercellular signalling networks, binding to their ligands and regulating their ability to interact productively with their receptors. Noggin acts as a potent antagonist to BMP-2 and BMP-4, binding both with high affinity, thereby preventing each ligand from binding to its receptor (Zimmerman *et al.* 1996). Noggin mutant embryos begin to show defects at embryonic day 8.5 and are characterised by a shortened body axis, loss of caudal vertebrae and malformed limbs (Smith 1999). Using a mouse model where the Noggin gene (*Nog*) has been replaced by a *β-galactosidase* gene (Zimmerman *et al.* 1996, Brunet *et al.* 1998), it has been shown that prior to implantation, Nog^{lacZ} is expressed in the stromal layer underlying the luminal epithelium, but its expression decreases with the initiation of implantation and BMP-2 expression (Paria *et al.* 2001). Further studies using such antagonists and mouse models need to be done to reveal the roles of BMPs in implantation.

The Wnt signalling pathway is another evolutionarily conserved signalling pathway recently examined in regard to implantation. The Wnt proteins have been recognised as one of the major families involved in embryonic induction, cell polarity generation and cell fate specification (Cadigan & Nusse 1997, Giles *et al.* 2003, Lloyd *et al.* 2003, Nusse 2003). These proteins comprise a family of secreted glycoproteins and to date, at least 19 *Wnt* genes have been discovered in mouse and vertebrates, with 7 in invertebrates (Gavin *et al.* 1990, Bergstein *et al.* 1997). Wnt proteins bind and act through cell surface receptors, Frizzled (Fzd), a large family of seven membrane-spanning domain receptors with a long N-terminal cysteine-rich domain (CRD), also known as Frizzled domain (Nusse 2003). Targeted deletion of several *Wnt* and *Fzd* genes in mice leads to specific developmental defects (Wodarz & Nusse 1998, Nusse 2003).

The canonical Wnt signalling pathway, highly conserved between *Drosophila* and vertebrates, involves the following sequence of events. In the mouse, after Wnt binds to the CRD of the Frizzled receptor (Fzd), associated with its co-receptors low-density lipoprotein receptor-related protein-5 (LRP-5) or LRP-6 (Nusse 2003), the cytoplasmic protein Disheveled (Dvl) is recruited to the cell membrane. Through an unknown mechanism, Dvl binds to axin, thereby inhibiting the constitutively expressed axin/β-catenin complex. The free, unphosphorylated β-catenin protein binds to Armadillo, translocates to the nucleus and acts as a cofactor for transcription factors of the T-cell factor/lymphoid enhancing factor (TCF/LEF) family to coactivate Wnt target genes. In the absence of Wnt, TCF-targeted gene transcription is actively repressed by negative regulators. Some of these negative regulators include corepressors of the Groucho (Grg) family and histone acetyltransferase CREB binding protein (CBP)/p300 (Bienz & Clevers 2000). Signalling through the canonical Wnt signalling pathway is present during embryogenesis, where it regulates many developmental patterning effects. Wnt proteins can also signal through non-canonical pathways including Wnt/Ca^{2+} and Wnt/Jun N-terminal kinase (JNK) pathways (Wodarz & Nusse 1998).

Secreted frizzled-related proteins (sFRPs) have strong homology with the CRD of Fzd proteins, but lack the transmembrane domain. Evidence suggests that sFRPs inhibit Wnt signalling directly by competing with Fzds for Wnt ligands or in a dominant-negative fashion by forming a non-signalling complex with Fzds (Fujita *et al.* 2002). Five sFRPS (sFRPs 1–5) have been identified in the mouse. Recently it has been shown that Wnt4 and sFRP4 show unique expression patterns in the uterus during the peri-implantation period. Low levels of Wnt4 were expressed in the luminal epithelium on day 1, while the expression was undetectable in any major uterine cell types on day 4 of pregnancy (Daikokua *et al.* 2004). On day 5, Wnt4 is expressed in stromal cells surrounding the implanting blastocyst, followed by expression in the deciduum (Paria *et al.* 2001). Expression of Wnt4 increased through day 8, expanding into the SDZ. In contrast, sFRP4 expression was limited to the connective tissue in the myometrial bed on day 1; on day 4, the expression was localised to a select population of stromal cells, and following implantation on day 5 and thereafter, sFRP4 expression became more intense but was restricted to the undifferentiated stromal cells forming a dividing zone between the circular muscle layer and the deciduum (Daikokua *et al.* 2004).

In mice, Wnt7a signalling is crucial for the female reproductive tract development along the anteroposterior axis during postnatal development. Targeted deletion of the *Wnt7a* gene has shown that cellular characteristics of the oviduct, uterus, cervix and vagina become aberrant along the anteroposterior axis resulting in global posterior shifting of the reproductive tract. This implies a role for Wnt signalling in the maintenance of molecular and morphological boundaries of specific cell populations along the anteroposterior and radial axes of the female reproductive tract (Cadigan & Nusse 1997). A recent report describes that Wnt signalling becomes aberrant in *Lif* mutant or *Hoxa10* mutant mice that exhibit implantation defects, again suggesting the importance of this signalling pathway in implantation (Daikokua *et al.* 2004).

Other developmental genes influential in implantation include the homeobox-containing transcription factors, the *Hox* genes. The *Hox* genes are developmentally regulated and share a common highly conserved sequence element, termed homeobox, that encodes a 61-amino acid helix-turn-helix DNA-binding domain (Krumlauf 1994). The *Hox* genes are organised in four clusters (A, B, C and D) on four different chromosomes in mice and humans, and follow a stringent pattern of spatial and temporal colinearity during embryogenesis (Krumlauf 1994). Several *Hox* genes at the 5'-end of each cluster are classified as *AbdB-like Hox* genes, because of their homology with the *Drosophila AbdB* gene. In vertebrates, *AbdB-like Hox* genes are expressed in developing genitourinary systems (Benson *et al.* 1996). For example, *Hoxa10* and *Hoxa11* are highly expressed in developing genitourinary tracts and adult female reproductive tract, suggesting their roles in reproductive events (Hsieh-Li *et al.* 1995, Benson *et al.* 1996, Gendron *et al.* 1997). *Hoxa10* mutant mice exhibit oviductal transformation of the proximal third of the uterus. Furthermore, adult female mice deficient in *Hoxa10* show failures in blastocyst implantation and decidualisation unrelated to the oviductal transformation (Benson *et al.* 1996). Subsequent studies revealed that uterine stromal cells in these mice show reduced proliferation in response to progesterone, leading to decidualisation defects (Lim *et al.* 1999b). Since several progesterone-responsive genes are dysregulated in the uterine stroma of $Hoxa10^{-/-}$ mice (Lim *et al.* 1999b), Hoxa10 may convey progesterone-responsiveness in the uterus by regulating gene expression as a transcription factor. A similar but more severe phenotype was also noted in *Hoxa11*-deficient female mice (Gendron *et al.* 1997). Defective proliferation of stromal cells in $Hoxa10^{-/-}$ female mice suggests that Hoxa-10 is involved in the local events of cellular proliferation by regulating cell cycle molecules. Indeed cyclin D3 is aberrantly expressed in *Hoxa10* mutant uteri in response to a decidualising stimulus (Das *et al.* 1999). Also among the genes that were up-regulated in *Hoxa10*-deficient uteri, two cell-cycle molecules, *p15* and *p57*, were notable. These two genes are both cyclin-dependent kinase inhibitors (CKIs), suggesting that the observed defect in stromal cell proliferation in *Hoxa10* mutant mice could be associated with the up-regulation of CKIs (Yao *et al.* 2003). In humans, both *HOXA10* and *HOXA11* genes are markedly up-regulated in the uterus during the mid-secretory phase in steroid hormone-dependent manner (Taylor *et al.* 1998), suggesting their roles in implantation.

Gene targeting experiments in mice have already identified a large number of genes that are important for female fertility; yet our understanding of the implantation process is still far from complete. Many of the genes that are expressed in an implantation-specific manner and appear to be important for implantation cannot be studied in depth, because deletion of these genes results in embryonic lethality. Uterine- or embryo-specific conditional knockout models for genes of interest are urgently needed to better understand the definitive roles of these genes in uterine biology and implantation. Although the mechanics and cellular architecture of implantation proves to vary among species, certain similarities do exist. For example, implantation occurs at the blastocyst stage, there is a defined 'window' of uterine receptivity for implantation, a reciprocal interaction between the blastocyst and the uterus is essential for implantation, and a localised increase in uterine vascular permeability occurs at the site of the blastocyst during the attachment reaction. It has become even more apparent from recent genetic studies that any deviation from this defined 'window' of receptivity for implantation not only affects the implantation process itself, but also can lead to subsequent developmental anomalies and loss of pregnancy. Therefore, the early embryo–uterine dialogue during implantation can determine the subsequent developmental programming. Recognition and characterisation of the signalling pathways in this cross-talk can give rise to a unifying scheme relevant to understanding the mechanism of human implantation and can therefore lead to strategies for correcting implantation and pregnancy losses.

ACKNOWLEDGEMENTS

Work embodied in this review was supported by NIH grants (HD12304, HD33994).

REFERENCES

Aono, A. M., Hazama, K., Notoya, S. *et al.* (1995). Potent ectopic bone-inducing activity of bone morphogenetic protein-4/7 heterodimer. *Biochem. Biophys. Res. Commun.*, **210**, 670–7.

Barak, Y., Liao, D., He, W. *et al.* (2002). Effects of peroxisome proliferator-activated receptor delta on placentation, adiposity, and colorectal cancer. *Proc. Natl. Acad. Sci. U.S.A.*, **99**, 303–8.

Beer, A. E., & Billingham, R. E. (1978). Immunoregulatory aspects of pregnancy. *Fed. Proc.*, **37**, 2374–8.

Benson, G. V., Lim, H., Paria, B. C. et al. (1996). Mechanisms of reduced fertility in Hoxa-10 mutant mice: uterine homeosis and loss of maternal Hoxa-10 expression. *Development*, 122, 2687–96.

Bergstein, I., Eisenberg, L. M., Bhalerao, L. et al. (1997). Isolation of two novel WNT genes, WNT14 and WNT15, one of which (WNT15) is closely linked to WNT3 on human chromosome 17q21. *Genomics*, 46, 450–8.

Bhatt, H., Brunet, L. J. & Stewart, C. L. (1991). Uterine expression of leukemia inhibitory factor coincides with the onset of blastocyst implantation. *Proc. Natl. Acad. Sci. U.S.A.*, 88, 11408–12.

Bienz, M. & Clevers, H. (2000). Linking colorectal cancer to Wnt signaling. *Cell*, 103, 311–20.

Bonventre, J. V., Huang, Z., Taheri, M. R. et al. (1997). Reduced fertility and postischaemic brain injury in mice deficient in cytosolic phospholipase A2. *Nature*, 390, 622–5.

Brunet, L. J., McMahon, J. A., McMahon, A. P. & Harland, R. M. (1998). Noggin, cartilage morphogenesis, and joint formation in the mammalian skeleton. *Science*, 280, 1455–7.

Cadigan, K. M. & Nusse, R. (1997). Wnt signaling: a common theme in animal development. *Genes Dev.*, 11, 3286–3305.

Carson, D. D., Bagchi, I., Dey, S. K. et al. (2000). Embryo implantation. *Dev. Biol.*, 223, 217–37.

Chakraborty, I., Das, S. K., Wang, J. & Dey, S. K. (1996). Developmental expression of the cyclo-oxygenase-1 and cyclo-oxygenase-2 genes in the periimplantation mouse uterus and their differential regulation by the blastocyst and ovarian steroids. *J. Mol. Endocrinol.*, 16, 107–22.

Chard, T. (1995). Cytokines in implantation. *Hum. Reprod. Update*, 1, 385–96.

Chobotova, K., Spyropoulou, I., Carver, J. et al. (2002). Heparin-binding epidermal growth factor and its receptor ErbB4 mediate implantation of the human blastocyst. *Mech. Dev.*, 119, 137–44.

Daikokua, T., Guo, Y., Rieseqijk, A. et al. (2004). Uterine Msx-1 and Wnt signaling becomes aberrant in mice with the loss of leukemia inhibitory factor or Hoxa-10: Evidence for a novel cytokine-homeobox-Wnt signaling in implantation. *Mol. Endocrinol.*, 18, 1238–50.

Das, S. K., Tsukamura, H., Paria, B. C., Andrews, G. K. & Dey, S. K. (1994a). Differential expression of epidermal growth factor receptor (EGF-R) gene and regulation of EGF-R bioactivity by progesterone and estrogen in the adult mouse uterus. *Endocrinology*, 134, 971–81.

Das, S. K., Wang, X. N., Paria, B. C. et al. (1994b). Heparin-binding EGF-like growth factor gene is induced in the mouse uterus temporally by the blastocyst solely at the site of its apposition: a possible ligand for interaction with blastocyst EGF-receptor in implantation. *Development*, 120, 1071–83.

Das, S. K., Chakraborty, I., Paria, B. C. et al. (1995). Amphiregulin is an implantation-specific and progesterone-regulated gene in the mouse uterus. *Mol. Endocrinol.*, 9, 691–705.

Das, S. K., Das, N., Wang, J. et al. (1997). Expression of betacellulin and epiregulin genes in the mouse uterus temporally by the blastocyst solely at the site of its apposition is coincident with the 'window' of implantation. *Dev. Biol.*, 190, 178–90.

Das, S. K., Lim, H., Paria, B. C. & Dey, S. K. (1999). Cyclin D3 in the mouse uterus is associated with the decidualization process during early pregnancy. *J. Mol. Endocrinol.*, 22, 91–101.

De Feo, V. (1967). Decidualization. In R. M. Wynn, ed., *Cellular Biology of the Uterus*. Amsterdam: North-Holland, pp. 191–290.

Dey, S. K. (1996). Implantation. In R. J. Adashi & E. Y. Rosenwaks, eds., *Reproductive Endocrinology, Surgery and Technology*. New York: Lippincott-Raven, pp. 421–34.

Dinchuk, J. E., Car, B. D., Focht, R. J. *et al.* (1995). Renal abnormalities and an altered inflammatory response in mice lacking cyclooxygenase II. *Nature*, **378**, 406–9.

Ernst, M., Inglese, M., Waring, P. *et al.* (2001). Defective gp130-mediated signal transducer and activator of transcription (STAT) signaling results in degenerative joint disease, gastrointestinal ulceration, and failure of uterine implantation. *J. Exp. Med.*, **194**, 189–203.

Escary, J. L., Perreau, J., Dumenil, D., Ezine, S. & Brulet, P. (1993). Leukaemia inhibitory factor is necessary for maintenance of haematopoietic stem cells and thymocyte stimulation. *Nature*, **363**, 361–4.

Fujita, M., Ogawa, S., Fukuoka, H. *et al.* (2002). Differential expression of secreted frizzled-related protein 4 in decidual cells during pregnancy. *J. Mol. Endocrinol.*, **28**, 213–23.

Gavin, B. J., McMahon, J. A. & McMahon, A. P. (1990). Expression of multiple novel Wnt-1/int-1-related genes during fetal and adult mouse development. *Genes Dev.*, **4**, 2319–32.

Gendron, R. L., Paradis, H., Hsieh-Li, H. M. *et al.* (1997). Abnormal uterine stromal and glandular function associated with maternal reproductive defects in Hoxa-11 null mice. *Biol. Reprod.*, **56**, 1097–105.

Giles, R. H., van Es, J. H. & Clevers, H. (2003.). Caught up in a Wnt storm: Wnt signaling in cancer. *Biochim. Biophys. Acta*, **1653**, 1–24.

Hambartsoumian, E. (1998). Endometrial leukemia inhibitory factor (LIF) as a possible cause of unexplained infertility and multiple failures of implantation. *Am. J. Reprod. Immunol.*, **39**, 137–43.

Hogan, B. L. (1996). Bone morphogenetic proteins: multifunctional regulators of vertebrate development. *Genes Dev.*, **10**, 1580–94.

Hogan, B., Constantini, F. & Lacy, E. (1994). *Manipulating the Mouse Embryo: A Laboratory Manual*. New York: Cold Spring Harbor Press.

Hsieh-Li, H. M., Witte, D. P., Weinstein, M. *et al.* (1995). Hoxa 11 structure, extensive antisense transcription, and function in male and female fertility. *Development*, **121**, 1373–85.

Huet, Y. M., Andrews, G. K. & Dey, S. K. (1989). Modulation of c-myc protein in the mouse uterus during pregnancy and by steroid hormones. *Prog. Clin. Biol. Res.*, **294**, 401–12.

Ingham, P. W. (1998). Transducing Hedgehog: the story so far. *EMBO J.*, **17**, 3505–11.

Israel, D. I., Nove, J., Kerns, K. M. *et al.* (1996). Heterodimeric bone morphogenetic proteins show enhanced activity in vitro and in vivo. *Growth Factors*, **13**, 291–300.

Iwamoto, R., Yamazaki, S., Asakura, M. *et al.* (2003). Heparin-binding EGF-like growth factor and ErbB signaling is essential for heart function. *Proc. Natl. Acad. Sci. U.S.A.*, **100**, 3221–6.

Kawabata, M., Imamura, T. & Miyazono, K. (1998). Signal transduction by bone morphogenetic proteins. *Cytokine Growth Factor Rev.*, **9**, 49–61.

Kennedy, T. G. (1985). Evidence for the involvement of prostaglandins throughout the decidual cell reaction in the rat. *Biol. Reprod.* **33**, 140–6.

Kingsley, D. M. (1994). The TGF-beta superfamily: new members, new receptors, and new genetic tests of function in different organisms. *Genes Dev.*, **8**, 133–46.

Kirby, D. R. S. & Cowell, T. (1968). Trophoblast – host interactions. In B. R. Fleischmeyer, ed., *Epithelial–Mesenchymal Interactions*. Baltimore: Williams & Wilkins, pp. 64–77.

Kishimoto, T., Taga, T. & Akira, S. (1994). Cytokine signal transduction. *Cell*, **76**, 253–62.

Kliewer, S. A., Umesono, K., Noonan, D. J., Heyman, R. A. & Evans, R. M. (1992). Convergence of 9-cis retinoic acid and peroxisome proliferator signaling pathways through heterodimer formation of their receptors. *Nature*, **358**, 771–4.

Kliewer, S. A., Forman, B. M., Blumberg, B. *et al.* (1994). Differential expression and activation of a family of murine peroxisome proliferator-activated receptors. *Proc. Natl. Acad. Sci. U.S.A.*, **91**, 7355–9.

Krumlauf, R. (1994). Hox genes in vertebrate development. *Cell*, **78**, 191–201.

Langenbach, R., Morham, S. G., Tiano, H. F. *et al.* (1995). Prostaglandin synthase 1 gene disruption in mice reduces arachidonic acid-induced inflammation and indomethacin-induced gastric ulceration. *Cell*, **83**, 483–92.

Leach, R. E., Khalifa, R., Ramirez, N. D. *et al.* (1999). Multiple roles for heparin-binding epidermal growth factor-like growth factor are suggested by its cell-specific expression during the human endometrial cycle and early placentation. *J. Clin. Endocrinol. Metab.*, **84**, 3355–63.

Lim, H. & Dey, S. K. (2000). PPAR delta functions as a prostacyclin receptor in blastocyst implantation. *Trends Endocrinol. Metab.*, **11**, 137–42.

Lim, H., Paria, B. C., Das, S. K. *et al.* (1997). Multiple female reproductive failures in cyclooxygenase 2-deficient mice. *Cell*, **91**, 197–208.

Lim, H., Das, S. K. & Dey, S. K. (1998). erbB genes in the mouse uterus: cell-specific signaling by epidermal growth factor (EGF) family of growth factors during implantation. *Dev. Biol.*, **204**, 97–110.

Lim, H., Gupta, R. A., Ma, W. G. *et al.* (1999a). Cyclo-oxygenase-2-derived prostacyclin mediates embryo implantation in the mouse via PPARdelta. *Genes Dev.*, **13**, 1561–74.

Lim, H., Ma, L., Ma, W. G., Maas, R. L. & Dey, S. K. (1999b). Hoxa-10 regulates uterine stromal cell responsiveness to progesterone during implantation and decidualization in the mouse. *Mol. Endocrinol.*, **13**, 1005–17.

Lim, H., Song, H., Paria, B. C. *et al.* (2002). Molecules in blastocyst implantation: uterine and embryonic perspectives. *Vitam. Horm.*, **64**, 43–76.

Lloyd, S., Fleming, T. P. & Collins, J. E. (2003). Expression of Wnt genes during mouse pre-implantation development. *Gene Expr. Patterns*, **3**, 309–12.

Luetteke, N. C., Qiu, T. H., Peiffer, R. L., *et al.* (1993). TGF alpha deficiency results in hair follicle and eye abnormalities in targeted and waved-1 mice. *Cell*, **73**, 263–78.

Luetteke, N. C., Qiu, T. H., Fenton, S. E. *et al.* (1999). Targeted inactivation of the EGF and amphiregulin genes reveals distinct roles for EGF receptor ligands in mouse mammary gland development. *Development*, **126**, 2739–50.

Ma, W. G., Song, H., Das, S. K., Paria, B. C. & Dey, S. K. (2003). Estrogen is a critical determinant that specifies the duration of the window of uterine receptivity for implantation. *Proc. Natl. Acad. Sci. U.S.A.*, **100**, 2963–8.

Mangelsdorf, D. J. & Evans, R. M. (1995). The RXR heterodimers and orphan receptors. *Cell*, **83**, 841–50.

Martin, K. L., Barlow, D. H. & Sargent, I. L. (1998). Heparin-binding epidermal growth factor significantly improves human blastocyst development and hatching in serum-free medium. *Hum. Reprod.*, **13**, 1645–52.

Massague, J. & Chen, Y. G. (2000). Controlling TGF-beta signaling. *Genes Dev.*, **14**, 627–44.

McLaren, A. (1990). The Embryo. In C. R. Austin, ed., *Reproduction in Mammals*. Cambridge: Cambridge University Press, pp. 1–26.

Mead, R. A. (1993). Embryonic diapause in vertebrates. *J. Exp. Zool.* **266**, 629–41.

Michalik, L., Desvergne, B., Tan, N. S. *et al.* (2001). Impaired skin wound healing in peroxisome proliferator-activated receptor (PPAR)alpha and (PPAR)beta mutant mice. *J. Cell Biol.*, **154**, 799–814.

Negishi, M., Sugimoto, Y. & Ichikawa, A. (1995). Molecular mechanisms of diverse actions of prostanoid receptors. *Biochim. Biophys. Acta*, **1259**, 109–19.

Ni, H., Sun, T., Ding, N. Z., Ma, X. H. & Yang, Z. M. (2002). Differential expression of microsomal prostaglandin E synthase at implantation sites and in decidual cells of mouse uterus. *Biol. Reprod.*, **67**, 351–8.

Ni, H., Sun, T., Ma, X. H. & Yang, Z. M. (2003). Expression and regulation of cytosolic prostaglandin E synthase in mouse uterus during the periimplantation period. *Biol. Reprod.*, **68**, 744–50.

Nusse, R. (2003). Wnts and Hedgehogs: lipid-modified proteins and similarities in signaling mechanisms at the cell surface. *Development*, **130**, 5297–305.

Onagbesan, O. M., Bruggeman, V., Van As, P. *et al.* (2003). BMPs and BMPRs in chicken ovary and effects of BMP-4 and -7 on granulosa cell proliferation and progesterone production in vitro. *Am. J. Physiol. Endocrinol. Metab.*, **285**, E973–83.

Paria, B. C., Huet-Hudson, Y. M. & Dey, S. K. (1993). Blastocyst's state of activity determines the 'window' of implantation in the receptive mouse uterus. *Proc. Natl. Acad. Sci. U.S.A.*, **90**, 10159–62.

Paria, B. C., Ma, W., Tan, J. *et al.* (2001). Cellular and molecular responses of the uterus to embryo implantation can be elicited by locally applied growth factors. *Proc. Natl. Acad. Sci. U.S.A.*, **98**, 1047–52.

Paria, B. C., Reese, J., Das, S. K. & Dey, S. K. (2002). Deciphering the crosstalk of implantation: advances and challenges. *Science*, **296**, 2185–8.

Peters, J. M., Lee, S. S., Li, W. *et al.* (2000). Growth, adipose, brain, and skin alterations resulting from targeted disruption of the mouse peroxisome proliferator-activated receptor beta (delta). *Mol. Cell. Biol.*, **20**, 5119–28.

Petraglia, F., Santuz, M., Florio, P. *et al.* (1998). Paracrine regulation of human placenta: control of hormonogenesis. *J. Reprod. Immunol.*, **39**, 221–33.

Pollard, J. W., Hunt, J. S., Wiktor-Jedrzejczak, W. & Stanley, E. R. (1991). A pregnancy defect in the osteopetrotic (op/op) mouse demonstrates the requirement for CSF-1 in female fertility. *Dev. Biol.*, **148**, 273–83.

Psychoyos, A. (1973a). Endocrine control of egg implantation. In R. O. Greep & S. R. Geiger, eds. *Handbook of Physiology*. Washington, DC: American Physiological Society, pp. 187–215.

    (1973b). Hormonal control of ovoimplantation. *Vitam. Horm.*, **31**, 201–56.

Reddy, S. T. & Herschman, H. R. (1997). Prostaglandin synthase-1 and prostaglandin synthase-2 are coupled to distinct phospholipases for the generation of prostaglandin D2 in activated mast cells. *J. Biol. Chem.*, **272**, 3231–7.

Robb, L., Li, R., Hartley, L. *et al.* (1998). Infertility in female mice lacking the receptor for interleukin 11 is due to a defective uterine response to implantation. *Nat. Med.*, **4**, 303–8.

Roberts, R. M., Ealy, A. D., Alexenko, A. P., Han, C. S. & Ezashi, T. (1999). Trophoblast interferons. *Placenta*, **20**, 259–64.

Salamonsen, L. A., Doughton, B. W. & Findlay, J. K. (1986). The effects of the pre-implantation blastocyst in vivo and in vitro on protein synthesis and secretion by cultured epithelial cells from sheep endometrium. *Endocrinology*, **119**, 622–8.

Sharkey, A. (1998). Cytokines and implantation. *Rev. Reprod.*, **3**, 52–61.

Smith, W. C. (1999). TGF beta inhibitors. New and unexpected requirements in vertebrate development. *Trends Genet.*, **15**, 3–5.

Smith, W. L., Garavito, R. M. & DeWitt, D. L. (1996). Prostaglandin endoperoxide H synthases (cyclooxygenases)-1 and -2. *J. Biol. Chem.*, **271**, 33157–60.

Song, H., Lim, H., Das, S. K., Paria, B. C. & Dey, S. K. (2000). Dysregulation of EGF family of growth factors and COX-2 in the uterus during the preattachment and attachment reactions of the blastocyst with the luminal epithelium correlates with implantation failure in LIF-deficient mice. *Mol. Endocrinol.*, **14**, 1147–61.

Song, H., Lim, H., Paria, B. C. *et al.* (2002). Cytosolic phospholipase A2alpha is crucial [correction of A2alpha deficiency is crucial] for 'on-time' embryo implantation that directs subsequent development. *Development*, **129**, 2879–89.

Spencer, A. G., Woods, J. W., Arakawa, T., Singer, I. I. & Smith, W. L. (1998). Subcellular localization of prostaglandin endoperoxide H synthases-1 and -2 by immunoelectron microscopy. *J. Biol. Chem.* **273**, 9886–93.

Stewart, C. L. & Cullinan, E. B. (1997). Pre-implantation development of the mammalian embryo and its regulation by growth factors. *Dev. Genet.*, **21**, 91–101.

Stewart, C. L., Kaspar, P., Brunet, L. J. *et al.* (1992). Blastocyst implantation depends on maternal expression of leukaemia inhibitory factor. *Nature*, **359**, 76–9.

Takano, T., Panesar, M., Papillon, J. & Cybulsky, A. V. (2000). Cyclooxygenases-1 and 2 couple to cytosolic but not group IIA phospholipase A2 in COS-1 cells. *Prostaglandins Other Lipid Mediat.*, **60**, 15–26.

Tan, J., Raja, S., Davis, M. K. *et al.* (2002). Evidence for coordinated interaction of cyclin D3 with p21 and cdk6 in directing the development of uterine stromal cell decidualization and polyploidy during implantation. *Mech. Dev.*, **111**, 99–113.

Taylor, H. S., Arici, A., Olive, D. & Igarashi, P. (1998). HOXA10 is expressed in response to sex steroids at the time of implantation in the human endometrium. *J. Clin. Invest.*, **101**, 1379–84.

Uozumi, N., Kume, K., Nagase, T. *et al.* (1997). Role of cytosolic phospholipase A2 in allergic response and parturition. *Nature*, **390**, 618–22.

Wang, H., Ma, W. G., Tejada, L. *et al.* (2003). Rescue of female infertility from the loss of cyclooxygenase-2 by compensatory upregulation of cyclooxygenase-1 is a function of genetic background. *J. Biol. Chem.*, **279**, 10649–58.

Wilcox, A. J., Baird, D. D. & Weinberg, C. R. (1999). Time of implantation of the conceptus and loss of pregnancy. *New Engl. J. Med.*, **340**, 1796–99.

Winnier, G., Blessing, M., Labosky, P. A. & Hogan, B. L. (1995). Bone morphogenetic protein-4 is required for mesoderm formation and patterning in the mouse. *Genes Dev.*, **9**, 2105–16.

Wodarz, A. & Nusse, R. (1998). Mechanisms of Wnt signaling in development. *Annu. Rev. Cell. Dev. Biol.*, **14**, 59–88.

Yang, Z. M., Das, S. J., Wang, J. *et al.* (1997). Potential sites of prostaglandin actions in the periimplantation mouse uterus: differential expression and regulation of prostaglandin receptor genes. *Biol. Reprod.*, **56**, 368–79.

Yao, M. W., Lim, H., Schust, D. J. *et al.* (2003). Gene expression profiling reveals progesterone-mediated cell cycle and immunoregulatory roles of Hoxa-10 in the preimplantation uterus. *Mol. Endocrinol.*, **17**, 610–27.

Yoo, H. J., Barlow, D. H. & Mardon, H. J. (1997). Temporal and spatial regulation of expression of heparin-binding epidermal growth factor-like growth factor in the human endometrium: a possible role in blastocyst implantation. *Dev. Genet.*, **21**, 102–8.

Yoshinaga, K. & Adams, C. E. (1966). Delayed implantation in the spayed, progesterone treated adult mouse. *J. Reprod. Fertil.*, **12**, 593–5.

Zhang, H. & Bradley, A. (1996). Mice deficient for BMP2 are nonviable and have defects in amnion/chorion and cardiac development. *Development*, **122**, 977–86.

Zimmerman, L. B., De Jesus-Escobar, J. M. & Harland, R. M. (1996). The Spemann organizer signal noggin binds and inactivates bone morphogenetic protein 4. *Cell*, **86**, 599–606.

DISCUSSION

McLaren What do you think is the signal from the blastocyst that actually stimulates the HB-EGF in the uterus?

Dey It has been a puzzling question. Recently we did a microarray experiment comparing dormant and activated blastocysts, using the template that Minoru Ko at the NIA/NIH developed containing about 30 000 genes. We found that HB-EGF transcript levels significantly increased in activated blastocysts. We thought that HB-EGF might be inducing its own gene in the uterus, creating an autoinduction loop. This is what we found. If we take Affi-gel Blue beads, pre-soak them in HB-EGF and transfer them into uterine lumens of day 4 pseudopregnant recipient mice, they induce HB-EGF expression in the endometrium surrounding the beads preloaded with HB-EGF. I think this could initiate the whole cascade. We now have the floxed HB-EGF knockout mice and we will be trying more experiments on them. We will attempt to silence the *HB-EGF* gene in the uterus by using adenoviral Cre and see what effect it has.

McLaren That will be a very interesting experiment.

Sharkey You said you see altered trophoblast development in some of your mutants. You implied that even in the wild-type mice, when implantation occurs late, similar kinds of problems are seen in the placenta. Can you tell us what you think is going on there?

Dey   If you alter the attachment timing, this somehow creates a problem. The decidual response remains more or less unaltered, but the feto–placental growth becomes defective. We have observed this in wild-type and transgenic mice (Song *et al.* 2002). This is very important. We know in the literature that mutation of some genes causes embryonic lethality, but it is not clear whether this is a direct effect on fetal development or an indirect effect mediated via defective embryo–uterine interaction. Often, people don't look at the timing of implantation in these mice, which may be different.

Cross   So there are placental defects. Just along the line of it being a ripple effect, have you looked at the stages of placental development and transitions from the yolk sac placenta, to chorioallantoic placenta?

Dey   Not really. We'd like to look at this more carefully, but my work normally stops by day 8.

Lever   How do you envisage the compensatory up-regulation of COX-1?

Dey   That's a million dollar question. We are baffled why this is induced just like COX-2.

Lever   Is there a generalised up-regulation?

Dey   No. It mainly happens at the implantation sites, just like COX-2.

Lever   Can you get a similar sort of result using pharmacological COX inhibitors?

Dey   Yes, we have some evidence. This raises an interesting question. People are now using COX-2 inhibitors as anti-inflammatory drugs. This could be a function of genetic make-up. There is now some discussion that COX-2 selective inhibitors are not effective in certain individuals. I wonder whether COX-1 compensates for the loss of COX-2 activity in these individuals.

Sharkey Do you think this mechanism of delayed implantation operates in humans? I was thinking of the human chorionic gonadotrophin (HCG) paper where they looked at the rates of miscarriage compared with the time at which they first detected HCG. If I recall correctly, if HCG was first detected after day 10 or 11 of ovulation, the miscarriage rate went rocketing upwards. The implication was that if you missed the window, even if the pregnancy starts, it then fails subsequently.

Dey   That could be one of the causes.

McLaren There was a point in the discussion yesterday, suggesting that abnormalities were occurring possibly because implantation was happening towards the end of the window. That would certainly fit in with what you are saying now.

Kunath   How does this work relate to human implantation? Are these molecules also involved?

Dey   Investigators at UK and USA have looked at this. They found that HB-EGF is the most potent growth factor in IVF programmes. Heparin-binding EGF-like growth factor is also expressed during the window of implantation in humans. When the transmembrane form of HB-EGF is expressed in cells in culture, the embryo can attach onto these cells. This attachment is through ErbB4. Cyclooxygenase-2 has been shown to be expressed in the uterus or embryo during implantation in various animals, including minks, ferrets, skunks, pigs, baboons and humans. There are some epidemiological studies that suggest that women who chronically use NSAIDS (non-steroidal anti-inflammatory drugs, which inhibit COX-1 and COX-2) have problems with fertility. One such article appeared recently in the *British Medical Journal* (Li *et al.* 2003).

Braude   This probably refers to the inhibition of ovulation (Stone *et al.* 2002).

Dey   In this recent paper they thought that the failure occurred at a time after fertilisation.

Braude   Do we have any evidence about the effects of prostaglandin synthase inhibitors generally? One of the important factors in attempting to prevent miscarriages is the idea that inadvertently people have been given aspirin. There is a recent paper suggesting that the use of aspirin increased the risk of miscarriage rather than decreasing it, although it was a very poorly put-together paper. But there is this disparity at the moment. One of the suggestions for people who have anti-phospholipid syndrome is that they should have aspirin or heparin. The way that this has been taken forward is that if this helps those people, it can't be a bad thing to give everyone aspirin, and that is what is happening to a large degree. It is not clear whether this is a good or a bad thing. Certainly, from what you are saying – if it does inhibit the enzymes – then it may not be a good thing.

McLaren   Prostaglandin does seem to have an extraordinary variety of different effects in the course of reproduction.

Keverne   If the HB-EGF signal from the blastocyst is to induce HB-EGF production by the uterus, this will be a powerful amplifying feed-forward effect. Do you see this as a way of spreading the decidual response in some way? Something then has to change or it would just amplify for ever.

Dey   We don't know what happens after embryo attachment takes place. Is HB-EGF expression shut off or does it still continue?

Braude   Presumably the decidual reaction doesn't have to be purely local in humans. If you have a pregnancy in the tube, you still get a marked decidual reaction in the uterus, even though the embryo is somewhere else.

McLaren   Yes, the human is different from the mouse, because the decidual reaction is not related to the implantation stimulus from the embryo. In the mouse it is directly related, forming at the point where the blastocyst attaches and spreading out from there. In the human, whether you get an embryo there or not, at the right stage of the cycle you get a decidual reaction. I am not surprised that ectopic implantation in the Fallopian tube would give you the same decidual reaction in the uterus.

This was one of the things that made me think that perhaps implantation in the mouse was not a terribly good model for implantation in the human. But at the molecular level I suspect that it may still be.

Dey   We can take this information, apply it to humans and see whether it holds true or not.

Braude   I don't see how you do the experiment.

Dey   Many of the molecules seen involved in mouse implantation have been proven to work in humans also. Of course, you can't do extensive studies with human embryos, especially in USA.

Braude   What is the question you are going to be asking? Are you going to do this in vitro?

Dey   The IVF programmes have shown that HB-EGF may be one of the most potent growth factors for stimulating embryonic growth up to the blastocyst stage. Many years ago we showed that if you culture mouse embryos individually or in groups, those in groups grow much better. This is now practised in IVF programmes. It came from mouse work.

Moffett   If you put blastocysts somewhere else in the mouse, do you see the same up-regulation?

Dey   We haven't checked this but it would be interesting to see.

McLaren   I bet you won't see it. There is no decidual reaction elsewhere, and there is growth of the embryo from the blastocyst whatever the hormonal status of the mouse.

Moffett   How are they attaching then?

McLaren   They are not. They are simply going through embryonic development. David Kirby, who I mentioned earlier, had a paper at a Scottish conference that I attended in the 1960s in which he described how he put mouse blastocysts under the kidney, spleen or testis capsule, or in the brain. In all those locations the trophoblast invaded aggressively irrespective of the oestrous cycle (Kirby 1965).

Dey   And then they invade like trophoblasts. We have a model we discovered by accident in CB1 knockout mice. Embryos develop to the blastocyst stage in the oviduct and remain trapped therein for several days. We thought this would be a model for ectopic pregnancy but we don't know whether we can induce implantation-like reactions in the oviduct.

McLaren   You can get a delayed blastocyst sitting in the uterus not implanting and not developing while the blastocysts elsewhere are developing happily. In order to develop the blastocyst has to be put into a solid tissue where it can have space to develop. It can't get through an epithelium. If you put it into the peritoneal cavity it won't do anything, nor will it if you leave it in the oviduct.

Moffett   But it will in humans, so again there is a difference here.

Hemberger   In normally occurring delay of implantations, for example when the mother is lactating, how is this HB-EGF signalling deferred? Is it blocked initially and then catches on?

Dey	If we induce delayed implantation we don't see that signal any more.
McLaren	But you still get a decidual reaction.
Dey	In delayed implantation we don't see induction of HB-EGF. As soon as we give oestrogen to reactivate the blastocyst, within 12 hours we see signals, and by 24 hours it is fairly strong. We know that during this time the embryo doesn't have the EGF receptor. It is down-regulated. Gene array experiments also suggest that in dormant blastocysts HB-EGF is not induced.
McLaren	Have you looked for the HB-EGF in the uterine epithelium at the time when implantation would have occurred normally but the mouse is in delay? Is it possible that the luminal epithelium has already been stimulated?
Dey	No.
McLaren	If you looked at day 4, when the blastocysts would normally be expected to signal to the luminal epithelium, you might see a transient rise in HB-EGF.
Dey	No, we don't see this.

REFERENCES

Kirby, D. R. S. (1965). The 'invasiveness' of the trophoblast. In W. W. Park, ed., *The Early Conceptus, Normal and Abnormal*. Edinburgh: University of St Andrews Press, pp. 68–74.

Li, D. K., Liu, L. & Odouli, R. (2003). Exposure to non-steroidal anti-inflammatory drugs during pregnancy and risk of miscarriage: population based cohort study. *BMJ*, **327**, 368.

Song, H., Lim, H., Paria, B. C. *et al.* (2002). Cytosolic phospholipase A2alpha is crucial for 'on-time' embryo implantation that directs subsequent development. *Development*, **129**, 2879–89 (Erratum in *Development*, **129**, 3761).

Stone, S., Khamashta, M. A. & Nelson-Piercy, C. (2002). Nonsteroidal anti-inflammatory drugs and reversible female infertility: is there a link? *Drug Safety*, **25**, 545–51.

10

Trophoblast and pre-eclampsia

C. W. G. Redman, I. L. Sargent and E. A. Linton

Nuffield Department of Obstetrics and Gynaecology, University of Oxford, UK

Introduction

In this chapter, the importance of trophoblast in generating the maternal signs and symptoms that comprise the syndrome of pre-eclampsia will be discussed, but not the processes of placentation in early pregnancy that may be important in the preclinical phases of the disorder. Pre-eclampsia is a potentially dangerous and highly variable complication of the second half of pregnancy, labour or the early puerperium. It has been known for nearly 100 years that it originates in the placenta (Holland 1909). The presence of a placenta is both necessary and sufficient to cause the disorder (Redman 1991). A fetus is not required as pre-eclampsia can occur with hydatidiform mole (Chun *et al.* 1964). A uterus is probably not required because pre-eclampsia may develop with abdominal pregnancy (Piering *et al.* 1993). Central to management is delivery, which removes the causative organ, namely the placenta.

The maternal illness of pre-eclampsia was originally thought to be caused primarily by generalised maternal endothelial activation and dysfunction (Roberts *et al.* 1989). Later this concept was broadened by incorporating endothelial dysfunction as one of several components of a maternal systemic inflammatory response in pre-eclampsia (Redman *et al.* 1999).

A key feature is that systemic inflammation is not only characteristic of the pre-eclamptic woman but an intrinsic part of every normal pregnancy, which becomes most evident in the third trimester (Redman *et al.* 1999). The inflammatory response of pre-eclampsia does not differ in type, but only in degree, being more intense.

Biology and Pathology of Trophoblast, eds. Ashley Moffett, Charlie Loke and Anne McLaren.
Published by Cambridge University Press © Cambridge University Press 2005.

Definition of the syndrome: maternal or placental pre-eclampsia

The processes driving maternal systemic inflammation in pregnancy, whether normal or pre-eclamptic, must originate in the placenta, specifically from the syncytiotrophoblast in direct contact with maternal blood or extravillous cytotrophoblast in direct contact with decidua. Today, the challenge for understanding pre-eclampsia is to identify the relevant trophoblast factors and to know why they are released in greater abundance in pre-eclampsia. We have previously referred to these factors in sum as 'Factor x' (Redman 1992).

The concept of the involvement of maternal systemic inflammation has clarified the issues by a modest amount. For there are two components that make the systemic inflammatory response abnormally intense: an excessive placental stimulus or an overactive maternal response to a normal placental stimulus. These two situations are termed 'Placental' and 'Maternal' pre-eclampsia respectively (Ness & Roberts 1996) and are deemed to operate by the common mechanism of systemic inflammatory dysfunction. Placental pre-eclampsia represents a disorder that is specific to pregnancy whereas maternal pre-eclampsia is specific to the woman. The two types are often mixed together to varying degrees.

Placental pre-eclampsia: the problem of uteroplacental perfusion and spiral artery disease

In placental pre-eclampsia the placenta is considered to suffer from the consequences of inadequate perfusion secondary to spiral artery dysfunction (Brosens et al. 1972, Pijnenborg et al. 1991), which leads to placental hypoxia, oxidative stress and, in the most severe cases, infarction. Two abnormalities affect the spiral arteries, which are the end-arteries that supply the intervillous space: the arteries may be either too small or obstructed. They are too small if they fail to undergo the structural (physiological) modifications that are largely achieved in the first half of pregnancy and depend on invasive extravillous cytotrophoblast infiltrating the tissues of the placental bed. This is a highly active process, which dies down in the second half of pregnancy. With poor placentation the depth of invasion is too shallow and the arteries are too small. This process has been reconstructed from placental bed biopsies taken at therapeutic abortion or at delivery.

Acute atherosis (Hertig 1945) affects mainly the spiral arteries and is most closely associated with placental infarction (Zeek & Assali 1950). It comprises necrosis (necrotising arteriopathy) (Robertson et al. 1976), particularly affecting the media. The lesions in their early stages are characterised by endothelial damage (De Wolf et al. 1975, 1982). As with poor placentation, they may occur in the absence of maternal hypertension (Sheppard & Bonnar 1976, De Wolf et al. 1980, Khong

1991) although some authors disagree (Brosens *et al.* 1977). Little work has been done on the pathogenesis of acute atherosis.

Neither of the two lesions – deficient placentation (Robertson *et al.* 1985, Naicker *et al.* 2003) or spiral artery obstruction from acute atherosis (Robertson *et al.* 1976) – are invariably identified in pre-eclampsia (Pijnenborg *et al.* 1991). Whether this is because the lesions have been missed or because they are not always present is not known.

It has been taken for granted that pre-eclampsia originates with deficient placentation occurring during the first half of pregnancy and this has led to the concept of a 'two stage disease' (Redman 1991). In this model the seeds for pre-eclampsia are sown in the first half of pregnancy when full placentation fails. The disease evolves over the second half of pregnancy when the signs of pre-eclampsia are caused directly or indirectly by increasing uteroplacental ischaemia.

We now propose that poor placentation should be classified as a separate problem which powerfully predisposes to, but is not the same as, pre-eclampsia (Redman *et al.* 1999). Early onset pre-eclampsia, which is most associated with fetal growth impairment (Douglas & Redman 1994), is likely to be the end point of poor placentation and is an example of placental pre-eclampsia. Not all small for gestational age neonates are the consequence of poor placentation since there are, of course, several other causes.

Maternal pre-eclampsia

In its purest form, maternal pre-eclampsia results from the interaction of a normal pregnancy and placenta with an 'abnormal' maternal constitution. Some medical conditions are well known to predispose to pre-eclampsia, including obesity (Ros *et al.* 1998), diabetes (Garner *et al.* 1990) and chronic hypertension (Sibai *et al.* 1995). Because it is now known that pre-eclampsia results from an excessive systemic inflammatory response it is important and relevant that low-grade systemic inflammation is a feature of all these conditions in men or non-pregnant women. It also is evident in chronic arterial disease such as ischaemic heart disease (Hansson *et al.* 2002), to which pre-eclampsia sufferers seem to be susceptible in later life (Smith *et al.* 2001).

The effect of such medical problems is to elevate the baseline of systemic inflammation upon which the changes of pregnancy are superimposed (Fig. 10.1). We propose that, in pregnancy, the decompensation from excessive systemic inflammation will happen earlier and at a lower threshold accounting for the predisposition of affected women to pre-eclampsia.

Since it is postulated that circulating factors derived from the placenta are the stimuli to these responses (Redman 1992), the questions that need to be addressed

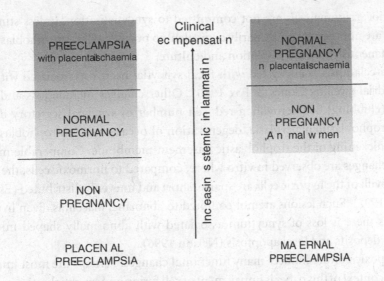

Figure 10.1 Placental and maternal pre-eclampsia. On the left an ischaemic placenta generates an intense enough maternal systemic inflammatory response to cause maternal decompensation and clinical signs. On the right is what can occur with pregnant women with chronic systemic inflammation associated with obesity, chronic hypertension, diabetes and other medical problems. The response to a normal pregnancy may be enough to cause clinical decompensation.

are: what are these factors and how do they cause the maternal systemic features of pre-eclampsia?

Placental pre-eclampsia with ischaemia: trophoblast hypoxia

Placental ischaemia would be expected to cause hypoxia. The increased occurrence of placental infarcts in pre-eclampsia (Zeek & Assali 1950, Little 1960, Wentworth 1967, Boyd & Scott 1985), which are secondary to obstruction of the spiral arteries (Brosens & Renaer 1972, Wallenburg et al. 1973) is consistent with the concept. Therefore the effect of hypoxia on villous trophoblast has received extensive attention.

The problems can be studied ex vivo in the pre-eclampsia placenta or in vitro in cultured trophoblast cells. The latter may be choriocarcinoma cell lines, or cytotrophoblasts purified from enzymically dispersed chorionic villi, using one of the many variants of the method first published by Kliman et al. (1986). Some investigators culture explants of chorionic villi. In these circumstances, changes in the contents of the culture medium induced by hypoxia may be due to other cell types such as endothelium or macrophages. Hence, the results need to be interpreted with care.

Choriocarcinoma cells are not committed to syncytialisation, unless stimulated. They are not therefore necessarily equivalent to purified villous trophoblast, which spontaneously fuse after isolation and culture.

Pre-eclampsia is associated with focal syncytial necrosis associated with mitochondrial swelling (Jones & Fox 1980). Other changes include loss and distortion (clubbing) of microvilli, a reduced number of syncytial secretory droplets, cytotrophoblastic hyperplasia, degeneration of occasional cytotrophoblastic cells and thickening of the trophoblastic basement membrane. Comparable microvillous changes are observed in vitro where, compared to normoxic cells, the surface microvilli of the hypoxic cells are sparse, short and unevenly distributed (Esterman et al. 1997). Such lesions are not confined to abnormal placentas. Even in normal tissues there is loss of syncytium associated with abnormally shaped microvilli, fibrin deposits and local apoptosis (Nelson 1996).

Hypoxic culture induces many functional changes. Perhaps the most important in the context of this paper is impairment of cell fusion and syncytialisation, as well as induction of apoptosis. Spontaneous fusion of cultured cytotrophoblast is reduced when the ambient oxygen concentration is lowered (Alsat et al. 1996, Hardy & Yang 2002). In a comparable way forskolin-induced fusion of choriocarcinoma cell lines is also suppressed (reversibly) in 2% oxygen compared with 20% oxygen. Trophoblast fusion depends on expression of the highly fusogenic membrane glycoprotein, called syncytin (Mi et al. 2000), which is the product of a human endogenous retrovirus gene, termed HERV-W (Blond et al. 2000). Its mRNA is specifically expressed in trophoblast (Mi et al. 2000). The gene for the syncytin receptor has also been identified as ASCT2 (Blond et al. 2000, Lavillette et al. 2002), whose protein is the system B0 amino acid transporter that has long been known to be expressed in the basal plasma membrane of syncytiotrophoblast (Kudo & Boyd 1990).

Hypoxia causes dysregulation of trophoblast expression of syncytin and its receptor (Kudo et al. 2003), which may suppress the normal processes of cell fusion and so inhibit syncytialisation (Knerr et al. 2003, Kudo et al. 2003). It is consistent with this concept that cytotrophoblast prepared from pre-eclampsia (i.e. hypoxic) placentas have lower rates of syncytialisation than those prepared from the placentas of normotensive women (Pijnenborg et al. 1996, Li et al. 2003) and, in limited studies, evidence for suppressed expression of syncytin (Knerr et al. 2002). Its distribution in pre-eclampsia placentas seems to be apical rather than basal (Lee et al. 2001), which may also impede the interaction of syncytin with its receptor, which is expressed on the basal membrane.

Hypoxia also triggers trophoblast apoptosis to which cytotrophoblast seem to be more sensitive than syncytiotrophoblast, probably because of its higher activity of caspases 3, 6, 8 and 9, which execute programmed cell death (Levy et al. 2000,

Table 10.1 Naturally occurring antioxidants

Non-enzymatic	Enzymatic
Alpha-tocopherol (vitamin E)	Superoxide dismutases (CuZn-SOD, Mn-SOD)
Ascorbate (vitamin C)	Catalase
β-carotene (vitamin A)	Glutathione peroxidases
Urate	Thioredoxin peroxidase
Peptides such as glutathione, thioredoxin	
Proteins such as caeruloplasmin, transferrin	

Yusuf *et al.* 2002). In pre-eclampsia placentas, trophoblast apoptosis is significantly increased (Leung *et al.* 2001, Ishihara *et al.* 2002), especially when the fetus is small for dates (Austgulen *et al.* 2004). The possible sequence of events caused by trophoblast hypoxia has been clarified by studying explanted villi from late first and third trimester placentas. Culture in 2% oxygen increased cytotrophoblast proliferation. The proteins necessary for execution of apoptosis were mostly retained in the cytotrophoblast due to lack of syncytial fusion. Culture in higher concentrations of oxygen reduced cytotrophoblast proliferation and enhanced syncytial fusion. Severe hypoxia causes necrosis rather than apoptosis (Huppertz *et al.* 2003) as observed in ex vivo specimens by Jones & Fox (1980).

The ways in which trophoblast hypoxia can lead to release of factors that generate the systemic inflammatory response of pre-eclampsia need to be considered. First, oxidative stress in the placenta will be discussed.

Oxidative stress

During aerobic respiration, the final enzyme of the electron transport chain that donates electrons to oxygen is cytochrome oxidase. Normally, oxygen is reduced completely to water but accidental release of a single electron results in the formation of superoxide anion, which is highly reactive chemically because of its single unpaired electron. The danger of superoxide anion is that it can trigger self-perpetuating chain reactions of chemical destruction involving cell lipids, DNA and proteins, which, if unchecked, lead to tissue degradation and cell death. Antioxidants are a variety of enzymes, peptides and other biochemical substances that remove these highly reactive products and protect the integrity of the organism (see Table 10.1).

Oxidative stress is a disequilibrium between antioxidant defences and production of reactive oxygen species in favour of the latter. It cannot be easily demonstrated directly in tissues. Evidence of oxidative damage can be found in terms of excess

Table 10.2 Markers of oxidative stress are increased in placentas of pre-eclamptic women

Marker	Direction of changes	Reference
Lipid peroxides	Increased	Walsh & Wang 1993
	Increased (TBARS[a])	Gratacos et al. 1998
	Increased – spectrophotometric method; homogenised tissue	Serdar et al. 2003
	No change – chromogenic assay; homogenised tissue	Bowen et al. 2001
MDA-modified proteins	Increased – mitochondria prepared from homogenised whole placental tissue	Wang & Walsh 1998
	Increased – release from cultured chorionic villi	Wang & Walsh 2001
	Increased – isolated microvillous membranes – PIH[b]	Cester et al. 1994
	No change – homogenised tissue: specific TBARS method	Bowen et al. 2001
HNE-modified proteins	No change – immunocytochemistry of syncytiotrophoblast	Santoso et al. 2002
	Increased – immunoblotting (tissue) and immunocytochemistry (syncytiotrophoblast)	Shibata et al. 2001
	Increased (inconsistently) – immunocytochemistry of syncytiotrophoblast	Morikawa et al. 1997
Superoxide	Increased levels – chorionic villi	Sikkema et al. 2001
	Increased generation – purified trophoblast	Wang & Walsh 2001
Protein carbonyls	Increased – homogenised whole placental tissue: HELLP syndrome[c]	Zusterzeel et al. 2001

[a]TBARS: thiobarbituric acid reacting substances (see text)

[b]PIH: Pregnancy-induced hypertension; a general term that includes pre-eclampsia and reversible hypertension without proteinuria

[c]HELLP syndrome: severe variant of pre-eclampsia (Weinstein 1982)

malondialdehyde (MDA), or proteins modified by 4-hydroxy-nonenal (HNE), which are both by-products of lipid peroxidation. Measurements of thiobarbituric acid reacting substances (TBARS), which releases a chromogen by reacting with MDA, have also been used. It is a simple assay but non-specific and for that reason is not used now. Protein carbonyls are products of oxidation of proteins, which are measured by a colorimetric procedure that involves dinitrophenylhydrazine or by ELISA. The subject has been recently reviewed (Mayne 2003).

There is general agreement (with some exceptions) that markers of oxidative stress are increased in the placentas of pre-eclamptic women, which includes evidence of direct involvement of syncytiotrophoblast (see Table 10.2 for summary of reports). But there is less agreement about antioxidant levels or activity.

The major sources of oxidative stress in tissues are mitochondria, which are also the targets for its consequences. Mitochondria are more abundant in the pre-eclampsia placenta as determined by electron microscopy (Jones & Fox 1980) or amount of mitochondrial protein (Wang & Walsh 1998). But overall, the activity

Table 10.3 Antioxidant levels or activities in placentas of pre-eclamptic women

Antioxidant	Direction of changes	References
Activity of CuZn-SOD[a] and mRNA	Reduced in placental tissue homogenate	Wang & Walsh 1996
Immunohistochemistry (CuZn-SOD[a] and Mn-SOD[b])	No change in intensity of labelling in syncytiotrophoblast	Myatt et al. 1997
Activity of GSH-Px[c]	Reduced	Walsh & Wang 1993
	Increased – women with HELLP[d] syndrome	Knapen et al. 1999
	No change	Poranen et al. 1996
Vitamin E content of whole placenta	Reduced in placental tissue homogenate	Wang & Walsh 1996
Catalase activity	Increased in placental tissue homogenate	Wang & Walsh 1996
Thioredoxin and glutaredoxin reducing systems	Reduced – mRNA	Sahlin et al. 2000
	Increased – proteins	Shibata et al. 2001
	Increased mRNA and protein for periredoxin III/SP-22	Shibata et al. 2003

[a]CuZn-SOD, copper zinc superoxide dismutase
[b]Mn-SOD, manganese superoxide dismutase
[c]GSH-Px, glutathione peroxidase
[d]HELLP syndrome: severe variant of pre-eclampsia (Weinstein 1982)

of cytochrome c oxidase is reduced (Wang et al. 1999), the number of mitochondria expressing the enzyme is markedly lower (Matsubara et al. 1997) and this is matched by significantly reduced cytochrome c oxidase subunit I mRNA in syncytiotrophoblast in pre-eclamptic placentas compared to control placentas (Furui et al. 1994, He et al. 2004). One investigator finds no difference however (Vuorinen et al. 1998). The mitochondria also show more evidence of lipid peroxidation (Morikawa et al. 1997, Wang & Walsh 1998).

In contrast to the general consensus concerning increased markers of oxidative stress, there are variable reports concerning the levels of antioxidants in the pre-eclampsia placenta (Table 10.3).

Oxidative stress is not confined to trophoblast in the pre-eclampsia placenta. Other cell types such as endothelial cells are involved as judged, for example, by the presence of nitrotyrosine residues (Myatt et al. 1996). These are formed by reactive oxygen species such as peroxynitrite, which in turn is the product of the reaction between superoxide anion and nitric oxide (Patel et al. 1999). It is also a systemic problem for the mother. For example the decidua is also involved (Staff et al. 1999).

Oxidative stress in pre-eclampsia has been reviewed by Poston (2003). It is important because it is a major trigger to apoptosis, programmed cell death, which affects trophoblast in both normal and pre-eclampsia pregnancies.

Trophoblast apoptosis

As already mentioned normal human syncytiotrophoblast becomes apoptotic in relation to breaks in the syncytial layer (Nelson 1996). There are many characteristic features including loss of microvilli and blebbing of the surface membrane. It has been proposed that apoptosis plays a central role in turnover of cytotrophoblast and renewal of the syncytial surface of chorionic villi (Huppertz *et al.* 1998); that it causes controlled cell fragmentation, in order to allow continuous renewal of the syncytial surface of chorionic villi. Clustered nuclei (pre-apoptotic and apoptotic) in syncytial knots probably represent the extrusion component of normal, continuous epithelial turnover (Mayhew *et al.* 1999). Apoptosis rates are significantly increased in the syncytiotrophoblast in pre-eclampsia (Allaire *et al.* 2000, Leung *et al.* 2001), especially if there is also fetal growth retardation (Austgulen *et al.* 2004). It is also known that in vitro hypoxia induces apoptosis of cultured human cytotrophoblasts (Levy *et al.* 2000).

Oxidative stress has been shown to induce apoptotic cell death by targeting the mitochondria directly. Mitochondrial-dependent apoptosis requires release of cytochrome c from mitochondria and subsequent activation of caspases, which are specific aspartate proteases. The BCl2 protein, an anti-apoptotic protein localised to mitochondria, has been shown in other cell types to inhibit cytochrome c release and protect against oxidative stress-induced apoptosis and hypoxic necrosis (Kluck *et al.* 1997).

In trophoblast, BCl2 is expressed mainly in the syncytial layer (Sakuragi *et al.* 1994). Of cultured cytotrophoblasts, those that express the lowest levels of BCl2 appear to be most susceptible to apoptosis (Ho *et al.* 1999). In pre-eclampsia the expression of BCl2 protein in syncytiotrophoblast has been reported to be reduced (Ishihara *et al.* 2002).

The reduced mitochondrial content of BCl2 and cytochrome c in pre-eclampsia are both consistent with the observations of concurrent increases in syncytial apoptosis.

Apoptosis and release of trophoblast debris into the maternal circulation

Apoptosis amounts to controlled cell fragmentation with release of subcellular microparticles in forms that are easy to clear by macrophages and other components of the reticuloendothelial system. The shedding of microparticles is the hallmark of apoptosis (Aupeix *et al.* 1997). Various types of trophoblast debris that must originate in this way can be detected in the maternal circulation. They include syncytial membrane microparticles (Knight *et al.* 1998), cytokeratin of placental origin also known as tissue polypeptide antigen (Norman *et al.* 1989), soluble fetal

Table 10.4 Circulating placental factors that are increased in pre-eclampsia

Trophoblast factor	Reference
Activin A and inhibin A	Muttukrishna *et al.* 1997
CRH	Campbell *et al.* 1987
Leptin	Mise *et al.* 1998
Neurokinin B	Page *et al.* 2000
Soluble Flt-1	Maynard *et al.* 2003
Lipid peroxides (Malondialdehyde)	Takacs *et al.* 2001
Trophoblast debris	Redman & Sargent 2000

CRH, corticotrophin releasing hormone.

DNA (Lo *et al.* 1999) and soluble fetal RNA (Ng *et al.* 2003b). All such factors are increased in the circulation in pre-eclamptic women (Schrocksnadel *et al.* 1993, Lo *et al.* 1999, Zhong *et al.* 2001, Ng *et al.* 2003a).

Not only can such debris be detected as evidence of increased syncytiotrophoblast apoptosis but it represents one of the possible factors that may cause the maternal syndrome of the second stage of pre-eclampsia. The range of trophoblast-derived factors that could come under the rubric 'Factor x' is discussed in the next section.

Trophoblast factors that are increased in the circulation of the pre-eclamptic women

Pre-eclampsia is a systemic disorder, so the problem must be disseminated from the placenta. Most interest is focused on factors that enter the circulation from syncytiotrophoblast, which have the potential to cause or exacerbate systemic inflammatory responses and are increased in pre-eclampsia. Some are listed in Table 10.4.

The claims for neurokinin B have not yet been confirmed and will not be discussed further. The remainder are mostly involved in inflammatory processes or consequences of hypoxia, in line with the general thesis of this paper that the cause of the pre-eclampsia syndrome lies in the hypoxic placenta, and the expression of the maternal symptoms derives from systemic inflammation.

Circulating trophoblast factors in pre-eclampsia: soluble Flt-1

A strong candidate is the soluble receptor for vascular endothelial growth factor (VEGFR-1), also known as soluble (s)Flt-1. It is synthesised and released by endothelial cells and peripheral blood monocytes (Hornig *et al.* 2000, Barleon 2001).

In the circulation it binds to VEGF and inhibits its functions. Vascular endothelial growth factor is an important survival factor for endothelium so systemic inhibition would be expected to cause generalised endothelial dysfunction. This has been confirmed in human and animal studies. Clinical trials of a neutralising monoclonal antibody to VEGF for the treatment of metastatic colorectal or renal cancer have shown that hypertension and proteinuria are the commonest side effects (Kabbinavar et al. 2003, Yang et al. 2003). Likewise, the infusion of sFlt-1 into rats (Maynard et al. 2003) causes these signs to appear. In the latter study the associated glomerular lesions were the same as those seen specifically in pre-eclampsia, namely glomerular endotheliosis (Gaber et al. 1994).

Serum sFlt-1 is increased in pre-eclampsia (Maynard et al. 2003). Because it is complexed to VEGF, its high levels in pre-eclampsia can explain the variable reports of changes of plasma VEGF in this condition. If total VEGF is measured it is increased whereas if only free VEGF is assayed it is reduced. The origin of the circulating sFlt-1 is presumed to be the placenta although this has not yet been directly demonstrated (Clark et al. 1998, Maynard et al. 2003, Tsatsaris et al. 2003). The most compelling evidence is its rapid decline in concentration after delivery (Maynard et al. 2003).

If sFlt-1 were the main cause of pre-eclampsia this could explain the paradoxical protective effect of cigarette smoking on the occurrence of pre-eclampsia, which was first noted 40 years ago (Zabriskie 1963) and has been repeatedly confirmed. Non-pregnant cigarette smokers have lower levels of circulating sFlt-1 than controls who do not smoke (Belgore et al. 2000). The fact that fetuses with trisomy 13 are particularly likely to provoke pre-eclampsia in their mothers (Boyd et al. 1987) is consistent with the location of the gene for sFlt-1 on chromosome 13 (Barr et al. 1991).

Soluble Flt-1 seems to be predominantly produced by extravillous trophoblast in the decidua and by endothelial and stromal cells in the chorionic villi, but not by the villous trophoblast (Clark et al. 1998). Villous explants release sFlt-1 into the culture supernatant in significantly greater amounts when cultured under hypoxic conditions (Ahmed et al. 2000a), which is consistent with the view that placental hypoxia is an important part of the pathogenesis (Ahmed et al. 2000a). The fact that it is also released by endothelium and monocytes (Hornig et al. 2000, Barleon 2001) suggests that these inflammatory cells may be one source of this factor in pre-eclampsia. In non-pregnant individuals, chronic medical conditions that are associated with mild systemic inflammatory responses yield conflicting findings with sFlt-1 measured as increased (Belgore et al. 2001b) or decreased (Belgore et al. 2001a, Felmeden et al. 2003). However, until these uncertainties are resolved it cannot be concluded that sFlt-1 is the relevant placental factor in pre-eclampsia.

Circulating trophoblast factors in pre-eclampsia: trophoblast microparticles

Circulating placental debris is likely to be an important part of the systemic inflammatory stimulus associated with both normal and pre-eclamptic pregnancies. We have shown that they are directly damaging to endothelium (Smarason *et al.* 1993) and stimulate the release of pro-inflammatory substances (von Dadelszen *et al.* 1999). They display markers of apoptosis (Kumar *et al.* 2000). Our preliminary evidence is that they bind to monocytes both in vivo and in vitro (Germain *et al.* 2002) and are directly pro-inflammatory (Sacks *et al.*, unpublished observations; Branton *et al.*, unpublished observations). It is possible that it is this circulating debris which is the inflammatory stimulus that causes the maternal syndrome. It is present in greatest amounts in the third trimester (Knight *et al.* 1998) when pre-eclampsia is most common, it would be released in greater quantities from larger placentas as with multiple pregnancies and would regress after delivery as does pre-eclampsia.

Circulating trophoblast factors in pre-eclampsia: corticotrophin-releasing hormone

Pregnancy is the only common human condition where there are large amounts of circulating corticotrophin-releasing hormone (CRH), which is produced by the human placenta, specifically from the syncytiotrophoblast (Perkins & Linton 1995). The placental content of CRH mRNA and peptide (Robinson *et al.* 1989) progressively increase throughout normal pregnancy and this is reflected in increasing levels of maternal plasma CRH (Campbell *et al.* 1987, Sasaki *et al.* 1987). An excess of CRH circulating binding protein (CRHBP) buffers, at least partially, the rising plasma levels in the first 35 weeks (Linton *et al.* 1990). But in the last 5 weeks, levels of CRHBP fall as the concentrations of CRH in maternal blood continue to rise exponentially (Linton *et al.* 1993).

Circulating CRH is substantially higher in pre-eclampsia than in matched normal pregnancy (Perkins *et al.* 1995), reflecting increased placental production of the CRH precursor (proCRH) and its mRNA (Ahmed *et al.* 2000b).

Not much is reported about the effects of hypoxia on CRH secretion, but conditions that mimic hypoxia (incubation with cobalt chloride) stimulate CRH secretion from primary cultured human trophoblast by a pathway that probably depends on haemoxygenase (Navarra *et al.* 2001). Since the role of circulating CRH in normal pregnancy is not defined, its functions in pre-eclampsia are also obscure.

Experimental evidence suggests that CRH may modulate the immune and inflammatory responses via two pathways: anti-inflammatory via centrally released CRH, and pro-inflammatory through direct action of peripherally released CRH (Leu & Singh 1991, Karalis *et al.* 1997). Pro-inflammatory effects include activation of monocytes/macrophages (Paez Pereda *et al.* 1995). By this systemic action CRH could contribute to inflammatory activation of pregnancy peripheral blood leukocytes in both normal and pre-eclamptic pregnancies.

Circulating trophoblast factors in pre-eclampsia: leptin

Leptin is a small peptide mainly produced by adipose tissue, which has wide ranging effects on glucose and lipid metabolism including control of body weight and appetite (Coppack 2001). It has some similarities to interleukin 6. Obese individuals have higher circulating leptin concentrations than lean people. In the circulation a soluble leptin receptor is the major leptin binding protein (Lammert *et al.* 2001) and promotes leptin clearance from the circulation. It may be a key factor determining the amount of total leptin in circulation (Huang *et al.* 2001).

Leptin is also produced in relatively large amounts by the placenta, more specifically by trophoblast (Masuzaki *et al.* 1997). Circulating plasma concentrations increase during pregnancy (Mise *et al.* 1998), which is ascribed to leptin produced by syncytiotrophoblast (Masuzaki *et al.* 1997, Mise *et al.* 1998) and not by villous stromal cells (Senaris *et al.* 1997). Plasma leptin concentrations peak at around 20–30 weeks of gestation before declining towards term (Sattar *et al.* 1998). However, the proportion of free leptin relative to that which is bound (and inactive) remains constant. The soluble receptor is also produced and secreted by syncytiotrophoblast and is presumed to contribute to the plasma binding capacity (Gavrilova *et al.* 1997) but it is possible that during pregnancy it is only a minor component of total leptin binding capacity in the circulation (Nuamah *et al.* 2003).

Circulating total leptin concentrations are significantly higher in pre-eclampsia (Mise *et al.* 1998, McCarthy *et al.* 1999). There is strong evidence that this is a direct consequence of reduced oxygen tension (Mise *et al.* 1998). Hypoxia increases leptin mRNA and secretion in trophoblast-derived BeWo cells (Grosfeld *et al.* 2001). In the chronically hypoxic placenta of pre-eclampsia, leptin is one of the most up-regulated placental transcripts (Reimer *et al.* 2002).

Leptin is closely involved in regulation of the inflammatory response. It helps to regulate the metabolic response to sepsis and systemic inflammation (Arnalich *et al.* 1999, Fantuzzi & Faggioni 2000) and can be pro-inflammatory (Zarkesh-Esfahani *et al.* 2001). It is also angiogenic (Sierra-Honigmann *et al.* 1998, Park *et al.* 2001) and promotes wound healing and haematopoiesis (Fantuzzi & Faggioni 2000).

Circulating trophoblast factors in pre-eclampsia: activin A

Activin A is a dimeric, pluripotent growth factor, a member of the transforming growth factor (TGF)β super family, which interacts with various low- and high-affinity binding proteins, such as follistatin and α2-macroglobulin, that can reduce bioavailability. As are the other factors discussed here, it is produced by human trophoblast (Mohan *et al.* 2001) including syncytiotrophoblast (Schneider-Kolsky *et al.* 2002). But it can be secreted also by other cell types including inflammatory (Eramaa *et al.* 1992, Tannetta *et al.* 2003) and endothelial cells (de Waard *et al.* 1999, Tannetta *et al.* 2003), specifically with pro-inflammatory factors. Moreover, interaction with activated T cells is also potently stimulatory (Abe *et al.* 2002). It is entirely consistent therefore that circulating levels are increased in non-pregnancy individuals with septicaemia (Michel *et al.* 2003).

Given that pre-eclampsia is characterised by systemic inflammation it is not surprising that plasma activin A is increased in established pre-eclampsia (Muttukrishna *et al.* 1997) and in some cases, particularly of early onset, before the disease becomes manifest (Muttukrishna *et al.* 2000). Not all of the rise is necessarily derived from trophoblast because activated monocytes and endothelium (both components of the pre-eclampsia syndrome) are also potential sources (Tannetta *et al.* 2003).

What evidence there is suggests that activin A is anti- rather than pro-inflammatory (Ohguchi *et al.* 1998). There is modest in vitro evidence that it can suppress certain components of the acute phase response, which is a generalised metabolic response to stress, induced by pro-inflammatory factors (Russell *et al.* 1999).

Likewise, hypoxic culture of placental explants inhibits rather than increases its production (Blumenstein *et al.* 2002, Schneider-Kolsky *et al.* 2002). However, no effect could be detected in primary cytotrophoblasts cultured on their own. Activin A inhibits endothelial cell proliferation (McCarthy & Bicknell 1993), so like sFlt-1 it is anti-angiogenic.

Conclusion

Factors released by syncytiotrophoblast must be the direct cause of the maternal syndrome of pre-eclampsia, which presents before or at delivery. Because they circulate in all pregnant women in increasing amounts during the second half of pregnancy they can account for the systemic inflammatory response, which is common to all pregnant women. Pre-eclampsia is the extreme end of a continuum of systemic inflammation common to all pregnancies, which is why its clinical features always overlap with those of normal pregnancy.

Spiral artery insufficiency generating placental ischaemia and hypoxia is a critical event, which causes poor syncytialisation and syncytiotrophoblast apoptosis. The syncytiotrophoblast is stimulated by oxygen-sensitive or other mechanisms to release into maternal blood a number of factors that activate systemic inflammation and so cause the syndrome of pre-eclampsia. Some of the individual factors have been discussed. There is no reason to believe that there is exclusively one factor that contributes to the syndrome.

Poor placentation is an important cause of placental ischaemia, but not the only one. Its mechanisms are being elucidated by others and are not discussed in this chapter. It is not the exclusive cause of the syndrome nor is pre-eclampsia always present when it occurs. It is better considered as a separate condition which is a major predisposing factor to pre-eclampsia.

REFERENCES

Abe, M., Shintani, Y., Eto, Y. *et al.* (2002). Potent induction of activin A secretion from monocytes and bone marrow stromal fibroblasts by cognate interaction with activated T cells. *J. Leukocyte Biol.*, **72**, 347–52.

Ahmed, A., Dunk, C., Ahmad, S. & Khaliq, A. (2000a). Regulation of placental vascular endothelial growth factor (VEGF) and placenta growth factor (PIGF) and soluble Flt-1 by oxygen – a review. *Placenta*, **21** (Suppl A), S16–24.

Ahmed, I., Perkins, A. V., Glynn, B. P. *et al.* (2000b). Processing of procorticotrophin releasing hormone (proCRH): molecular forms of CRH in placentae from normal and pre-eclamptic pregnancies. *J. Clin. Endocrinol. Metab.*, **85**, 755–64.

Allaire, A. D., Ballenger, K. A., Wells, S. R., McMahon, M. J. & Lessey, B. A. (2000). Placental apoptosis in preeclampsia. *Obstet. Gynecol.*, **96**, 271–6.

Alsat, E., Wyplosz, P., Malassine, A. *et al.* (1996). Hypoxia impairs cell fusion and differentiation process in human cytotrophoblast, *in vitro*. *J. Cell. Physiol.*, **168**, 346–53.

Arnalich, F., Lopez, J., Codoceo, R. *et al.* (1999). Relationship of plasma leptin to plasma cytokines and human survival in sepsis and septic shock. *J. Infect. Dis.*, **180**, 908–11.

Aupeix, K., Hugel, B., Martin, T. *et al.* (1997). The significance of shed membrane particles during programmed cell death *in vitro*, and *in vivo*, in HIV-1 infection. *J. Clin. Invest.*, **99**, 1546–54.

Austgulen, R., Isaksen, C. V., Chedwick, L. *et al.* (2004). Preeclampsia: associated with increased syncytial apoptosis when the infant is small-for-gestational-age. *J. Reprod. Immunol.*, **61**, 39–50.

Barleon, B., Reusch, P., Totzke, F. *et al.* (2001). Soluble VEGFR-1 secreted by endothelial cells and monocytes is present in human serum and plasma from healthy donors. *Angiogenesis*, **4**, 143–54.

Barr, F. G., Biegel, J. A., Sellinger, B., Womer, R. B. & Emanuel, B. S. (1991). Molecular and cytogenetic analysis of chromosomal arms 2q and 13q in alveolar rhabdomyosarcoma. *Genes Chromosomes Cancer*, **3**, 153–61.

Belgore, F. M., Lip, G. Y. & Blann, A. D. (2000). Vascular endothelial growth factor and its receptor, Flt-1, in smokers and non-smokers. *Br. J. Biomed. Sci.*, **57**, 207–13.

Belgore, F. M., Blann, A. D., Li, S. H., Beevers, D. G. & Lip, G. Y. (2001a). Plasma levels of vascular endothelial growth factor and its soluble receptor (sFlt-1) in essential hypertension. *Am. J. Cardiol.*, **87**, 805–7.

Belgore, F.M., Blann, A.D. & Lip, G.Y. (2001b). Measurement of free and complexed soluble vascular endothelial growth factor receptor, Flt-1, in fluid samples: development and application of two new immunoassays. *Clin. Sci. (Lond.)*, **100**, 567–75.

Blond, J.L., Lavillette, D., Cheynet, V. *et al.* (2000). An envelope glycoprotein of the human endogenous retrovirus HERV-W is expressed in the human placenta and fuses cells expressing the type D mammalian retrovirus receptor. *J. Virol.*, **74**, 3321–9.

Blumenstein, M., Mitchell, M.D., Groome, N.P. & Keelan, J.A. (2002). Hypoxia inhibits activin A production by term villous trophoblast *in vitro*. *Placenta*, **23**, 735–41.

Bowen, R.S., Moodley, J., Dutton, M.F. & Theron, A.J. (2001). Oxidative stress in preeclampsia. *Acta Obstet. Gynecol. Scand.*, **80**, 719–25.

Boyd, P.A. & Scott, A. (1985). Quantitative structural studies on human placentae associated with preeclampsia, essential hypertension and intrauterine growth retardation. *Br. J. Obstet. Gynaecol.*, **92**, 714–21.

Boyd, P.A., Lindenbaum, R.H. & Redman, C.W.G. (1987). Preeclampsia and trisomy 13: a possible association. *Lancet*, **ii**, 425–7.

Brosens, I. & Renaer, M. (1972). On the pathogenesis of placental infarcts in preeclampsia. *J. Obstet. Gynaecol. Br. Commonw.*, **79**, 794–9.

Brosens, I.A., Robertson, W.B. & Dixon, H.G. (1972). The role of the spiral arteries in the pathogenesis of preeclampsia. *Obstet. Gynecol. Annu.*, **1**, 177–91.

Brosens, I., Dixon, H.G. & Robertson, W.B. (1977). Fetal growth retardation and the arteries of the placental bed. *Br. J. Obstet. Gynaecol.*, **84**, 656–63.

Campbell, E.A., Linton, E.A., Wolfe, C.D. *et al.* (1987). Plasma corticotropin-releasing hormone concentrations during pregnancy and parturition *J. Clin. Endocrinol. Metab.*, **64**, 1054–9.

Cester, N., Staffolani, R., Rabini, R.A. *et al.* (1994). Pregnancy induced hypertension: a role for peroxidation in microvillus plasma membranes. *Mol. Cell. Biochem.*, **131**, 151–5.

Chun, D., Braga, C., Chow, C. & Lok, L. (1964). Clinical observations on some aspects of hydatidiform moles. *J. Obstet. Gynaecol. Br. Commonw.*, **71**, 180–4.

Clark, D.E., Smith, S.K., He, Y. *et al.* (1998). A vascular endothelial growth factor antagonist is produced by the human placenta and released into the maternal circulation. *Biol. Reprod.*, **59**, 1540–8.

Coppack, S.W. (2001). Pro-inflammatory cytokines and adipose tissue. *Proc. Nutr. Soc.*, **60**, 349–56.

de Waard, V., van-den Berg, B., Veken, J. *et al.* (1999). Serial analysis of gene expression to assess the endothelial cell response to an atherogenic stimulus. *Gene*, **226**, 1–8.

De Wolf, F., Robertson, W.B. & Brosens, I. (1975). The ultrastructure of acute atherosis in hypertensive pregnancy. *Am. J. Obstet. Gynecol.*, **123**, 164–74.

De Wolf, F., Brosens, I. & Renaer, M. (1980). Fetal growth retardation and the maternal arterial supply of the human placenta in the absence of sustained hypertension. *Br. J. Obstet. Gynaecol.*, **87**, 678–85.

De Wolf, F., Brosens, I. & Robertson, W.B. (1982). Ultrastructure of uteroplacental arteries. *Contrib. Gynecol. Obstet.*, **9**, 86–99.

Douglas, K.A. & Redman, C.W. (1994). Eclampsia in the United Kingdom. *BMJ*, **309**, 1395–1400.

Eramaa, M., Hurme, M., Stenman, U.H. & Ritvos, O. (1992). Activin A/erythroid differentiation factor is induced during human monocyte activation. *J. Exp. Med.*, **176**, 1449–52.

Esterman, A., Greco, M.A., Mitani, Y. et al. (1997). The effect of hypoxia on human trophoblast in culture: morphology, glucose transport and metabolism. Placenta, 18, 129–36.

Fantuzzi, G. & Faggioni, R. (2000). Leptin in the regulation of immunity, inflammation, and hematopoiesis. J. Leukocyte Biol., 68, 437–46.

Felmeden, D.C., Spencer, C.G., Belgore, F.M. et al. (2003). Endothelial damage and angiogenesis in hypertensive patients: relationship to cardiovascular risk factors and risk factor management. Am. J. Hypertens., 16, 11–20.

Furui, T., Kurauchi, O., Tanaka, M., et al. (1994). Decrease in cytochrome c oxidase and cytochrome oxidase subunit I messenger RNA levels in preeclamptic pregnancies. Obstet. Gynecol., 84, 283–8.

Gaber, L.W., Spargo, B.H. & Lindheimer, M.D. (1994). Renal pathology in pre-eclampsia. Builliere's Clin. Obstet. Gynecol., 8, 443–68.

Garner, P.R., D'Alton, M.E., Dudley, D.K., Huard, P. & Hardie, M. (1990). Preeclampsia in diabetic pregnancies. Am. J. Obstet. Gynecol., 163, 505–8.

Gavrilova, O., Barr, V., Marcus, S.B. & Reitman, M. (1997). Hyperleptinemia of pregnancy associated with the appearance of a circulating form of the leptin receptor. J. Biol. Chem., 272, 30546–51.

Germain, S.J., Knight, M., Sooranna, S.R., Redman, C.W.G. & Sargent, I.L. (2002). Interaction of circulating syncytiotrophoblast microvillous fragments with maternal monocytes in normal and pre-eclamptic pregnancies. J. Soc. Gynecol. Invest., 9(Suppl), 259A.

Gratacos, E., Casals, E., Deulofeu R., et al. (1998). Lipid peroxide and vitamin E patterns in pregnant women with different types of hypertension in pregnancy. Am. J. Obstet. Gynecol., 178, 1072–6.

Grosfeld, A., Turban, S., Andre, J. et al. (2001). Transcriptional effect of hypoxia on placental leptin. FEBS Lett, 502, 122–6.

Hansson, G.K., Libby, P., Schönbeck, U. & Yan, Z.Q. (2002). Innate and adaptive immunity in the pathogenesis of atherosclerosis. Circ. Res., 91, 281–91.

Hardy, D.B. & Yang, K. (2002). The expression of 11 β-hydroxysteroid dehydrogenase type 2 is induced during trophoblast differentiation: effects of hypoxia. J. Clin. Endocrinol. Metab., 87, 3696–701.

He, L., Wang, Z. & Sun, Y. (2004). Reduced amount of cytochrome c oxidase subunit I messenger RNA in placentae from pregnancies complicated by preeclampsia. Acta Obstet. Gynecol. Scand., 83, 144–8.

Hertig, A.T. (1945). Vascular pathology in the hypertensive albuminuric toxemias of pregnancy. Clinics, 4, 602–14.

Ho, S., Winkler-Lowen, L.B., Morrish, D.W. et al. (1999). The role of Bcl-2 expression in EGF inhibition of TNF-alpha/IFN-gamma-induced villous trophoblast apoptosis. Placenta, 20, 423–30.

Holland, E. (1909). Recent work on the aetiology of eclampsia. J. Obstet. Gynaecol. Br. Emp., 16, 255–73.

Hornig, C., Barleon, B., Ahmad, S. et al. (2000). Release and complex formation of soluble VEGFR-1 from endothelial cells and biological fluids. Lab. Invest., 80, 443–54.

Huang, L., Wang, Z. & Li, C. (2001). Modulation of circulating leptin levels by its soluble receptor. *J. Biol. Chem.*, **276**, 6343–9.

Huppertz, B., Frank, H.G., Kingdom, J.C., Reister, F. & Kaufmann, P. (1998). Villous cytotrophoblast regulation of the syncytial apoptotic cascade in the human placenta. *Histochem. Cell Biol.*, **110**, 495–508.

Huppertz, B., Kingdom, J., Caniggia, I. *et al.* (2003). Hypoxia favours necrotic versus apoptotic shedding of placental syncytiotrophoblast into the maternal circulation. *Placenta*, **24**, 181–90.

Ishihara, N., Matsuo, H., Murakoshi, H. *et al.* (2002). Increased apoptosis in the syncytiotrophoblast in human term placentae complicated by either preeclampsia or intrauterine growth retardation. *Am. J. Obstet. Gynecol.*, **186**, 158–66.

Jones, C.J. & Fox, H. (1980). An ultrastructural and ultrahistochemical study of the human placenta in maternal preeclampsia. *Placenta*, **1**, 61–76.

Kabbinavar, F., Hurwitz, H.I., Fehrenbacher, L. *et al.* (2003). Phase II, randomized trial comparing bevacizumab plus fluorouracil (FU)/leucovorin (LV) with FU/LV alone in patients with metastatic colorectal cancer. *J. Clin. Oncol.*, **21**, 60–5.

Karalis, K., Muglia, J.L., Bae, D., Hilderbrand, H. & Majzoub, J.A. (1997). CRH and the immune system. *J. Neuroimmunol.*, **172**, 131–6.

Khong, T.Y. (1991). Acute atherosis in pregnancies complicated by hypertension, small-for-gestational-age infants, and diabetes mellitus. *Arch. Pathol. Lab. Med.*, **115**, 722–5.

Kliman, H.J., Nestler, J.E., Sermasi, E., Sanger, J.M. & Strauss, J.F. (1986). Purification, characterization, and *in vitro* differentiation of cytotrophoblasts from human term placentae. *Endocrinology*, **118**, 1567–82.

Kluck, R.M., Bossy, W.E., Green, D.R. & Newmeyer, D.D. (1997). The release of cytochrome c from mitochondria: a primary site for Bcl-2 regulation of apoptosis. *Science*, **275**, 1132–6.

Knapen, M.F., Peters, W.H., Mulder, T.P. *et al.* (1999). Glutathione and glutathione-related enzymes in decidua and placenta of controls and women with pre-eclampsia. *Placenta*, **20**, 541–6.

Knerr, I., Beinder, E. & Rascher, W. (2002). Syncytin, a novel human endogenous retroviral gene in human placenta: evidence for its dysregulation in pre-eclampsia and HELLP syndrome. *Am. J. Obstet. Gynecol.*, **186**, 210–13.

Knerr, I., Weigel, C., Linnemann, K. *et al.* (2003). Transcriptional effects of hypoxia on fusiogenic syncytin and its receptor ASCT2 in human cytotrophoblast BeWo cells and in ex vivo perfused placental cotyledons. *Am. J. Obstet. Gynecol.*, **189**, 583–8.

Knight, M., Redman, C.W., Linton, E.A. & Sargent, I.L. (1998). Shedding of syncytiotrophoblast microvilli into the maternal circulation in pre-eclamptic pregnancies. *Br. J. Obstet. Gynaecol.*, **105**, 632–40.

Kudo, Y. & Boyd, C.A. (1990). Characterization of amino acid transport systems in human placental basal membrane vesicles. *Biochim. Biophys. Acta*, **1021**, 169–74.

Kudo, Y., Boyd, C.A., Sargent, I.L. & Redman, C.W. (2003). Hypoxia alters expression and function of syncytin and its receptor during trophoblast cell fusion of human placental BeWo cells: implications for impaired trophoblast syncytialization in pre-eclampsia. *Biochim. Biophys. Acta*, **1638**, 63–71.

Kumar, S., Lo, D.Y.M., Smarason, A.K. *et al.* (2000). Pre-eclampsia is associated with increased levels of circulating apoptotic microparticles and fetal cell-free DNA. *J. Soc. Gynecol. Invest.*, 7(Suppl), 181a.

Lammert, A., Kiess, W., Bottner, A., Glasow, A. & Kratzsch, J. (2001). Soluble leptin receptor represents the main leptin binding activity in human blood. *Biochem. Biophys. Res. Commun.*, **283**, 982–8.

Lavillette, D., Marin, M., Ruggieri, A. *et al.* (2002). The envelope glycoprotein of human endogenous retrovirus type W uses a divergent family of amino acid transporters/cell surface receptors. *J. Virol.*, **76**, 6442–52.

Lee, X., Keith, J.-C.J., Stumm, N. *et al.* (2001). Downregulation of placental syncytin expression and abnormal protein localization in preeclampsia. *Placenta*, **22**, 808–12.

Leu, S.J. & Singh, V.K. (1991). Modulation of natural killer cell-mediated lysis by corticotropin-releasing neurohormone. *J. Neuroimmunol.*, **33**, 253–60.

Leung, D.N., Smith, S.C., To, K.F., Sahota, D.S. & Baker, P.N. (2001). Increased placental apoptosis in pregnancies complicated by preeclampsia. *Am. J. Obstet. Gynecol.*, **184**, 1249–50.

Levy, R., Smith, S.D., Chandler, K., Sadovsky, Y. & Nelson, D.M. (2000). Apoptosis in human cultured trophoblasts is enhanced by hypoxia and diminished by epidermal growth factor. *Am. J. Physiol. Cell. Physiol.*, **278**, C982–8.

Li, H., Dakour, J., Kaufman, S. *et al.* (2003). Adrenomedullin is decreased in preeclampsia because of failed response to epidermal growth factor and impaired syncytialization. *Hypertension*, **42**, 895–900.

Linton, E.A., Behan, D.P., Saphier, P.W. & Lowry, P.J. (1990). Corticotropin-releasing hormone binding protein: reduction in the ACTH releasing activity of placental but not hypothalamic CRF. *J. Clin. Endocrinol. Metab.*, **70**, 1574–80.

Linton, E.A., Perkins, A.V., Woods, R.J. *et al.* (1993). Corticotropin-releasing hormone-binding protein (CRH-BP) plasma levels decrease during the third trimester of normal human pregnancy. *J. Clin. Endocrinol. Metab.*, **76**, 260–2.

Little, W.A. (1960). Placental infarction. *Obstet. Gynecol.*, **15**, 109–30.

Lo, Y.M., Leung, T.N., Tein, M.S. *et al.* (1999). Quantitative abnormalities of fetal DNA in maternal serum in preeclampsia. *Clin. Chem.*, **45**, 184–8.

Masuzaki, H., Ogawa, Y., Sagawa, N. *et al.* (1997). Nonadipose tissue production of leptin: leptin as a novel placenta-derived hormone in humans. *Nat. Med.*, **3**, 1029–33.

Matsubara, S., Minakami, H., Sato, I. & Saito, T. (1997). Decrease in cytochrome c oxidase activity detected cytochemically in the placental trophoblast of patients with preeclampsia. *Placenta*, **18**, 255–9.

Mayhew, T.M., Leach, L., McGee, R. *et al.* (1999). Proliferation, differentiation and apoptosis in villous trophoblast at 13–41 weeks of gestation (including observations on annulate lamellae and nuclear pore complexes). *Placenta*, **20**, 407–22.

Mayne, S.T. (2003). Antioxidant nutrients and chronic disease: use of biomarkers of exposure and oxidative stress status in epidemiologic research. *J. Nutr.*, **133**, (Suppl 3), 933S–40S.

Maynard, S.E, Min, J.Y., Merchan, J. *et al.* (2003). Excess placental soluble fms-like tyrosine kinase 1 (sFlt1) may contribute to endothelial dysfunction, hypertension, and proteinuria in preeclampsia. *J. Clin. Invest.*, **111**, 649–58.

McCarthy, S.A. & Bicknell, R. (1993). Inhibition of vascular endothelial cell growth by activin-A. *J. Biol. Chem.*, **268**, 23066–71.

McCarthy, J.F., Misra, D.N. & Roberts, J.M. (1999). Maternal plasma leptin is increased in preeclampsia and positively correlates with fetal cord concentration. *Am. J. Obstet. Gynecol.*, **180**, 731–6.

Mi, S., Lee, X., Li, X. *et al.* (2000). Syncytin is a captive retroviral envelope protein involved in human placental morphogenesis. *Nature*, **403**, 785–9.

Michel, U., Ebert, S., Phillips, D. & Nau, R. (2003). Serum concentrations of activin and follistatin are elevated and run in parallel in patients with septicemia. *Eur. J. Endocrinol.* **148**, 559–64.

Mise, H., Sagawa, N., Matsumoto, T. *et al.* (1998). Augmented placental production of leptin in preeclampsia: possible involvement of placental hypoxia. *J. Clin. Endocrinol. Metab.*, **83**, 3225–9.

Mohan, A., Asselin, J., Sargent, I.L., Groome, N.P. & Muttukrishna, S. (2001). Effect of cytokines and growth factors on the secretion of inhibin A, activin A and follistatin by term placental villous trophoblasts in culture. *Eur. J. Endocrinol.*, **145**, 505–11.

Morikawa, S., Kurauchi, O., Tanaka, M. *et al.* (1997). Increased mitochondrial damage by lipid peroxidation in trophoblast cells of preeclamptic placentae. *Biochem. Mol. Biol. Int.*, **41**, 767–75.

Muttukrishna, S., Knight, P.G., Groome, N.P., Redman, C.W. & Ledger, W.L. (1997). Activin A and inhibin A as possible endocrine markers for preeclampsia. *Lancet*, **349**, 1285–8.

Muttukrishna, S., North, R.A., Morris, J. *et al.* (2000). Serum inhibin A and activin A are elevated prior to the onset of preeclampsia. *Hum. Reprod.*, **15**, 1640–5.

Myatt, L., Rosenfield, R.B., Eis, A.L. *et al.* (1996). Nitrotyrosine residues in placenta. Evidence of peroxynitrite formation and action. *Hypertension*, **28**, 488–93.

Myatt, L., Eis, A.L., Brockman, D.E. *et al.* (1997). Differential localization of superoxide dismutase isoforms in placental villous tissue of normotensive, pre-eclamptic, and intrauterine growth-restricted pregnancies. *J. Histochem. Cytochem.*, **45**, 1433–8.

Naicker, T., Khedun, S.M., Moodley, J. & Pijnenborg, R. (2003). Quantitative analysis of trophoblast invasion in preeclampsia. *Acta Obstet. Gynecol. Scand.*, **82**, 722–9.

Navarra, P., Miceli, F., Tringali, G. *et al.* (2001). Evidence for a functional link between the heme oxygenase-carbon monoxide pathway and corticotropin-releasing hormone release from primary cultures of human trophoblast cells. *J. Clin. Endocrinol. Metab.*, **86**, 317–23.

Nelson, D.M. (1996). Apoptotic changes occur in syncytiotrophoblast of human placental villi where fibrin type fibrinoid is deposited at discontinuities in the villous trophoblast. *Placenta*, **17**, 387–91.

Ness, R.B. & Roberts, J.M. (1996). Heterogeneous causes constituting the single syndrome of preeclampsia, a hypothesis and its implications. *Am. J. Obstet. Gynecol.*, **175**, 1365–70.

Ng, E.K., Leung, T.N., Tsui, N.B. *et al.* (2003a). The concentration of circulating corticotropin-releasing hormone mRNA in maternal plasma is increased in preeclampsia. *Clin. Chem.*, **49**, 727–31.

Ng, E.K.O., Tsui, N.B.Y., Lau, T.K. *et al.* (2003b). mRNA of placental origin is readily detectable in maternal plasma. *Proc. Natl. Acad. Sci. U.S.A.*, **100**, 4748–53.

Norman, M., Eriksson, C.G. & Eneroth, P. (1989). A comparison between the composition of maternal peripheral plasma and plasma collected from the retroplacental compartment at

Caesarean section. A study on protein and steroid hormones and binding proteins. *Arch. Gynecol. Obstet.*, **244**, 215–26.

Nuamah, M. A., Sagawa, N., Yura, S. *et al.* (2003). Free-to-total leptin ratio in maternal plasma is constant throughout human pregnancy. *Endocr. J.*, **50**, 421–8.

Ohguchi, M., Yamato, K., Ishihara, Y. *et al.* (1998). Activin A regulates the production of mature interleukin-1beta and interleukin-1 receptor antagonist in human monocytic cells. *J. Interferon Cytokine Res.*, **18**, 491–8.

Paez Pereda, M., Sauer, J., Perez-Castro, C. *et al.* (1995). Corticotropin-releasing hormone differentially modulates the interleukin-1 system according to the level of monocyte activation by endotoxin. *Endocrinology*, **136**, 5504–10.

Page, N. M., Woods, R. J., Gardiner, S. M. *et al.* (2000). Excessive placental secretion of neurokinin B during the third trimester causes preeclampsia. *Nature*, **405**, 797–800.

Park, H. Y., Kwon, H. M., Lim, H. J. *et al.* (2001). Potential role of leptin in angiogenesis: leptin induces endothelial cell proliferation and expression of matrix metalloproteinases *in vivo* and *in vitro*. *Exp. Mol. Med.*, **33**, 95–102.

Patel, R. P., McAndrew, J., Sellak, H. *et al.* (1999). Biological aspects of reactive nitrogen species. *Biochim. Biophys. Acta*, **1411**, 385–400.

Perkins, A. V. & Linton, E. A. (1995). Identification and isolation of corticotrophin-releasing hormone-positive cells from the human placenta. *Placenta*, **16**, 233–43.

Perkins, A. V., Linton, E. A., Eben, F. *et al.* (1995). Corticotrophin-releasing hormone and corticotrophin-releasing hormone binding protein in normal and pre-eclamptic human pregnancies. *Br. J. Obstet. Gynaecol.*, **102**, 118–22.

Piering, W. F., Garancis, J. G., Becker, C. G., Beres, J. A. & Lemann, J. (1993). Preeclampsia related to a functioning extrauterine placenta, report of a case and 25-year follow-up. *Am. J. Kidney Dis.*, **21**, 310–13.

Pijnenborg, R., Anthony, J., Davey, D. A. *et al.* (1991). Placental bed spiral arteries in the hypertensive disorders of pregnancy. *Br. J. Obstet. Gynaecol.*, **98**, 648–55.

Pijnenborg, R., Luyten, C., Vercruysse, L. & Van Assche, F. A. (1996). Attachment and differentiation *in vitro* of trophoblast from normal and preeclamptic human placentae. *Am. J. Obstet. Gynecol.*, **175**, 30–6.

Poranen, A. K., Ekblad, U., Uotila, P. & Ahotupa, M. (1996). Lipid peroxidation and antioxidants in normal and pre-eclamptic pregnancies. *Placenta*, **17**, 401–5.

Poston, L. (2003). The role of oxidative stress. In J. J. & Walker L. Poston, eds., *Preeclampsia, Proceedings of RCOG Study Group*. London: RCOG Press, pp. 134–46.

Redman, C. W. G. (1991). Current topic. Preeclampsia and the placenta. *Placenta*, **12**, 301–8.

(1992). The placenta and preeclampsia. In C. W. G. Redman, I. L. & Sargent, P. M. Starkey, eds., *The Human Placenta*. Oxford: Blackwell Scientific Publications, pp. 433–67.

Redman, C. W. G. & Sargent, I. L. (2000). Placental debris, oxidative stress and preeclampsia. *Placenta*, **21**, 597–602.

Redman, C. W. G., Sacks, G. P. & Sargent, I. L. (1999). Preeclampsia, an excessive maternal inflammatory response to pregnancy. *Am. J. Obstet. Gynecol.*, **180**, 499–506.

Reimer, T., Koczan, D., Gerber, B. *et al.* (2002). Microarray analysis of differentially expressed genes in placental tissue of preeclampsia: upregulation of obesity-related genes. *Mol. Hum. Reprod.*, **8**, 674–80.

Roberts, J.M., Taylor, R.N., Musci, T.J. *et al.* (1989). Preeclampsia, an endothelial cell disorder. *Am. J. Obstet. Gynecol.*, **161**, 1200–4.

Robertson, W.B., Brosens, I. & Dixon, G. (1976). Maternal uterine vascular lesions in the hypertensive complications of pregnancy. *Perspect. Nephrol. Hypertens.*, **5**, 115–27.

Robertson, W.B., Brosens, I. & Landells, W.N. (1985). Abnormal placentation. *Obstet. Gynecol. Annu.*, **14**, 411–26.

Robinson, B.G., Arbiser, J.L., Emanuel, R.L. & Majzoub, J.A. (1989). Species-specific placental corticotropin releasing hormone messenger RNA and peptide expression. *Mol. Cell. Endocrinol.*, **62**, 337–41.

Ros, H.S., Cnattingius, S. & Lipworth, L. (1998). Comparison of risk factors for preeclampsia and gestational hypertension in a population-based cohort study. *Am. J. Epidemiol.*, **147**, 1062–70.

Russell, C.E., Hedger, M.P., Brauman, J.N., de Krester, D.M. & Phillips, D.J. (1999). Activin A regulates growth and acute phase proteins in the human lives cell line, HepQ2. *Mol. Cell. Endocrinol.* **148**, 129–36.

Sahlin, L., Ostlund, E., Wang, H., Homgren, A. & Fried, G. (2000). Decreased expression of thioredoxin and glutaredoxin in placentae from pregnancies with preeclampsia and intrauterine growth restriction. *Placenta*, **21**, 603–9.

Sakuragi, N., Matsuo, H., Coukos, G. *et al.* (1994). Differentiation-dependent expression of the BCL-2 proto-oncogene in the human trophoblast lineage. *J. Soc. Gynecol. Invest.*, **1**, 164–72.

Santoso, D.I., Rogers, P., Wallace, E.M. *et al.* (2002). Localization of indoleamine 2,3-dioxygenase and 4-hydroxynonenal in normal and pre-eclamptic placentae. *Placenta*, **23**, 373–9.

Sasaki, A., Shinkawa, O., Margioris, A.N. *et al.* (1987). Immunoreactive corticotropin-releasing hormone in human plasma during pregnancy, labor, and delivery. *J. Clin. Endocrinol. Metab.*, **64**, 224–9.

Sattar, N., Greer, I.A., Pirwani, I., Gibson, J. & Wallace, A.M. (1998). Leptin levels in pregnancy: marker for fat accumulation and mobilization? *Acta. Obstet. Gynecol. Scand.*, **77**, 278–83.

Schneider-Kolsky, M.E., Manuelpillai, U., Waldron, K., Dole, A. & Wallace, E.M. (2002). The distribution of activin and activin receptors in gestational tissues across human pregnancy and during labour. *Placenta*, **23**, 294–302.

Schrocksnadel, H., Daxenbichler, G., Artner, E., Steckel-Berger, G. & Dapunt, O. (1993). Tumor markers in hypertensive disorders of pregnancy. *Gynecol. Obstet. Invest.*, **35**, 204–8.

Senaris, R., Garcia, C.T., Casabiell, X. *et al.* (1997). Synthesis of leptin in human placenta. *Endocrinology*, **138**, 4501–4.

Serdar, Z., Gur, E., Colakoethullary, M., Develioethlu, O. & Sarandol, E. (2003). Lipid and protein oxidation and antioxidant function in women with mild and severe preeclampsia. *Arch. Gynecol. Obstet.*, **268**, 19–25.

Sheppard, B.L. & Bonnar, J. (1976). The ultrastructure of the arterial supply of the human placenta in pregnancy complicated by fetal growth retardation. *Br. J. Obstet. Gynaecol.*, **83**, 948–59.

Shibata, E., Ejima, K., Nanri, H. *et al.* (2001). Enhanced protein levels of protein thiol/disulphide oxidoreductases in placentae from pre-eclamptic subjects. *Placenta*, **22**, 566–72.

Shibata, E., Nanri, H., Ejima, K. *et al.* (2003). Enhancement of mitochondrial oxidative stress and upregulation of antioxidant protein peroxiredoxin III/SP-22 in the mitochondria of human pre-eclamptic placentae. *Placenta*, **24**, 698–705.

Sibai, B. M., Gordon, T., Thom, E. *et al.* (1995). Risk factors for preeclampsia in healthy nulliparous women: a prospective multicenter study. The National Institute of Child Health and Human Development Network of Maternal-Fetal Medicine Units. *Am. J. Obstet. Gynecol.*, **172**, 642–8.

Sierra-Honigmann, M. R., Nath, A. K. Mwakami, C. *et al.* (1998). Biological action of leptin as an angiogenic factor. *Science*, **281**, 1683–6.

Sikkema, J. M., van Rijn, B. B., Franx, A. *et al.* (2001). Placental superoxide is increased in preeclampsia. *Placenta*, **22**, 304–8.

Smarason, A. K., Sargent, I. L., Starkey, P. M. & Redman, C. W.G. (1993). The effect of placental syncytiotrophoblast microvillous membranes from normal and pre-eclamptic women on the growth of endothelial cells *in vitro. Br. J. Obstet. Gynaecol.*, **100**, 943–9.

Smith, G. C., Pell, J. P. & Walsh, D. (2001). Pregnancy complications and maternal risk of ischaemic heart disease: a retrospective cohort study of 129,290 births. *Lancet*, **357**, 2002–6.

Staff, A. C., Ranheim, T., Khoury, J. & Henriksen, T. (1999). Increased contents of phospholipids, cholesterol, and lipid peroxides in decidua basalis in women with preeclampsia. *Am. J. Obstet. Gynecol.*, **180**, 587–92.

Takacs, P., Kauma, S. W., Sholley, M. M. *et al.* (2001). Increased circulating lipid peroxides in severe preeclampsia activate NF-KappaB and upregulate ICAM-1 in vascular endothelial cells. *FASEB J.*, **15**, 279–81.

Tannetta, D. S., Muttukrishna, S., Groome, N. P., Redman, C. W. & Sargent, I. L. (2003). Endothelial cells and peripheral blood mononuclear cells are a potential source of extraplacental activin a in preeclampsia. *J. Clin. Endocrinol. Metab.*, **88**, 5995–6001.

Tsatsaris, V., Goffin, F., Munaut, C. *et al.* (2003). Over-expression of the soluble vascular endothelial growth factor receptor in preeclamptic patients: pathophysiological consequences. *J. Clin. Endocrinol. Metab.*, **88**, 5555–63.

Von Dadelszen, P., Hurst, G. & Redman, C. W.G. (1999). The supernatants from co-cultured endothelial cells and syncytiotrophoblast microvillous membranes activate peripheral blood leucocytes *in vitro. Hum. Reprod.*, **14**, 919–24.

Vuorinen, K., Remes, A., Sormunen, R., Tapanainen, J. & Hassinen, I. E. (1998). Placental mitochondrial DNA and respiratory chain enzymes in the etiology of preeclampsia. *Obstet. Gynecol.*, **91**, 950–955.

Wallenburg, H. C., Stolte, L. A. M. & Janssens, J. (1973). The pathogenesis of placental infarction I. A morphologic study in the human placenta. *Am. J. Obstet. Gynecol.*, **116**, 835–40.

Walsh, S. W. & Wang, Y. (1993). Deficient glutathione peroxidase activity in preeclampsia is associated with increased placental production of thromboxane and lipid peroxides. *Am. J. Obstet. Gynecol.*, **169**, 1456–61.

Wang, Y. & Walsh, S. W. (1996). Antioxidant activities and mRNA expression of superoxide dismutase, catalase, and glutathione peroxidase in normal and preeclamptic placentae. *J. Soc. Gynecol. Inves.*, **3**, 179–84.

(1998). Placental mitochondria as a source of oxidative stress in preeclampsia. *Placenta*, **19**, 581–6.

(2001). Increased superoxide generation is associated with decreased superoxide dismutase activity and mRNA expression in placental trophoblast cells in preeclampsia. *Placenta*, **22**, 206–12.

Wang, Z., Zhang, G. & Lin, M. (1999). Mitochondrial tRNA(leu)(UUR) gene mutation and the decreased activity of cytochrome c oxidase in preeclampsia. *J. Tongji Med. Univ.*, **19**, 209–11.

Weinstein, L. (1982). Syndrome of hemolysis, elevated liver enzymes, and low platelet count: a severe consequence of hypertension in pregnancy. *Am. J. Obstet. Gynecol.*, **142**, 159–67.

Wentworth, P. (1967). Placental infarction and toxemia of pregnancy. *Am. J. Obstet. Gynecol.*, **99**, 318–26.

Yang, J.C., Haworth, L., Sherry, R.M. *et al.* (2003). A randomized trial of bevacizumab, an anti-vascular endothelial growth factor antibody, for metastatic renal cancer. *New Engl. J. Med.*, **349**, 427–34.

Yusuf, K., Smith, S.D., Sadovsky, Y. & Nelson, D.M. (2002). Trophoblast differentiation modulates the activity of caspases in primary cultures of term human trophoblasts. *Pediatr. Res.*, **52**, 411–15.

Zabriskie, J.R. (1963). Effect of cigarette smoking during pregnancy. Study of 2000 cases. *Obstet. Gynecol.*, **21**, 405–11.

Zarkesh-Esfahani, H., Pockley, G., Metcalfe, R.A. *et al.* (2001). High-dose leptin activates human leucocytes via receptor expression on monocytes. *J. Immunol.*, **167**, 4593–9.

Zeek, P.M. & Assali, N.S. (1950). Vascular changes with eclamptogenic toxemia of pregnancy. *Am. J. Clin. Pathol.*, **20**, 1099–109.

Zhong, X.Y., Laivuori, H., Livingston, J.C. *et al.* (2001). Elevation of both maternal and fetal extracellular circulating deoxyribonucleic acid concentrations in the plasma of pregnant women with preeclampsia. *Am. J. Obstet. Gynecol.*, **184**, 414–19.

Zusterzeel, P.L., Rutten, H., Roelofs, H.M., Peters, W.H. & Steegers, E.A. (2001). Protein carbonyls in decidua and placenta of pre-eclamptic women as markers for oxidative stress. *Placenta*, **22**, 213–19.

DISCUSSION

McLaren   I get the impression that the placental form of pre-eclampsia and the maternal form are rather different. Should they be given different names and not lumped together?

Redman   It is very difficult to separate them. From the clinician's point of view they look the same. They see exaggerated blood pressure elevation, proteinuria, disturbances of the clotting system and so on. The end point is a similarly exaggerated systemic inflammatory response. It makes sense to treat them as the same clinically. When it comes to research studies, some effort has to be made to separate them. The question is, how? The simplest way is to use the modern tools that are available to study what is going on in the placental circulation. This can now be done, but rarely is. In some cases of pre-eclampsia there is nothing wrong with the uteroplacental circulation or the fetal placental circulation.

Moffett   Is that in a minority of cases?

Redman   I don't know. The severest cases are a mixture of maternal and placental disease. These are the ones that occur very early. The very late onset disease is often not associated with any apparent placental problem. Where you can find a pure placental problem is probably in the disease with minimal maternal manifestations and maximum fetal manifestations.

Evain-Brion   From a clinical viewpoint, is the placental form of pre-eclampsia more often associated with severe intrauterine growth retardation?

Redman   I would imagine so. But when you look at the severe early onset disease with the maximum growth retardation, many of those women also have maternal conditions that would be predisposing. It seems to be a combination of the maternal and placental problems. I don't think this has been sorted out clearly. I can't be more precise than this.

Braude   In the theory that you put forward, with apoptosis in the syncytiotrophoblast, how does this square with the idea that pre-eclampsia tends not to occur in second pregnancies, or the fact that, of those who have had it severely, only a small percentage will get it in the next pregnancy? What is the modulating feature?

Redman   It is the uterine placental circulation, which is altered by pregnancy in some way.

Braude   It is a new placenta.

Redman   Yes, but it is the old maternal vessels. There is a wonderful radiograph that compares the uteri of a nulliparous and multiparous woman. The nulliparous woman has quite a sparse uterine circulation whereas the network is much more open and better developed in the multiparous woman. In general, multiparous women have not all just had a pregnancy. Their uteri have been examined years after the event yet retain the changes, which are presumably due to vascular remodelling. It is currently believed that when pre-eclampsia occurs in a woman who has had previously normal pregnancies, it is a long interpregnancy interval that is the relevant variable. This may mean that the vascular remodelling from a previous pregnancy is slowly lost over time. People used to emphasise the importance of a change of partner as a factor in atypical pre-eclampsia after previously normal pregnancies. But longer interpregnancy intervals are frequently associated with a change in partner, so the two factors have to be separated and currently it is the interval that seems the more important.

Smith   One of the epidemiological peculiarities of pre-eclampsia is that it is reduced among smokers. Comparing healthy smokers and non-smokers, do these circulating particles differ? Can you put your hypothesis into a context consistent with this association?

Redman	We don't know this. We do know that smoking affects the concentration of circulating soluble Flt-1 in non-pregnant individuals. It may be that this has a part to play in the process. We also know that carbon monoxide is used by the immune system as an antioxidant. There is lots of carbon monoxide in smokers' circulations.
S. Fisher	For many years we have been studying the effects of smoking on the placenta. One of the reasons was this enigmatic observation that smokers have much less pre-eclampsia. We couldn't figure this out. We did a VEGF molecule study. Trophoblast cells make every VEGF ligand and receptor. It is an amazing array of vasculogenic factors. We had several different groups of women, including those who were not exposed to smoke, those who were exposed to passive smoke and those who smoked up to two packs a day. There was a massive induction of VEGF, even in women who were just exposed to passive smoke. We thought that this effect might be attributable to VEGF.
Redman	That would fit with the Maynard model. I don't see why one should suppose otherwise than what they showed being part of the story.
Pijnenborg	I am still not sure about when the inflammatory response comes in during pregnancy. Has it anything to do with the failed invasion of the spiral arteries in the beginning of pregnancy?
Redman	We don't know. We have begun looking at the inflammatory response in very early pregnancy. There is a systemic inflammatory response well established early on in the first trimester. I suspect the origins are different. The provocative factors are to do with the growth in and remodelling of the decidua, and the effect of the placenta on the decidua, rather than the turnover of a large syncytial layer. However, Graham Burton disagrees with me: he has seen the sloughing trophoblast coming off his anoxic models in vitro.
Burton	There has been the regression of the villi over the chorion leave, which is a physiological event. One would expect some debris of the same sort to be released at that time.
Redman	I take your point, but we can't find it at the moment.
Burton	I wonder whether this is a sort of priming stimulus. Perhaps when you get a second stimulus coming along later this has a much greater effect.
Redman	A lot of events are taking place in the innate immune system of the mother right from the start. It remains to be seen what is the cause and time course.
Pijnenborg	Could acute atherosis be a direct consequence of the inflammatory reaction against invading trophoblast? I have been trying for a long time to spot remnants of trophoblastic cells in the walls of atherotic blood vessels. Sometimes we find cytokeratin-positive material buried in necrotic areas, but this is rare and difficult to find.

Lever   As a process, apoptosis is actually anti-inflammatory. Apoptotic cells don't trigger inflammation. This could either be one of those processes where excess apoptosis actually triggered inflammation, or it may be the necrotic debris that is causing the inflammation.

Redman   There is a spectrum of effects. Just by ingesting and processing any particle, cells like monocytes and dendritic cells will be moderately stimulated, but not enough to be classified as an inflammatory response. Although these changes occur in normal pregnant women, they are not ill with them. It is low key. Nevertheless there is a massive load of debris coming through, and the normal process of clearing it away provokes the modest inflammatory response that is readily measurable. It is reasonable to ascribe this to apoptotic particles. Abnormal systemic inflammation of pre-eclampsia would be much more likely to be due to necrotic debris.

Sharkey   You concentrated on membranes because these are accessible in terms of FACS analysis and quantitation. But the syncytiotrophoblast sloughs off and every antigen and cytoplasmic protein under the sun is then released. What sort of immune responses do you see to all those thousands of polymorphic proteins that the mother is subjected to?

Redman   If they are apoptotic, then they will be still inside the membrane. They are not going to be immunostimulatory.

Sharkey   You see DNA and RNA, so these have obviously been released. If apoptosis was completely efficient they would be encapsulated.

Redman   Yes. There is no evidence for a T cell-mediated response. We have just completed a study in which we have tried to work out the proposition that pregnancy itself is a T helper (Th)2 situation in which the immune responses are deviated away from cytotoxicity. Pre-eclampsia is a Th1 state in which cytotoxicity can develop. There is no evidence of any antigen-specific stimulation of T cells. When we looked at this Th1/Th2 balance we found that it doesn't involve T cells at all. It simply involves the natural killer (NK) cells. They are directing the balance either to Th2 or Th1. The NK cells are part of the inflammatory system. It does look as if immune-specific responses to the placenta aren't happening.

Loke   I see no reason why there should be a T cell response. I have a question. When you say 'acute inflammatory systemic response', I visualise phenomena such as vasodilatation and leukocyte emigration. Is this what is happening?

Redman   That is the extreme end. Mild inflammation, which is usually chronic, involves all the components of the innate immune system. It is not just leukocytes or monocytes, it is also the endothelium, platelets and complement. They are all part of the same network. In mild inflammation there will be low-grade activation of the endothelium. If the endothelium is activated it is going to produce

	vasoconstrictors. These are the factors that are known to be increased in pre-eclampsia.
Loke	Is there evidence of complement activation in pre-eclamptic women?
Redman	To a degree, yes. It is not as in major auto-immune illnesses. We published a paper showing that C4 is systematically lower in severe pre-eclampsia than in normal pregnant women (Hofmeyr *et al.* 1991).
Braude	I think it is important that people unfamiliar with clinical features of pre-eclampsia shouldn't go away thinking that this is very clear. There is no single marker for pre-eclampsia. It can't be diagnosed other than when a woman appears with some degree of hypertension plus or minus proteinuria and oedema, all of which cease when the fetus is delivered. The rest is all surmised.
Redman	No, it is not all surmised.
Braude	Even in your graphs which showed clear trends, usually you had significant outliers. There were many women with pre-eclampsia whose data were entirely the same as for normal pregnant women.
Redman	I showed you the reason why. Pre-eclampsia and normal pregnancy are part of the same spectrum of events. In the middle, where most of the clinical events are happening, whether or not there is decompensation is decided by just small changes in the normal spectrum. I would never suggest that this is a clearly distinct disease with features that separate it from normal pregnancy. If you take the extreme diseases, such as extreme pre-eclampsia and highly selected normal pregnant women, they would be separated. But we don't do that. We are working in the middle of a spectrum of changes where small differences move a woman from normal pregnancy to pre-eclampsia. The individual responsiveness to those changes will be idiosyncratic. With the same systemic changes a woman may or may not show the other signs.
Cross	What would the data look like if you separated the disease into a placental type and a maternal type, as Anne suggested? How many of the data points at the bottom are strictly maternal form or strictly placental form?
Redman	That's a good question. I don't know, but I would like to think that it would improve the separation.
Burton	In relation to that, the Hafner paper (Hafner *et al.* 2003), in which they looked at placental size by ultrasonography longitudinally, showed that in the early-onset intrauterine growth retardation (IUGR)-associated pre-eclampsia, placental size was small even at 12 weeks. Then it followed a different trajectory, whereas in the late-onset pre-eclampsia placental growth was increased in the second trimester and only tailed off in the start of the third.
Redman	That's a highly relevant point. Ultrasonographic examination of the placenta and its circulation is going to be the key to this separation. We haven't begun to do this

systematically. It is obviously very important to do this, and I just don't know how these results would change if we did this again using that technique.

Pijnenborg Why doesn't pre-eclampsia occur in other species? Is it something special about the human placenta?

Redman Spontaneous cases have been reported from zoos in gorillas and chimpanzees.

Cross It occurs in genetically modified mice through perturbations on the maternal side or the fetal placental side.

Redman There are apparently good models in rats and sheep, but the disease is not spontaneous.

REFERENCES

Hafner, E., Metzenbauer, M., Hofinger, D. *et al.* (2003). Placental growth from the first to the second trimester of pregnancy in SGA-foetuses and pre-eclamptic pregnancies compared to normal foetuses. *Placenta*, **24**, 336–42.

Hofmeyr, G.J., Wilkins, T. & Redman, C.W. (1991). C4 and plasma protein in hypertension during pregnancy with and without proteinuria. *BMJ*, **302**, 218.

11

Trophoblast and uterine mucosal leukocytes

Ashley Moffett

University of Cambridge, UK

Introduction

The mucosal lining of the uterus is transformed from endometrium in the non-pregnant state to the decidua of pregnancy. This transformation is induced under the influence of progesterone and is associated with leukocyte infiltration (Loke & King 1995, King 2000). In decidua, 70% of the infiltrating leukocytes are CD56[bright] natural killer (NK) cells together with some macrophages. Only small numbers of T cells are present (5%–15% of leukocytes) and B cells are virtually absent (King et al. 1989). Thus, at the site of trophoblast invasion in the first trimester, an influx of cells of the specific adaptive immune system does not occur so it seems unlikely that a maternal classical immune response to trophoblast is generated in the decidua. In contrast, there is an accumulation of innate immune cells, such as NK cells and macrophages at the implantation site. Recently, a population of dendritic cells (DCs) have been isolated and characterised from human decidua which have the phenotype of immature myeloid DCs (Gardner & Moffett 2003).

Uterine NK cells

The infiltration of uterine (u)NK cells is a part of the cyclical changes of the endometrium and it is clearly influenced by sex hormones, particularly progesterone. Recently, endometrial-derived interleukin (IL)15 and prolactin have been implicated in the proliferation and differentiation of these cells. Both of these hormones are produced by mucosal stromal cells and their production is up-regulated by progesterone as decidualisation occurs (Dunn et al. 2002, Gubbay et al. 2002). Uterine NK cells are small and agranular in the proliferative pre-ovulatory phase. They then proliferate, enlarge and become increasingly granulated in the post-ovulatory secretory phase (Spornitz 1992). About two days before

Table 11.1 Comparison of CD56$^+$ NK cells

Characteristic	Blood CD56^{dim}	Blood CD56^{bright}	Decidua CD56^{bright}
Phenotypic markers			
CD16	++	+/−	−
CD94	+/−	++	++
KIR	+	−	+
Cytoplasmic CD3	−	−	+
c-KIT	−	+	+/−
CD69	−	−	+
CD45RA	+	+	−
CD45RO	−	−	+
CD62L (L-selectin)	+/−	++	−
αεβ7	−	−	+
CD49a (α1-integrin)	−	−	+
CD49f (α6-integrin)	+	+	−
NK activity	High	Low	Low
Morphology	LGLs	Agranular small lymphocytes	Both agranular small lymphocytes and LGLs
Cytokines			
MIP1α	−	+	++++
GM-CSF	−	+	++++
CSF1	−	+	++++
IFN-γ	+	−	+/−

c-KIT, human c-kit oncoprotein (CD117); CSF1, colony-stimulating factor 1; GM-CSF, granulocyte-macrophage colony-stimulating factor; IFN-γ, interferon-γ; KIR, killer-cell immunoglobulin-like receptor; LGL, large granular lymphocyte; MIP1α, macrophage inflammatory protein 1α; NK, natural killer.

menstruation (when progesterone levels are falling as the corpus luteum involutes), nuclear changes in the uNK cells indicate that they may be dying, although classical features of apoptosis are absent. A form of caspase-independent cell death may be occurring that is the first morphological sign of impending menstrual breakdown. If pregnancy occurs, the NK cells accumulate as a dense infiltrate around the invading trophoblast cells in the decidua basalis but they progressively disappear from mid-gestation onwards and are absent at term. Therefore, their presence is coincident with the period of trophoblast invasion because placentation is complete by about 20 weeks' gestation. The unusual phenotypic and functional properties of uNK cells compared to NK cells in peripheral blood are shown in Table 11.1. The origin of uNK cells is unknown but because they closely resemble the minor agranular CD56^{bright} NK cell population in blood, one possibility is that these blood NK cells move into the uterus to proliferate, differentiate, enlarge and acquire cytoplasmic granules in the hormone-rich uterine mucosal environment.

The functions of uNK cells are unknown. Two possibilities are currently under investigation: (1) control of trophoblast invasion; and (2) regulation of menstruation and decidualisation.

Control of trophoblast invasion by uNK cells

In humans, since uNK cells are particularly abundant among the trophoblast cells as they invade the decidua, the question arises as to whether they can recognise paternal/trophoblast ligands and, as a result, control the extent of placental invasion. Trophoblast cells are inherently invasive and, in the absence of decidua in humans, their invasion is uncontrolled, as seen when the placenta implants over scar tissue from a previous Caesarian section or in an ectopic tubal pregnancy.

To date, the only potential trophoblast ligands found that could be recognised by uNK cells are the major histocompatibility complex (MHC) class I molecules human leukocyte antigen (HLA)-C, HLA-E and HLA-G (see Loke, Chapter 12, this book). The receptors for HLA-C and HLA-E are now well described (Braud et al. 1998, Lee et al. 1998, Boyington et al. 2001, Long et al. 2001, Vilches & Parham 2002) and they have been found to be expressed by uNK cells (Fig. 11.1). The presence of receptors on maternal NK cells which have ligands on trophoblast cells does provide a potential molecular mechanism for maternal–fetal recognition, although the functional consequences of this recognition are unclear. By contrast, in humans, maternal T cell or antibody responses to trophoblast (as opposed to fetal cells) have not been shown convincingly either in normal or abnormal pregnancies.

Closer inspection of the pattern of expression of receptors that are found on uNK cells has shown that it is different to the expression pattern of blood NK cells taken from the same woman at the same time. All uNK cells express high levels of the inhibitory receptor CD94/NKG2A (Fig. 11.1), the ligand for which is HLA-E (King et al. 2000a). As surrounding maternal cells and trophoblast both express HLA-E, this interaction might prevent lysis of any tissue cells (either maternal or fetal) in the vicinity. Tissue NK cells at other sites, such as the nasal mucosa, are also CD94[bright] (Haedlicke et al. 2000). Interestingly, the binding affinity of the inhibitory receptor CD94/NKG2A is higher than that of the activating CD94/NKG2C receptor. This latter is also transcribed on uNK cells but it is not known if the protein is expressed (Koopman et al. 2003). The nonamer peptide that is bound to HLA-E is derived from the signal peptide of other MHC class I molecules. The sequence of this leader sequence-derived peptide also influences the binding affinities of CD94/NKG2. Only the HLA-G leader-sequence peptide complexed with HLA-E binds CD94/NKG2C with an affinity that is great enough to trigger an NK

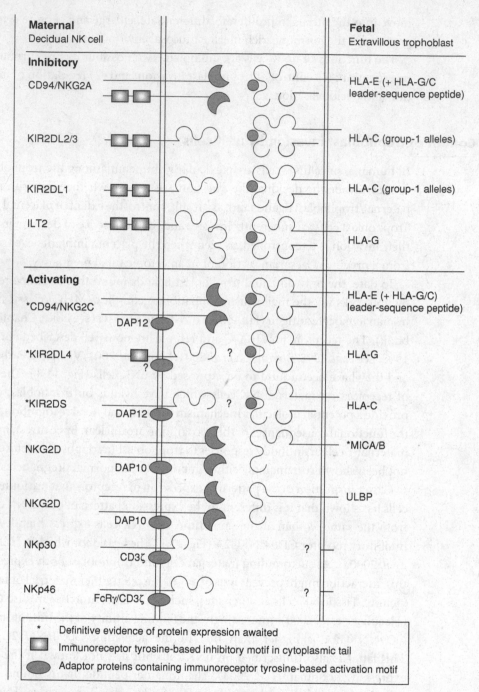

Figure 11.1 Maternal NK cell receptors for MHC class I molecules.

cell response (Llano *et al.* 1998, Vales-Gomez *et al.* 1999). This means that uNK cells could respond in utero differently to trophoblast HLA-E compared with other surrounding HLA-E-positive (but HLA-G-negative) maternal cells.

The NK cell receptors for HLA-C are members of the killer-cell immunoglobulin-like receptor (*KIR*) multigene family (Fig. 11.1). Individual KIR can distinguish between an epitope of all HLA-C allotypes, which is based on a dimorphism at position 80 of the α1 domain. This divides HLA-C alleles into Group 1 (C1) or Group 2 (C2). There is great diversity of KIR haplotypes in humans and primates, with variation in the number of genes, as well as polymorphism at individual loci (Vilches & Parham 2002). Some of the *KIR* genes encode an inhibitory receptor whilst others (with a similar extracellular domain) encode for a receptor that gives an activating signal (Uhrberg *et al.* 1997, Wilson *et al.* 2000, Rajalingam *et al.* 2001). Killer-cell immunoglobulin-like receptors that are specific for HLA-C are expressed by a greater proportion of uNK cells than by peripheral blood NK cells in pregnant women (Hiby *et al.* 1997, Verma *et al.* 1997). Furthermore, the CD56[bright] NK cell population in blood lacks expression of KIR (Jacobs *et al.* 2001). If blood CD56[bright] NK cells are the source of CD56[bright] uNK cells, then this observation indicates that KIR expression is induced in utero. Because both *HLA-C* and *KIR* genes are polymorphic, the interaction between paternal trophoblast HLA-C and maternal uNK cell KIR might result in different outcomes in each pregnancy. Some of these interactions could be disadvantageous for implantation and might contribute to the underlying pathogenesis of important diseases, such as pre-eclampsia, for which partner specificity, correlation with first pregnancies and oocyte donation are all features that indicate there is an 'immunological' basis. We have recently tested the hypothesis that certain combinations of maternal KIR and fetal HLA-C may be associated with an increased risk of pre-eclampsia. The *KIR* genes were typed as AA (only inhibitory KIR) or AB/BB (additional activating KIR present) genotypes. Human leukocyte antigen-C alleles were assigned to either C1 or C2 supertypic group. A significantly increased risk of developing pre-eclampsia was found for one particular maternal KIR–fetal HLA-C combination. This is when mothers have an AA KIR genotype in combination with an HLA-C2 group in the fetus. The combination of the maternal AA genotype with a C2 group in the fetus is increased in frequency in pre-eclampsia even when the C2 group is also present in the mother and therefore not either a 'non-self' or 'missing-self' molecule in the fetus. Thus, this maternal–fetal immunological interaction involves a novel type of allogeneic recognition, which is not based on either classical T 'non-self' or NK cell 'missing-self' discrimination (see Loke, Chapter 12, this book). Intriguingly, an inverse relationship between the prevalence of HLA-C2 and KIR AA genotypes is found in different populations, indicating that combinations of innate immune genes may be selected to influence reproductive outcome.

The identity of a specific receptor for HLA-G on NK cells is still being debated. Early reports that implicated CD94/NKG2 as the HLA-G receptor were shown subsequently to be due to the co-expression of HLA-E (Lanier 1999). Soluble fusion proteins of KIR2DL4 – a member of the KIR family that is present in all individuals and that is transcribed in all NK cells – bind HLA-G transfectants (Ponte *et al.* 1999, Rajagopalan & Long 1999). However, binding of KIR2DL4 to HLA-G has not been confirmed using other assays. For example, HLA-G tetramers failed to bind any KIR molecules, including KIR2DL4 (Allan *et al.* 1999).

Of the immunoglobulin-like transcript (ILT) or leukocyte immunoglobulin-like receptors (LILR), ILT2 and ILT4 bind a wide range of HLA class I molecules, including HLA-G (Allan *et al.* 1999, Navarro *et al.* 1999, Shiroishi *et al.* 2003), but of these, only ILT2 is found on a small percentage of uNK cells. Immunoglobulin-like transcript 2 and ILT4 are, however, expressed by macrophages, so there is a potential for HLA-G to interact with decidual macrophages although no binding of HLA-G tetramers to any decidual leukocytes was detected (Allan & Moffett, unpublished). Interestingly, ILT4-expressing monocytes and DCs have reduced expression of co-stimulatory molecules and are tolerogenic (Chang *et al.* 2002).

One reason why the search for an HLA-G receptor has been so problematic is that the characteristics of trophoblast HLA-G might not be the same as those of other HLA class I molecules – for example, in terms of the degree of glycosylation, the nature of the bound peptide and the existence of non-β2-microglobulin-associated forms (Loke *et al.* 1997, McMaster *et al.* 1998, King *et al.* 2000b). Complexes of disulphide-linked HLA-G dimers have indeed now been demonstrated (Boyson *et al.* 2002, Gonen-Gross *et al.* 2003) and may provide an explanation for why tetramers of classic β2-microglobulin-associated HLA-G bound no uterine leukocytes. In addition, the unusual phenotype and functional properties of uNK cells also need to be considered. The uterine microenvironment in early pregnancy is unique.

Role of uNK cells in decidualisation and menstruation

Despite the central importance of the process of decidualisation in normal pregnancy, remarkably little is known about why and how decidua forms. The central role of progesterone acting on an oestrogen-primed tissue is well-known (Masler 1988). In humans, unlike other species, there is no need for the stimulus of blastocyst attachment to induce decidualisation which already commences in the luteal phase and continues if pregnancy occurs (Finn 1996, 1998). The period between implantation and menstruation (i.e. 7–14 days after the luteal hormone (LH) surge) is critical for the endometrium to make the decision whether to continue the process of decidualisation or to break down and be shed at menstruation. The progesterone concentrations parallel this decision and either plummet or rapidly rise.

There are several observations that support that uterine NK cells may be associated with the decidualisation process, but whether as chicken or egg is unresolved. Natural killer cells begin to increase in number around LH surge + 2 and are therefore present before pre-decidualisation occurs. The coexistence of NK cells with decidual change is also always observed in ectopic foci of decidua, such as in the Fallopian tube, cervix, ovary or in foci of endometriosis (Massi *et al.* 1995). In contrast, NK cells are absent from non-decidualised tubal wall in ectopic pregnancy even at sites of trophoblast invasion (Bulmer *et al.* 1988). Persistent infiltration of NK cells was also seen in the pseudo-decidualised endometrium associated with levonorgestrel intrauterine devices (Critchley *et al.* 1998).

Uterine NK cells are probably a feature of the pregnant uterine mucosa of many species although they have been most studied in rodents. The abnormalities seen in the implantation sites of mice with no systemic or uNK cells indicate that the decidua is 'acellular and oedematous'. Furthermore, the decidual arteries remain similar in appearance to those in the non-pregnant uterus with a well-developed media, suggesting that the dilatation required for the increased blood flow of pregnancy does not occur. These findings indicate that the absence of uNK cells leads to failure of proper development and maintenance of the decidua and maternal arteries.

In humans the first morphological signs that menstruation rather than decidualisation is to occur are nuclear changes in NK cells. These may represent caspase-independent cell death (King *et al.* 1989, Trundley & Moffett, 2004). These changes are seen on LH surge + 12–13 and are, therefore, present before any other features of menstrual breakdown such as neutrophil infiltration, clumping of stromal cells and interstitial haemorrhage are present. The association of falling progesterone levels with the death of NK cells suggests that their survival is hormonally regulated. This does not appear to be a direct effect of progesterone because uNK cells do not express the progesterone receptor (King *et al.* 1996). The indirect effects may be exerted via cytokines or other soluble factors produced by stromal cells which do express progesterone receptors at this time (Loke & King 1995). Human uNK cells produce a combination of cytokines that are involved in angiogenesis and vascular stability, such as vascular endothelial growth factor C (VEGF-C) (Sharkey *et al.* 1993), placental growth factor (PlGF) and angiopoietin 2 (Ang2) (Li *et al.* 2001). The absence of these factors due to the demise of the uNK cells might be expected to lead to menstrual breakdown (for which vascular collapse is the initial event).

We believe that there is a role for NK cells in the process of decidualisation and menstruation as well as in the control of trophoblast invasion (King 2000). When reproduction is viewed from an evolutionary standpoint, there must have been mucosal leukocytes in the oviduct that were responsible for mucosal integrity, renewal and differentiation just as there were in any invertebrate surface location (Loke & King 1996). In mammalian species that have evolved an invasive form of

Table 11.2 Differences between human and mouse implantation

Human	Mouse
NK cells present in non-pregnant endometrium	NK cells not present in non-pregnant endometrium
Decidualisation commences in each non-pregnant cycle	Decidualisation occurs only after implantation
NK cells infiltrate diffusely throughout the decidua	NK cells are confined to central decidua basalis and the mesometrial triangle
Extensive trophoblast invasion into decidual stroma and arteries	Minimal trophoblast invasion of stroma and arteries

NK, natural killer.

placentation where the uterine epithelium is breached, these mucosal leukocytes could then have been co-opted for a further additional role monitoring trophoblast invasion, ensuring that a balance between adequate fetal nourishment and maternal survival is achieved.

Animal models

The extraordinary species diversity in the anatomy of placentation (Steven 1975) means that animal models are of only limited value for understanding human pregnancy. One common requirement, though, is that the blood flow to the site of maternal–placental exchange must always increase throughout gestation to supply sufficient nutrients and oxygen to the growing fetus. The strategies that different species use to achieve this increase in blood flow are markedly different. In humans, there is extensive invasion and destruction of pre-existing arteries by trophoblast, whereas in species that have epitheliochorial placentation, no invasion of the uterine wall (even the surface epithelium) occurs and the blood flow is increased by angiogenesis. Mice are the obvious animal model, but although humans and mice have many features in common, there are also substantial differences that are often ignored (Liu & Young 2001, Rossant & Cross 2001, Georgiades *et al.* 2002) (Table 11.2).

Nevertheless, there are obviously experiments in mice that cannot be done in humans that can offer an insight into some aspects of uNK cell biology. It has been shown that CD56[bright], but not CD56[dim], NK cells from human peripheral blood selectively adhere to mouse uteri in a Stamper–Woodruff Assay, and that splenic lymphocytes from pregnant mice can reconstitute uNK cells in NK cell-deficient mice (Chantakru *et al.* 2002). In both rodents and humans, different vascular addressins are found in different anatomical locations at different stages of gestation in the pregnant uterus, with endothelial vascular cell adhesion molecule 1 (VCAM1) being expressed particularly at the site of trophoblast infiltration (Burrows *et al.* 1993, 1994, Kruse *et al.* 2002). These observations indicate that uNK cells might be constantly replenished by active recruitment from the blood.

There are particular difficulties in using mouse models to test the hypothesis that uNK cells modify trophoblast cell invasion. The surprising lack of information about MHC expression by different mouse trophoblast populations and about whether mouse uNK cells express receptors such as CD94/NKG2 and Ly49 (killer-cell lectin-like receptors) is an obvious problem. In addition, there is only minimal interstitial trophoblast invasion in the mouse and virtually no endovascular invasion. Examination of the implantation sites of mice that are deficient in uNK cells shows that the arterial changes that are typical of the decidua basalis do not occur, which indicates that an important function of mouse uNK cells is to directly modify decidual blood vessels. The effects on feto–placental growth in these uNK cell-deficient mice are minimal and inconsistent, which might reflect the use of inbred strains (Guimond *et al.* 1998, Greenwood *et al.* 2000, Ashkar & Croy 2001, Barber & Pollard 2003).

Even when compared with our close relatives, the primates, marked differences in the extent of trophoblast invasion are found. In species such as the Rhesus macaque and baboon, there is minimal interstitial invasion of decidual stroma and the modification of uterine arteries occurs only as a result of infiltration by endovascular trophoblast. The HLA-C locus has evolved recently and is found in humans, the African great apes and some (but not all) orang-utans (Adams & Parham 2002). Likewise, there are species-specific features of the KIR family of receptors, which indicates that there has been rapid evolution of this gene family in primates (Khakoo *et al.* 2000, Rajalingam *et al.* 2001, 2004, Vilches & Parham 2002). It will be interesting to see if the selective pressures on reproductive success have contributed to the restless change of *HLA*-C and *KIR* genes in primates.

Such observations indicate that the mechanisms of attachment of the placenta and subsequent acquisition of maternal nutrients by trophoblast are remarkably divergent. The maternal mechanisms that have evolved to cope with these diverse placental morphologies will also be plastic. However, in all cases, the ultimate requirement is a regulated increase of uterine blood flow. In some species, this might be achieved by the direct action of uNK cells on the uterine arteries, whereas in other species, this is mediated indirectly by the influence of uNK cells on trophoblast invasiveness.

It seems therefore that maternal uNK cells might have evolved in different mammals to have differing functions. In humans it is proposed that in addition to any direct effect on arteries they mediate a mucosal immunological balancing act that prevents trophoblast over-invasion, but also allows a degree of placental access to the maternal blood supply. A compromise is reached and both maternal and fetal polymorphic gene systems (particularly *MHC/MHC-like* genes and *NK cell receptor* genes) might affect this compromise. Gene polymorphisms could influence reproductive outcome in subclinical and subtle ways that might be important over many generations of breeding.

Uterine macrophages and dendritic cells (DCs)

In humans, immunohistological studies have shown that about 20% of leukocytes in both the endometrium and decidua are $CD14^+$ macrophages (King *et al.* 1989). These cells do not appear to be under hormonal control as their numbers are relatively constant throughout the menstrual cycle unlike the variation in numbers of NK cells. They are present in decidua but are particularly abundant at the implantation site. Whether decidual macrophages have any specific immunological functions related to pregnancy is unknown. Macrophages are capable of producing and responding to a wide range of soluble products. They express several cytokine receptors, such as the granulocyte-macrophage colony stimulating factor receptor (GM-CSF-R) (Jokhi *et al.* 1994), colony stimulating factor-1 receptor (CSF-1R) (Jokhi *et al.* 1993) and interferon-γ receptor (IFN-γR) (Jokhi 1994). In addition, apparently uniquely among tissue macrophages, all decidual macrophages express c-*kit*. The kit ligand (KL), also known as stem cell factor (SCF), is secreted by extravillous trophoblast (Sharkey *et al.* 1992, 1994).

Recently, our laboratory has also identified a population of $HLA-DR^+$, $CD11c^+$, lin^- ($CD3^-$, $CD19^-$, $CD56^-$, $CD14^-$) DCs by three-colour flow cytometry (Gardner & Moffett 2003). They account for about 1.7% of the $CD45^+$ decidual leukocytes. Virtually all the DCs isolated from decidua were $CD11c^+$ and had other phenotypic features suggestive of immature myeloid DCs typical of most non-lymphoid tissues (Bancherau & Steinman 1998). We never detected any $CD11c^-$ or $CD123^+$ cells in this population, indicating that IFN-α/-β-producing plasmacytoid DCs are not present in decidua. This is in keeping with observations that these cells are mainly a feature of T cell areas of secondary lymphoid tissue (Liu *et al.* 2001). The $CD11c^+$ cells were further characterised with other markers. No CD1a cells were detected and, thus, Langerhans cells typical of squamous epithelium (Hart 1997) are not a feature of the uterus.

Similar findings have been found by others (Miyazaki *et al.* 2003) although the increased CD80, CD86 and CD83 expression in this study could reflect maturation of DCs induced by their extraction method. The phenotype of $CD14^-$ DCs and $CD14^+$ macrophages in the first trimester shows considerable overlap (Gardner & Moffett 2003). The relationship of these two similar populations is unknown but there is evidence that $CD14^+$ cells can differentiate into DCs in vivo and in vitro (Szabolcs *et al.* 1996, Hart 1997, Bell *et al.* 2001). In addition, $CD14^+$ $CD16^-$ cells (similar to the decidual macrophage phenotype) have been found subepidermally and defined as a subset of DCs (Turville *et al.* 2002). Thus, the functional capabilities of the two subsets of HLA-DR⁺ cells in decidua may show considerable overlap.

At present, however, the functions of HLA-DR⁺ cells in decidua are still unknown. At other epithelial surfaces, notably the gut, DCs may be pivotal in directing either the induction of tolerance to food antigens and commensals or the initiation of immune responses to pathogenic bacteria (Nagler-Anderson 2001). The continuous steady-state migration from the gut, lung and skin that occurs with sampling of apoptotic cells and luminal antigens in the absence of inflammation results in only a partial maturation of DC with up-regulation of MHC class I molecules but no induction of high levels of co-stimulatory molecules (Huang *et al.* 2000, Steinman & Nussenzweig 2002, Rolph 2002). In these situations DCs secrete IL10 or transforming growth factor (TGF)β resulting in induction of regulatory T cells (Akbari *et al.* 2001). Migration without full maturation may result either from failure of activation of appropriate Toll-like receptor (TLR) and other receptors or because of the local environmental milieu where the immature DCs contact antigen. Reduction of IL12 secretion has been reported in decidual DCs (Miyazaki *et al.* 2003). It is interesting that many other factors described to induce a 'tolerogenic' type of DC or 'alternatively activated' macrophages are present in abundance in the decidua. These include prostaglandin E2, Vitamin D, TGFβ and IL10 (Kennedy 1988, Goerdt & Orfanos 1999, Roth & Fisher 1999, Griffin *et al.* 2001, Harizi *et al.* 2002, Zehnder *et al.* 2002).

The most interesting and unique function that decidual DCs may perform is in the sampling, processing and presentation of trophoblast antigens that express unusual MHC and possibly MHC-like molecules as well as other paternally derived alloantigens. The older literature has suggested that decidua provides an 'immunosuppressive' environment or that the hormonal state of pregnancy induces maternal T helper (Th)2 responses. However, in mice, although there are several different models indicating T cell maternal tolerance to fetal antigens, the nature of the trophoblast MHC class I antigenic stimuli and the function of uterine DCs have not been studied. Indeed, the Th2 hypothesis must now be questioned given a recent report that mice lacking four Th2 type cytokines can reproduce normally (Fallon *et al.* 2002). Other murine models have shown that blockage of the enzyme indoleamine 2,3-dioxygenase (IDO) causes fetal demise and it has also been demonstrated recently that regulatory IDO-producing DCs inhibited T cell proliferation in humans (Mellor & Munn 1999, Finger & Bluestone 2002). Indeed, it is striking that in both humans and mice classical T cells are not recruited to the implantation site even in failing or 'rejecting' pregnancies. Stimulation of immature as opposed to mature DCs with alloantigens results in early up-regulation of the inhibitory CTLA-4 on the responding T cells and production of IL10 (Jonuleit *et al.* 2000). The nature and maturation state of the decidual DCs may thus be critical in T cell allorecognition of trophoblast. Alloantigen-specific T suppressor cells can also induce up-regulation of ILT3 and ILT4, inhibitory members of the ILT family, rendering the DCs tolerogenic (Chang *et al.* 2002). The trophoblast-specific class I molecule, HLA-G, can also inhibit murine DC function via interaction with paired immunoglobulin-like receptor (PIR)-B, a homologue of ILT4 (Liang *et al.* 2002). Thus several mechanisms involving decidual dendritic cells may operate to prevent maternal T cell activation to trophoblast.

In addition, decidual DCs may interact with the CD56[bright] NK cells in first trimester decidua. Dendritic cells can prime innate immunity by triggering NK cell functions and decidual DCs could be important in activation of NK cells in the presence of trophoblast. Alternatively, DCs may be alerted to the presence of the 'stress' of the implanting placenta by signals derived from NK cell recognition of specific trophoblast ligands (Moffett-King 2002). The ability of DCs and NK cells to influence each other provides a link between the innate adaptive immune responses depending on the density of NK cells and the state of DC maturation (Zivogel 2002). Our demonstration of small numbers of immature DCs in the decidua in areas of dense NK cell infiltration provides a basis for exploration of DC function in utero in early pregnancy in relation to both maternal uterine NK cells and T cells.

Conclusion

Like other mucosal surfaces, the uterus must be able to respond to antigenic challenge. However, the uterus is unique in that it is required to deal with three different types of antigens. These are pathogenic organisms, seminal plasma including spermatozoa and placental trophoblast during pregnancy. The immune response to pathogens is likely to be similar to that encountered at other mucosal sites such as the respiratory tract or the gut. Seminal plasma and spermatozoa do not appear to initiate any immune or inflammatory responses in the human endometrium. The immune response to trophoblast is still being investigated, but available data suggest that this response is a highly unusual one. Thus, it is not surprising to find that these diverse functions are reflected in the different types of immune effector cells present in the uterine mucosa.

REFERENCES

Adams, E. J. & Parham, P. (2002). Species-specific evolution of MHC class I genes in the higher primates. *Immunol. Rev.*, **183**, 41–64.

Akbari, O., DeKruyff, R. H. & Umetsu, D. T. (2001). Pulmonary dendritic cells producing IL-10 mediate tolerance induced by respiratory exposure to antigen. *Nat. Immun.*, **2**, 725–31.

Allan, D.S., Colonna, M., Lannier, L.L. *et al.* (1999). Tetrameric complexes of human histocompatibility leukocyte antigen (HLA-G)-G bind to peripheral blood myelomonocytic cells. *J. Exp. Med.*, **189**, 1149–56.

Ashkar, A.A. & Croy, B.A. (2001). Functions of uterine natural killer cells are mediated by interferon-γ production during murine pregnancy. *Semin. Immunol.*, **13**, 235–41.

Bancherau, J. & Steinman, R.M. (1998). Dendritic cells and the control of immunity. *Nature*, **392**, 245–52.

Barber, E.M. & Pollard, J.W. (2003). The uterine NK cell population requires IL-15 but these cells are not required for pregnancy nor the resolution of a *Listeria monocytogenes* infection. *J. Immunol.*, **171**, 37–46.

Bell, S.J., Rigby, R., English, N. *et al.* (2001). Migration and maturation of human colonic dendritic cells. *J. Immunol.* **166**, 4958–67.

Braud, V.M., Allan, D.S., O'Callaghan, C.A. *et al.* (1998). HLA-E binds to natural killer cell receptors CD94/NKG2A, B and C. *Nature*, **391**, 795–9.

Boyington, J.C., Brooks, A.G. & Sun, P.D. (2001). Structure of killer cell immunoglobulin-like receptors and their recognition of the class I MHC molecules. *Immunol. Rev.*, **181**, 62–5.

Boyson, J.E., Erskine. R., Whitman, M.C. *et al.* (2002) Disulphide bond-mediated dimerization of HLA-G on the cell surface. *Proc. Natl. Acad. Sci. U.S.A.*, **99**, 16180–5.

Bulmer, J.N., Pace, D. & Ritson, A. (1988). Immunoregulatory cells in human decidua: morphology, immunohistochemistry and function. *Reprod. Nutr. Dev.*, **28**, 1599–614.

Burrows, T.D., King, A. & Loke, Y.W. (1993). Expression of adhesion molecules by human decidual large granular lymphocytes. *Cell. Immunol.*, **147**, 81–94.

(1994). Expression of adhesion molecules by endovascular trophoblast and decidual endothelial cells: implications for vascular invasion during implantation. *Placenta*, **15**, 21–33.

Chang, C.C., Ciubotariu, R., Manavalan, J.S. *et al.* (2002). Tolerization of dendritic cells by T cells: the crucial role of inhibitory receptors ILT3 and ILT4. *Nat. Immun.*, **3**, 237–43.

Chantakru, S., Miller, C., Roach, L.E. *et al.* (2002). Contributions from self-renewal trafficking to the uterine NK-cell population of early pregnancy. *J. Immunol.*, **168**, 22–8.

Critchley, H.O.D., Wang, H., Jones, R.L. *et al.* (1998). Morphological and functional features of endometrial decidualisation following long-term intrauterine levonorgestrel delivery. *Hum. Reprod.*, **13**, 1218–24.

Dunn, C.L., Critchley, H.O.D. & Kelly, R. (2002). IL-15 regulation in human endometrial stromal cells. *J. Clin. Endocrinol. Metab.*, **87**, 1896–901.

Fallon, P.G., Jolin, H.E., Smith, P. *et al.* (2002). IL-4 induces characteristic Th2 responses even in the combined absence of IL-5, IL-9, and IL-13. *Immunity*, **17**, 7–17.

Finger, E.B. & Bluestone, J.A. (2002). When ligand becomes receptor – tolerance via B7 signaling on DCs. *Nat. Immun.*, **2**, 1056–7.

Finn, C.A. (1996). Why do women menstruate? Historical and evolutionary review. *Eur. J. Obstet. Gynecol. Reprod. Biol.*, **70**, 3–8.

(1998). Menstruation: a nonadaptive consequence of uterine evolution. *Q. Rev. Biol.*, **73**, 163–73.

Gardner, L. & Moffett, A. (2003). Dendritic cells in the human decidua. *Biol. Reprod.*, **69**, 1438–46.

Georgiades, P., Ferguson-Smith, A.C. & Burton, G.J. (2002). Comparative developmental anatomy of the murine and human definitive placentae. *Placenta*, **23**, 3–19.

Goerdt, W. & Orfanos, C.E. (1999). Other functions, other genes: alternative activation of antigen-presenting cells. *Immunity*, **10**, 137–42.

Gonen-Gross, T., Achdout, H., Gazit, R. *et al.* (2003). Complexes of HLA-G protein on the cell surface are important for leukocyte Ig-like receptor-1 function. *J. Immunol.*, **171**, 1343–51.

Greenwood, J.D., Minnas, K., di Santo, J.P. *et al.* (2000). Ultrasound studies of implantation sites from mice deficient in uterine natural killer cells. *Placenta*, **120**, 693–702.

Griffin, M.D., Lutz, W., Phan, V.A. *et al.* (2001). Dendritic cell modulation by 1alpha,25 dihydroxyvitamin D3 and its analogs: a vitamin D receptor-dependent pathway that promotes a persistent stage of immaturity *in vitro* and *in vivo*. *Proc. Natl. Acad. Sci. U.S.A.*, **98**, 6800–5.

Gubbay, O., Critchley, H.O.D., King, A., Bowen, J.M. & Jabbour, H.N. (2002) Prolactin induces ERK phosphorylation in epithelial CD56[+] natural killer cells of the human endometrium. *J. Clin. Endocrinol. Metab.*, **87**, 2329–35.

Guimond, M.-J., Wang, B. & Croy, B.A. (1998). Engraftment of bone marrow from severe combined immunodeficient (SCID) mice reverses the reproductive deficit in natural killer cell-deficient tge26 mice. *J. Exp. Med.*, **187**, 217–23.

Haedlicke, W., Ho, F.C.S., Chott, A. *et al.* (2000). Expression of CD94/NKG2A and killer immunoglobulin-like receptors in NK cells and a subset of extranodal cytotoxic T-cell lymphomas. *Blood*, **95**, 3628–30.

Harizi, H., Juzan, M., Pitard, V., Moreau, J.-F. & Gualde, N. (2002). Cyclooxygenase-2-issued prostaglandin E2 enhances the production of endogenous IL-10, which down-regulates dendritic cell functions. *J. Immunol.*, **168**, 2255–63.

Hart, D.N. (1997). Dendritic cells: unique leukocyte populations which control the primary immune response. *Blood*, **90**, 3245–87.

Hiby, S.E., King, A., Sharkey, A.M. & Loke, Y.W. (1997). Human uterine cells have a similar repertoire of killer inhibitory and activatory receptors to those found in blood as demonstrated by RT-PCR and sequencing. *Mol. Immunol.*, **34**, 419–30.

Huang, F.-P., Platt, N., Wykes, M. *et al.* (2000). A discrete subpopulation of dendritic cells transports apoptotic intestinal epithelial cells to T cell areas of mesenteric lymph nodes. *J. Exp. Med.*, **191**, 435–43.

Jacobs, R., Hintzen, G., Kemper, A. *et al.* (2001). CD56[bright] cells differ in the KIR repertoire and cytotoxic features from CD56[dim] NK cells. *Eur. J. Immunol.*, **31**, 3121–3126.

Jokhi, P.P. (1994). Cytokines and their receptors in human placental implantation. Unpublished Ph.D. thesis, University of Cambridge.

Jokhi, P.P., Chumbley, G., Gardner, L., King, A. & Loke, Y.W. (1993). Expression of the colony stimulating factor-1 receptor (c-fms product) by cells at the human uteroplacental interface. *Lab. Invest.*, **68**, 308–20.

Jokhi, P.P., King, A., Jubinsky, P. & Loke, Y.W. (1994). Demonstration of the low affinity subunit of the granulocyte-macrophage colony-stimulating factor receptor (GM-CSF-Ra) on human trophoblast and uterine cells. *J. Reprod. Immunol.*, **26**, 147–64.

Jonuleit, H., Schmitt, E., Schuler, G., Knop, J. & Enk, A. H. (2000). Induction of interleukin 10-producing, non-proliferating CD4$^+$ T cells with regulatory properties by repetitive stimulation with allogeneic immature human dendritic cells. *J. Exp. Med.*, **192**, 1213–22.

Kennedy, T. G. (1988). Prostaglandins and other non-steroidal mediators at and immediately after implantation. In R. W. Beard & F. Sharp, eds., *Early Pregnancy Loss: Mechanisms and Treatment*. London: RCOG Press, pp. 249–58.

Khakoo, S. I., Rajalingam, R., Shum, B. P. *et al.* (2000). Rapid evolution of NK-cell receptor systems demonstrated by comparison of chimpanzees and humans. *Immunity*, **12**, 687–98.

King, A. (2000). Uterine leucocytes and decidualisation. *Hum. Reprod. Update*, **6**, 28–36.

King, A., Wellings, V., Gardner, L. & Loke, Y. W. (1989). Immunocytochemical characterisation of the unusual large granular lymphocytes in human endometrium throughout the menstrual cycle. *Hum. Immunol.*, **24**, 195–205.

King, A., Gardner, L. & Loke, Y. W. (1996). Evaluation of oestrogen and progesterone receptor expression in uterine mucosal lymphocytes. *Hum. Reprod.*, **11**, 1079–82.

King, A., Allan, D. S. J., Joseph, S. *et al.* (2000a). HLA-E is expressed on trophoblast and interacts with CD94/NKG2 receptors on decidual NK cells. *Eur. J. Immunol.*, **30**, 1623–31.

King, A., Burrows, T. D., Hiby, S. E. *et al.* (2000b). Surface expression of HLA-C antigen by human extravillous trophoblast. *Placenta*, **21**, 376–87.

Koopman, L. A., Kopcow, H. D., Rybalov, B. *et al.* (2003). Human decidual natural killer cells are a unique NK cell subset with immunomodulatory potential. *J. Exp. Med.*, **198**, 1201–12.

Kruse, A., Martens, N., Gemekom, U., Hallmann, R. & Butcher, E. C. (2002). Alterations in the expression of homing-associated molecules at the maternal/fetal interface during the course of pregnancy. *Biol. Reprod.*, **66**, 333–45.

Lanier, L. L. (1999). Natural killer cells fertile with receptors for HLA-G? *Proc. Natl. Acad. Sci. U.S.A.*, **96**, 5343–5.

Lee, N., Llano, M., Carretero, M. *et al.* (1998). HLA-E is a major ligand for the natural killer inhibitory receptor CD94/NKG2A. *Proc. Natl. Acad. Sci. U.S.A.*, **95**, 5199–204.

Li, X. F., Charnock-Jones, S., Zhang, E. *et al.* (2001). Angiogenic growth factor mRNAs in uterine natural killer cells. *J. Clin. Endocrinol. Metab.*, **86**, 1823–34.

Liang, S., Baibakov, B. & Horuzsko, A. (2002). HLA-G inhibits the functions of murine dendritic cells via the PIR-B immune inhibitory receptor. *Eur. J. Immunol.*, **32**, 2418–26.

Liu, C.-C. & Young, J. D. E. (2001). Uterine natural killer cells in the pregnant uterus. *Adv. Immunol.*, **79**, 297–329.

Liu, Y.-J., Kanzler, H., Souvelis, V. & Gilliet, M. (2001). Dendritic cell lineage, plasticity and cross-regulation. *Nat. Immun.*, **2**, 585–9.

Llano, M., Lee, N., Navarro, F. *et al.* (1998). HLA-E bound peptides influence recognition by inhibitory and triggering CD94/NKG2 receptors: preferential response to an HLA-G derived nonamer. *Eur. J. Immunol.*, **28**, 2854–63.

Loke, Y. W. & King, A. (1995). *Human Implantation: Cell Biology and Immunology*. Cambridge: Cambridge University Press.

(1996). Immunology of human implantation: an evolutionary perspective. *Hum. Reprod.*, **11**, 283–6.

Loke, Y. W., King, A., Burrows, T. *et al.* (1997). Evaluation of trophoblast HLA-G antigen with a specific monoclonal antibody. *Tissue Antigens*, **50**, 135–46.

Long, E. O., Barber, D. F., Burshtyn, D. N. *et al.* (2001). Inhibition of natural killer cell activation signals by killer cell immunoglobulin-like receptors (CD158). *Immunol. Rev.*, **181**, 223–33.

Masler, I. A. (1988). The progestational endometrium. *Semin. Reprod. Endocrinol.*, **6**, 115–28.

Massi, D., Susini, T., Paglierani, M., Salvadori, A. & Giannini, A. (1995). Pregnancy-associated ectopic decidua. *Acta Obstet. Gynecol. Scand.*, **74**, 568–71.

McMaster, M., Zhou, Y., Shorter, S. *et al.* (1998). HLA-G isoforms produced by placental cytotrophoblasts and found in amniotic fluid are due to unusual glycosylation. *J. Immunol.*, **160**, 5992–8.

Mellor, A. L. & Munn, D. H. (1999). Tryptophan catabolism and T-cell tolerance: immunosuppression by starvation? *Immunol. Today*, **20**, 469–73.

Moffett-King, A. (2002). Natural killer cells and pregnancy. *Nat. Rev. Immunol.*, **2**, 656–63.

Miyazaki, S., Tsuda, H., Sakai, M. *et al.* (2003). Predominance of Th2-promoting dendritic cells in early human pregnancy *J. Leukocyte Biol.*, **74**, 514–22.

Nagler-Anderson, C. (2001). Man the barrier! Strategic defences in the intestinal mucosa. *Nat. Rev. Immunol.*, **1**, 59–67.

Navarro, F., Llano, M., Bellon, T. *et al.* (1999). The ILT2(LIR1) and CD94/NKG2A NK cell receptors respectively recognize HLA-G1 and HLA-E molecules co-expressed on target cells. *Eur. J. Immunol.*, **29**, 277–83.

Ponte, M., Cantoni, C., Biassoni, R. *et al.* (1999). Inhibitory receptors sensing HLA-G1 molecules in pregnancy: decidua-associated natural killer cells express LIR-1 and CD94/NKG2A and acquire p49, an HLA-G1-specific receptor. *Proc. Natl. Acad. Sci. U.S.A.*, **96**, 5674–9.

Rajagopalan, S. & Long, E. O. (1999). A human histocompatibility leukocyte antigen (HLA)-G-specific receptor expressed on all natural killer cells. *J. Exp. Med.*, **189**, 1093–100.

Rajalingam, R., Hong, M., Adams, E. J. *et al.* (2001). Short KIR haplotypes in pygmy chimpanzee (bonobo) resemble the conserved framework of diverse human KIR haplotypes. *J. Exp. Med.*, **193**, 135–46.

Rajalingam, R., Parham, P. & Abi-Rached, L. (2004). Domain shuffling has been the main mechanism forming new hominoid killer cell Ig-like receptors. *J. Immunol.*, **172**, 356–69.

Rolph, G. J. (2002). Is maturation required for Langerhans cell migration? *J. Exp. Med.*, **196**, 413–16.

Rossant, J. & Cross, J. C. (2001). Placental development: lessons from mouse mutants. *Nat. Rev. Genet.*, **2**, 538–48.

Roth, I. & Fisher, S. J. (1999). IL-10 is an autocrine inhibitor of human placental cytotrophoblast MMP-9 production and invasion. *Dev. Biol.*, **205**, 194–204.

Sharkey, A. M., Charnock-Jones, D. S., Brown, K. D. & Smith, S. K. (1992). Expression of messenger RNA for kit-ligand in human placenta: localization by *in situ* hybridisation and identification of alternatively spliced variants. *Mol. Endocrinol.*, **6**, 1235–41.

Sharkey, A. M., Charnock-Jones, D. S., Boocock, C. A., Brown, K. D. & Smith, S. K. (1993). Expression of mRNA for vascular endothelial growth factor in human placenta. *J. Reprod. Fertil.*, **99**, 609–15.

Sharkey, A. M., Jokhi, P. P., King, A. *et al.* (1994). Expression of c-kit and kit ligand at the human materno-fetal interface. *Cytokine*, **6**, 195–205.

Shiroishi, M., Tsumoto, K., Amano, K. *et al.* (2003). Human inhibitory receptors Ig-like transcript 2 (ILT2) and ILT4 compete with CD8 for MHC class I binding and bind preferentially to HLA-G. *Proc. Natl. Acad. Sci. U.S.A.*, **100**, 8856–61.

Spornitz, U. M. (1992). The functional morphology of the human endometrium and decidua. *Adv. Anat. Embryol. Cell Biol.*, **124**, 1–99.

Steinman, R. M. & Nussenzweig, M. C. (2002). Avoiding horror autotoxicus: the importance of dendritic cells in peripheral T cell tolerance. *Proc. Natl. Acad. Sci. U.S.A.*, **99**, 351–8.

Steven, D. H. (1975). *Comparative Placentation. Essays in Structure and Function*. London: Academic Press.

Szabolcs, P., Avigan, D., Gezelter, S. *et al.* (1996). Dendritic cells and macrophages can mature independently from a human bone marrow-derived post-colony-forming unit intermediate. *Blood*, **87**, 4520–30.

Trundley, A. & Moffett, A. (2004). Human uterine leukocytes and pregnancy. *Tissue Antigens*, **63**, 1–12.

Turville, S. G., Cameron, P. U., Handley, A. *et al.* (2002). Diversity of receptors binding HIV on dendritic cell subsets. *Nat. Immun.*, **3**, 975–83.

Uhrberg, M., Valiante, N. M., Shun, B. P. *et al.* (1997). Human diversity in killer cell inhibitory genes. *Immunity*, **7**, 753–63.

Vales-Gomez, M., Reburn, H. T., Erskine, R. A., Lopez-Botet, M. & Strominger, J. L. (1999). Kinetics and peptide dependency of the binding of the inhibitory NK receptor CD94/NKG2-A and the activating receptor CD94/NKG2-C to HLA-E. *EMBO J.*, **18**, 4250–60.

Verma, S., King, A. & Loke, Y. W. (1997). Expression of killer-cell inhibitory receptors (KIR) on human uterine NK cells. *Eur. J. Immunol.*, **27**, 979–83.

Vilches, C. & Parham, P. (2002). KIR: diverse, rapidly evolving receptors of innate adaptive immunity. *Annu. Rev. Immunol.*, **20**, 217–51.

Wilson, M., Torkar, M., Haude, A. *et al.* (2000). Plasticity in the organization and sequences of human KIR/ILT gene families. *Proc. Natl. Acad. Sci. U.S.A.*, **97**, 4778–83.

Zehnder, D., Evans, K. N., Kilby, M. D. *et al.* (2002). The ontogeny of 25-hydroxyvitamin D(3) 1alpha-hydroxylase expression in human placenta decidua. *Am. J. Pathol.*, **161**, 105–14.

Zivogel, L. (2002). Dendritic and natural killer cells cooperate in the control/switch of innate immunity. *J. Exp. Med.*, **195**, F9–14.

DISCUSSION

Keverne   You said that the NK cells that you find in the placenta are specific. Do they take their origin from a common stem cell population and then acquire this specificity by virtue of interacting with trophoblast? If this is the case, what is it that switches them on to become special cells?

Moffett   We don't know their origin. We don't know whether they are derived from stem cells that are seeded early in life, or whether they continually migrate from the blood throughout life. There is a cell in blood that has many similarities to a uNK cell. It is more common in women than men. It is possible that this cell differentiates uniquely in the uterine environment.

Keverne   Do you already find these specific uterine-type NK cells in the bone marrow stem cell population?

Moffett   There are cells that are similar, but not identical. The only other place that you would find cells similar to uNK cells is the nose.

Keverne   The nose is very much like the endometrium.

Moffett   I did put a question into our Cambridge Part II exam saying 'what do the nose and uterus have in common? Discuss,' and the examiners threw it out!

Keverne   In some of the old literature they used to do diagnosis of women's disorders by looking at the blood supply in the nose.

Redman   Anne Croy and her group have shown that there are homing receptors in the decidua that attract NK cells of this particular phenotype. She thinks there is trafficking going on that could explain their build-up in the late luteal phase and their continuation in pregnancy.

Moffett   However, they do proliferate *in situ* in the uterus.

McLaren   So is the phenotypic difference between the uNK cells and the somatic NK cells in the blood due to selection? Are the uNK cells in the blood attracted to the uterus?

Moffett   There may be a tiny subset of NK cells that selectively migrate into the uterus. We don't know this but it is the most likely scenario.

S. Fisher   We showed a few years ago that if we take trophoblast-conditioned media and peripheral blood leukocytes, we can get migration of the $CD56^+CD16^-$ population. We showed that MIP1α is responsible. In pregnancy, the trophoblast cells are in the uterus and they keep the NK cells going. At least with HLA-G, trophoblast cells fit a different carbohydrate chain on that molecule. It may be that HLA-C is polylactose mitoylated. This would be something that could easily be studied.

Moffett   That is another possibility, although I don't think that KIR has been shown to be affected by carbohydrates.

S. Fisher   It has never been tested. An ex-student of mine is now putting polylactosamine structures on HLA-G tetramers to ask this question. It is technically very difficult. Peter Parham showed that all the class I molecules are glycosylated similarly in a very boring way.

Moffett   C is glycosylated differently from A and B.

S. Fisher   In what way?

Moffett   A and B have just two possibilities for side sugars. C can have four or five.

Trowsdale   There may well be different forms of C. There is evidence from a number of studies that there may be odd dimers of class I molecules expressed on trophoblast. I don't think we know yet, but there could be novel forms of class I that are seen by some of these receptors, or novel modifications including these large sugars.

Surani   I noticed that the UK population is not as skewed as the Japanese and Indian populations for the frequency of the AA genotype. Why?

Moffett   I don't think we know. But if we work out in these two populations what is the frequency of mothers with an AA genotype combining with a group 2 HLA-C in the baby, it is roughly the same. In all populations we have information on, there is roughly the same possibility of this combination happening. This is because of the inverse relationship between the frequency of the AA phenotype and HLA-C group 2 allotypes.

Sibley   I have a general comment about fetal growth. You linked pre-eclampsia, change in blood flow and change in fetal growth. A change in fetal growth doesn't come about just because of a change in blood flow. This is the classic statement in the literature: small babies result from altering uterine flow, which decreases oxygen delivery. We have shown that in the syncytiotrophoblast there are abnormalities of transporter proteins in our uterine growth retardation. We think of pre-eclampsia as an extravillous trophoblast type of problem because of the invasion into the arteries, but Chris has raised the point about deportation of villous trophoblast, suggesting there might be something going on with villous trophoblast in pre-eclampsia. Alongside that, there is our observation on villous trophoblast that there is this transporter pathology in the disease.

Moffett   We need to think of them as operating in stages.

12

Immunology of trophoblast: a reappraisal

Y. W. (Charlie) Loke

University of Cambridge, UK

Introduction

In the light of the discovery of the major histocompatibility complex (MHC) and its role in transplantation, the seminal essay written by Medawar drew a logical comparison between an allograft and a fetus (Medawar 1953). Despite being non-self, the fetus survives while the transplant is rejected. Medawar himself pointed out that the placenta must play a central role in fetal acceptance as it is the placental trophoblast cells that interface with the mother. Now, over 50 years later, the question how the allogeneic trophoblast survives in the potentially immunological hostile uterine environment remains unanswered. Why is the solution to this problem so elusive? I would argue that comparing the placental/maternal relationship with the graft/host relationship is misleading because the analogy between the two is not as close as it appears to be.

The extent of cellular contact between trophoblast and maternal tissue will vary significantly between species depending on the type of placentation. The immunological problem is likely to be most acute in the deeply invasive haemochorial placenta used in humans so that the adaptation required and the strategy employed in human reproduction would be expected to be different from those of other species. For this reason, animal models are not very useful and extrapolation of data between species has led to much confusion. The present paper is focused on human placentation.

Models of immune recognition

The cellular basis of the classical 'self/non-self' model formulated by Burnet (1959) proposed that each lymphocyte (T cell) expresses a single receptor for a foreign antigen. Signalling through this receptor triggers an immune response.

Biology and Pathology of Trophoblast, eds. Ashley Moffett, Charlie Loke and Anne McLaren.
Published by Cambridge University Press © Cambridge University Press 2005.

Lymphocytes with receptors for non-self in the form of pathogens or allogeneic cells from another individual will be present in the host and will eliminate the infectious agent or reject the allograft (Billingham *et al.* 1953). The cell surface molecules responsible for allogeneic recognition are the HLA (human leukocyte antigen) class I and class II antigens of the MHC. These are highly polymorphic and are, therefore, likely to differ among individuals (Fig. 12.1a).

An alternative mechanism of detecting self depends on the presence of inhibiting receptors on certain leukocytes which, on recognition of self MHC class I, transmit an inhibitory signal preventing an immune response. If these self molecules are missing, the lack of inhibitory signals allows the leukocytes to kill. This is the 'missing-self' model proposed by Karre in relation to natural killer (NK) cells, which are prevented from cytolytic activity by binding to self MHC class I molecules on target cells (Karre *et al.* 1986). In this way, NK cells survey the levels of class I molecules on host's own cells. Any aberrant cell where there is down-regulation of class I molecules (e.g. viral infection or neoplastic transformation) will be eliminated (Fig. 12.1c). Thus, MHC antigens influence immune recognition in two ways – one is by the presence of difference (T cells) and the other by the absence of similarity (NK cells). Besides MHC antigens, there are other examples that fall into the 'missing-self' model, such as Siglecs (sialic acid-binding Ig-like lectins) and CD47. Siglecs are receptors found on myeloid cells and NK cells which are inhibited by binding to sialylated glycoproteins (Crocker & Varki 2001). CD47, which is expressed on all cells including red blood cells, binds to an inhibitory receptor signal regulatory protein (SIRP)α, preventing phagocytosis by macrophages (Oldenburg *et al.* 2000). As these markers of self are found on normal healthy cells, they will prevent killing by NK cells and phagocytosis by macrophages but their absence on microbes and infected, transformed or senescent cells will render these susceptible to attack.

A third model of immune recognition was proposed by Medzhitov & Janeway (2002) who showed that microbes can be detected by the conserved molecular patterns essential to their survival, somewhat akin to the barcode system used to identify goods in shops. These are known as pathogen-associated molecular patterns (PAMPs). Since PAMPs are not present in the vertebrate hosts, this system permits the host to distinguish between 'self/infectious non-self' (Fig. 12.1b). The receptor for PAMPs, known as pattern recognition receptors (PRRs) are germline encoded and are found mainly on antigen-presenting cells (APCs), such as dendritic cells and macrophages. Once a PRR is engaged by a PAMP, the APC is induced to mature, processes the microbial antigen and up-regulates co-stimulatory ligands for presentation to T cells. It is thus the APC and not a lymphocyte that initially detects the microbial non-self. One type of PRR is a toll-like receptor (TLR) similar

(a)   Self/non-self   *(Burnet)*

Each T and B lymphocyte expresses a single clonally distributed receptor that is generated by gene rearrangement and which is specific for a foreign entity. Self-reactive lymphocytes are deleted in fetal life.

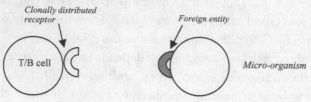

(b)   Self/infectious non-self   *(Janeway)*

Germline-encoded pattern recognition receptors (PRRs) expressed by antigen-presenting cells (APC) recognise pathogen-associated molecular patterns (PAMP) characteristic of particular classes of micro-organisms.

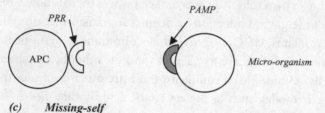

(c)   Missing-self   *(Karre)*

Activation of NK cells and other cells of innate system is inhibited by receptors which recognise ligands found on normal healthy cells (e.g. MHC class I).

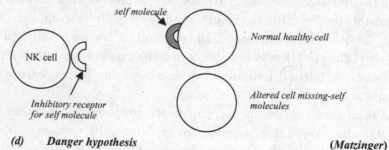

(d)   Danger hypothesis   *(Matzinger)*

APCs and other immune cells discern damaged cells in injured tissues.

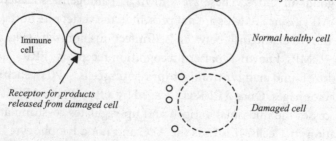

Figure 12.1 Models of immunological recognition.

to that used by *Drosophila* so this immune recognition system is an ancient one in evolutionary terms.

Finally, Matzinger (1994) has introduced a broader model to understand how the immune system discerns any unhealthy cell and this has moved away from the concept of self/non-self, foreign or microbial. Her 'danger' model proposes that the host is alerted by the presence of alarm signals released by damaged cells and tissues. The insult may be exogenous (e.g. microbes) or endogenous (e.g. virus, necrosis) that will not emanate from healthy tissue. (Fig. 12.1d). This proposal is attractive in its simplicity as it turns around the problem of defining all the agents and situations to which the immune system will react against towards the concept that normal healthy cells and tissues will not stimulate leukocyte activation.

Expression of MHC antigens by trophoblast

Since HLA class I and class II antigens of the MHC feature so prominently in allogeneic recognition, it is useful to have a clear view of the expression of these antigens by trophoblast. In humans, there are two trophoblast–maternal interfaces. One is between the layer of villous syncytiotrophoblast which lies in direct contact with maternal blood in the intervillous space. The other is between the extravillous trophoblast (EVT) cells which bud off from the tips of chorionic villi to invade into maternal uterine decidua (Loke & King 1995). The expression of MHC antigens is different in these two trophoblast populations. Villous syncytiotrophoblast does not express either HLA class I or class II antigens. It is this observation that has given rise to the original hypothesis that the placenta is lined by a layer of trophoblast cells which is immunologically neutral. This, therefore, explains why the placenta is not rejected by the mother. Unfortunately, this rather neat solution to the problem was undermined by the subsequent demonstration that EVT, in contrast, does express HLA class I although not class II antigens. Furthermore, the combination of HLA class I antigens expressed by EVT is somewhat unusual compared to a normal somatic cell. Nearly all somatic cells express the products of the three classical loci: HLA-A, -B, -C. These are highly polymorphic and are responsible for triggering graft rejection. This is in accordance with the 'self/non-self' model of Burnet. In contrast, EVT expresses not only one classical locus product, HLA-C, but also two non-classical locus products, HLA-E and HLA-G (Loke & King 2001).

It has taken a considerable time to establish the identity of these antigens. There have been two major constraints. One is the difficulty in isolating EVT with a sufficient degree of homogeneity for experimentation. This has now been achieved either by differential binding to substrates of extracellular matrix proteins or by FACS sorting using appropriate surface markers expressed by EVT (Loke & King

1995). The other constraint has been the lack of a locus-specific HLA antibody which can discriminate between the different class I antigens. Because of the structural similarity of the class I molecules, such antibodies are difficult to generate. Conventional procedures merely result in the production of pan-class I antibodies, which react with *all* HLA class I antigens. Special regimes are required. We have generated a monoclonal antibody (Mab) to HLA-G by the strategy of using HLA-G/β2 microglobulin (β2m)-transfected cells to immunise HLA-A2/β2m double transgenic mice, the rationale being that these animals would be tolerant to the major components of the HLA class I molecule and produce antibodies with a narrow specificity reactive only against HLA-G-specific epitopes (Loke *et al.* 1997).

The functions of these trophoblast class I molecules are not known and are presently the focus of much research interest.

Trophoblast HLA-G

This molecule has commanded centre stage among reproductive immunologists because its expression is restricted to extravillous trophoblast (Loke *et al.* 1999). It has not been convincingly demonstrated in any other fetal or adult tissue with the exception of the fetal thymus where HLA-G is found in certain epithelial cells late in gestation and in the first year of life (Crisa *et al.* 1997, Mallet *et al.* 1999). This could be responsible for the induction of tolerance to this antigen. There had been isolated reports that HLA-G is also expressed by some tumour cells but this is not confirmed in subsequent studies (Frumento *et al.* 2000, Davies *et al.* 2001).

The function of HLA-G is not known. There is a wide spectrum of views ranging from those who are sceptical that this antigen has any function at all in reproduction to those who are confident that this molecule is pivotal in determining the success of pregnancy. We ourselves subscribe to the latter view. Although there is some variation at the nucleotide level, there is remarkable conservation of the protein sequence. Therefore, HLA-G is non-polymorphic and will not transmit any paternal allogeneic signals. Based on the 'missing-self' model of immune recognition, we have proposed that HLA-G might protect trophoblast cells from attack by maternal uterine NK cells (King & Loke 1991) by acting as a kind of 'surrogate' self that would trigger inhibitory receptors on NK cells. Cytotoxicity experiments seem to support this hypothesis (King *et al.* 2000a). Decidual NK cells are able to kill an HLA class I$^-$ cell line LCL.221. Transfection of HLA-G into this cell line protected them from NK cell cytolysis and this protection is partially reversed in the presence of HLA-G antibody. However, the results of similar cytotoxicity experiments using isolated trophoblast cells as targets are more difficult to interpret (King *et al.* 2000a). Trophoblast cells are indeed resistant to killing by decidual NK cells, but this protection does not appear to be due to HLA-G (nor indeed to any HLA class I) because removal of these molecules on the surface of trophoblast by acid treatment or by masking with specific HLA-G antibody did not induce lysis. In vitro cytotoxic assays may not be a valid measure of what happens in vivo. The term 'natural killer' cells gives the impression that the predominant activity of these cells is killing. This is misleading as a major function of NK cells is production of cytokines, which have a variety of functions (Guidotti & Chisari 2001). Perhaps the outcome of the contact between decidual NK cells and trophoblast HLA-G is production of cytokines by the former, which then influence trophoblast differentiation and invasion (Loke & King 2000).

An important piece of jigsaw that is still missing is the receptor for HLA-G. It has not yet been identified. Certain members of the immunoglobulin-like transcript (ILT) family of receptors (ILT2) or the killer-cell immunoglobulin-like receptor (KIR) family (KIR2DL4) have been suggested but not confirmed (Moffett-King 2002). Since HLA-G is expressed only by EVT, its receptor is likely to be found on the immune cells infiltrating the uterine mucosa. While the KIR family of receptors are confined to decidual NK cells, members of the ILT family are found also on decidual macrophages, so both these cell types are potential candidates where the HLA-G receptor could reside.

Human leukocyte antigen-G is unusual among class I molecules in that the primary transcripts can be alternatively spliced to yield different isoforms including soluble variants (Hiby *et al.* 1999). The functions of these soluble isoforms are also not known. The existence of an individual homozygous for a null allele which precludes the transcription of the full length transmembrane form of HLA-G1 (Ober *et al.* 1998) suggests that at least this variant of HLA-G is not essential for reproduction. Interestingly, there is a gene (*Mamu-AG*) in the rhesus monkey that produces transcriptional variants like those of human HLA-G (Slukvin *et al.* 2000). This points to evolutionary convergence of this process of alternative splicing of placental MHC genes.

Trophoblast HLA-E

This class I antigen is also monomorphic. Unlike HLA-G, the expression of HLA-E is not restricted to trophoblast but is present in a variety of other cell types. An interesting feature of HLA-E is that its cell surface expression requires binding to peptides derived from the leader sequence of other HLA class I molecules within the cell (Lee *et al.* 1998a). Thus, HLA-E could be regarded as a 'sentinel' molecule which reflects the expression of the other class I antigens. Since HLA-G is present only in trophoblast, the HLA-E expressed on the surface of trophoblast in conjunction with the leader sequence peptide from HLA-G will be unique to this cell type. In this way, HLA-G could influence maternal immune response indirectly through presentation by HLA-E. This would still occur even if the fetus is homozygous for the HLA-G1 null allele because the leader peptide will continue to be translated.

The receptor for HLA-E has been identified. It belongs to the C-type lectin superfamily and is a heterodimer made up of two subunits CD94/NKG2 (Lee *et al.* 1998b). The CD94 subunit is invariant while there are multiple variants of NKG2. The vast majority of decidual NK cells (93%–97%) are found to express CD94/NKG2A (King *et al.* 2000a). Using HLA-E tetrameric complexes unfolded with the leader sequence of HLA-G (to reflect the dominant sources of HLA-E-binding peptide in trophoblast), we have demonstrated that 89%–96% (mean 93%) of decidual NK cells bound these complexes (King *et al.* 2000a). This pattern differs markedly from that observed in the peripheral blood of non-pregnant women where a smaller proportion of CD56$^+$ CD3$^-$ NK cells (35%–77%) are found to bind the HLA-E tetramers. Furthermore, the intensity of HLA-E tetramer staining on decidual NK cells is considerably higher than that of peripheral blood NK cells. Thus, virtually all decidual NK cells are able to bind HLA-E as a result of very high expression of CD94/NKG2A receptors. Such uniform high expression of HLA-E specific receptors implies that HLA-E recognition is functionally important.

What this function is remains unclear. The NKG2A receptor contains an immunoreceptor tyrosine-based inhibition motif (ITIM) in its cytoplasmic domain so that binding of HLA-E to this receptor would be expected to induce an inhibitory signal. This is confirmed by cytotoxicity experiments using HLA-E transfectants as targets and blocking with anti-CD94 Mab, which show that, for decidual NK cells, the overall effect of HLA-E recognition is indeed inhibition of killing (King *et al.* 2000a). Thus, HLA-E expression might protect trophoblast cells from lysis by maternal NK cells. However, as already described previously for HLA-G, decidual NK cells are unable to kill isolated trophoblast cells even when CD94/NKG2A receptors or MHC class I molecules are masked by appropriate Mabs. Trophoblast cells appear to escape decidual NK cell lysis even without HLA-NK receptor interaction, implying that other inhibitory pathways exist in vivo. Alternatively, trophoblast may lack appropriate surface molecules necessary for initiation of killing.

Signals from HLA-E through CD94/NKG2 may lead to other effects beside inhibition of killing, such as regulation of cytokine production. Decidual NK cells also express the activating receptor CD94/NKG2C as detected by reverse transcriptase (RT)-PCR although the proportion of NK cells that bear this receptor is not known (Koopman *et al.* 2003). This could be of importance as it has been shown that HLA-E bound to the HLA-G leader peptide has a particularly high affinity for CD94/NKG2C.

At present, therefore, it is still unclear what is the outcome of maternal recognition of either trophoblast HLA-E or HLA-G. The role of these two HLA class I molecules in pregnancy awaits clarification.

Trophoblast HLA-C

Human leukocyte antigen-C has been demonstrated on the surface of EVT both as free heavy chains or in the conventional form complexed with β2m (King *et al.* 1996, 2000b). Both paternal and maternal alleles are expressed so HLA-C is not subjected to imprinting. Unlike HLA-E or HLA-G, HLA-C is polymorphic although the number of alleles is fewer than in the other classical class I molecules HLA-A and HLA-B. Thus, HLA-C is potentially able to transmit paternal allogeneic signals to the mother.

The HLA-C locus products are dominant ligands for the KIR family of receptors. However, recognition is not directed at individual HLA-C alleles but distinguishes between two groups of HLA-C (group 1 and group 2) based on dimorphism in amino acid residue at position 80 of the molecule. These two groups interact with different KIRs. There is great diversity of KIR haplotypes with variations in the number of genes as well as polymorphism at individual loci (Vilches & Parham 2002).

The KIRs specific for HLA-C are expressed by a greater proportion of decidual NK cells than in peripheral blood NK cells in pregnant women (Hiby *et al.* 1997) indicating that the NK cell receptor repertoire is skewed towards recognition of HLA-C in the uterus. This is rather surprising since KIR expression by peripheral NK cells has been shown to be remarkably stable in individuals. Furthermore, the CD56[bright] NK cell subset in blood, which most resembles those in decidua, lacks expression of KIRs. If blood CD56[bright] NK cells are the source of similar cells in decidua (as is thought to be the case by some investigators), then this observation indicates that KIR expression is induced in utero.

All women express KIRs for both groups of HLA-C alleles (Hiby *et al.* 1997). Since HLA-C is polymorphic, recognition of paternal non-self trophoblast HLA-C by maternal decidual NK cell KIRs should occur during pregnancy. Furthermore, each pregnancy will involve different combinations of paternal HLA-C and maternal KIR. Each pregnancy will therefore be different. Some combinations may be less optimal for implantation and these pregnancies will be less successful. This might explain the underlying pathogenesis of important diseases of pregnancy, such as pre-eclampsia.

To date, direct experimental evidence for a role of trophoblast HLA-C in pregnancy is lacking. While KIR soluble fusion proteins have been observed to bind to group 1 and group 2 HLA-C transfectants, no binding is seen with trophoblast cells

(King *et al.* 2000b). One possible explanation is that, unlike transfectants, the HLA-C expressed by trophoblast is in a form not recognisable by these KIRs. The KIR fusion proteins used in the above experiments are representative of the inhibitory forms of KIR (KIR2DL3 and KIR2DL1). It may be that trophoblast HLA-C is recognised only by activating forms of KIR (KIR2DS2 or KIR2DS3). These activating forms are also expressed by decidual NK cells. This possibility is supported by cytotoxicity assays using HLA-C transfectants and decidual NK cell effectors. Preincubation of NK cells with appropriate Mabs directed against the inhibitory KIRs (KIR2DL3 or KIR2DL1) have no effects on the levels of killing (King *et al.* 2000b).

The function of HLA-C in pregnancy, therefore, remains unestablished. Indeed, in a recent study on the association of HLA-C and pre-eclampsia, the interaction between trophoblast HLA-C and the mother appears to be more complex than previously envisaged (see Moffett, Chapter 11, this book).

Expression of endogenous retroviral products by trophoblast

The 'self/infectious non-self' model of Janeway proposes that the vertebrate host recognises microbes by their conserved molecular patterns (PAMPs). At first sight, this model might not seem to be relevant to pregnancy as trophoblast is clearly not microbial. However, there is the interesting finding that trophoblast cells express endogenous retroviral products (Harris 1998), so in some respects, trophoblast might be considered to be an 'infected' cell and could be discerned by PRR such as TLR3, which binds to double-stranded RNA (Akira & Hemmi 2003).

Endogenous retrovirus (ERVs) sequences with retroviral characteristics are normal components of the DNA of all vertebrate cells. They are thought to be remnants of ancient germ cell infections by now-extinct exogenous retroviruses. Phylogenetic analyses indicate that integrations occurred early in primate evolution. The largest wave of insertion of the various human endogenous retrovirus (HERV) families occurred approximately 30 million years ago after separation of the old and New World monkeys (Sverdlov 2000). The RNA expression of various HERV families has been studied in an extensive range of cell types and it is apparent that the placenta is unique amongst normal tissues in both the diverse range of HERV transcripts and their high level of expression. Indeed, some are expressed exclusively by the placenta, such as HERV-W.

The significance and consequence of the presence of HERVs in our genome has been the subject of intense speculation. Since the placenta is the major site of HERV expression, their potential function in reproduction has received much attention. In the context of 'self/infectious non-self' model, HERVs could act like PAMPs and exert effects on uterine dendritic cells (DCs) and macrophages via PRR.

For example, TLR3 detects viral double-stranded RNA and TLR4, which normally responds to bacterial lipopolysaccharide, can be directly activated by the envelope (EnV) protein of murine leukaemia virus (MuLV) and mouse mammary tumour virus (MMTV). To date, however, it has not yet been demonstrated that trophoblast HERV proteins can act in this way, nor have TLRs been demonstrated on decidual immune cells.

Other functions have also been proposed. The conserved immunosuppressive region of the EnV protein shared by several HERVs has a broad range of immunological effects that are pertinent to the decidua, such as suppression of NK cell cytolysis. This could contribute to the acceptance of the allogeneic invading EVT. Can HERV protein provide a peptide for trophoblast MHC class I? Although elution studies of trophoblast HLA-G have resulted in a variety of peptides with nonameric motif, none so far appear to be HERV-derived. Interestingly, the most abundant peptide presented by trophoblast HLA-G (Lee *et al.* 1995) is the Epstein–Barr virus induced gene 3 (EBI3), which is a soluble haemapoietin receptor related to the p40 subunit of interleukin (IL)12 (Devergne *et al.* 2001). The EBI3 can form heterodimers with members of the IL12 family so this trophoblast-derived cytokine might direct the nature of the maternal immune response by acting on decidual immune cells.

The most positive finding so far is for the EnV protein of HERV-W, also known as syncytin. Its name is derived from the observation that this protein has fusogenic properties and causes cell fusion to form a syncytium in vitro (Blond *et al.* 2000, Mi 2000, Frendo *et al.* 2003). Whether syncytin exerts a similar effect on trophoblast to direct terminal differentiation into syncytiotrophoblast or placental bed giant cells is now under investigation.

In addition to the potential functional importance of HERV proteins, the powerful transcriptional regulatory properties of their long terminal repeat (LTRs) should not be overlooked. For example, an HERV-E insertion in the 5′ untranslated region of the growth factor pleiotropin (PTN) created a trophoblast-specific promoter and the expression of HERV-E PTN, which has been linked with the invasive phenotype of trophoblast (Schulte *et al.* 2000). The placenta-specific expression of the insulin-like growth factor INSL4 also appears to be driven by an HERV insertion (Bieche *et al.* 2003). Thus, it is possible that some of the unique gene expression of the placenta could be retrovirally controlled, such as the abundance of proto-oncogene products, the expression of IgG-Fc and even the unusual array of MHC class I antigens.

Some proponents of the importance of HERVs argue that they have been instrumental in the evolution of the placental form of reproduction and the development of viviparity (Harris 1998). Others, however, believe that the abundance of HERVs in the placenta simply reflects the selection advantage to the virus of expression in an immune-privileged site during the period most expedient for transmission to the next generation (Fox 1999). The inter-species difference in ERV families and placental structures could be due to niche functions for different proviruses which conferred evolutionary benefits on different species at various times. The diversity of placental structures may then reflect the use of different EnV products in different mammals (Stoye & Coffin 2000). So the story of HERVs and the placenta is just beginning with the exciting possibility of other products and functions awaiting discovery (Muir *et al.* 2004).

The implantation site – is it 'dangerous'?

Matzinger has considered the problem of the fetal allograft in terms of the 'danger' model and suggested that the difference in outcome is because the surgical trauma and hypoxia of the iatrogenic transplant situation result in tissue damage and necrosis whereas with pregnancy, being a natural phenomenon with intermingling of normal healthy cells, no alarm signals are sent. At the cellular level, the placental bed cannot be considered to be a harmonious site. Indeed, it has been described as a 'battle-ground' (Robertson 1987). There is necrosis at the uterine surface where the anchoring villi attach (Nitabuch's layer) as well as the 'fibrinoid' necrosis of the spiral arterial media (Kaufmann & Burton 1994). The trophoblast cells around these arteries have a spidery appearance when stained for cytokeratin, suggesting cell damage (Loke & King 1995). Thus, both trophoblast and maternal cells show signs of damage although it is remarkable how the invasion through the decidua basalis between the spiral arteries is accompanied by relatively little necrosis compared with that seen in tumour invasion. It is only at specific anatomical sites in the placental bed that necrosis is seen. The implantation site, therefore, is not 'danger' free and from the viewpoint of the 'danger' model, leukocytes should be alerted.

Conclusion

The immunology of implantation is unique and cannot readily be fitted into any of the prevailing models of immune recognition. It is, therefore, unwise to design experiments exploring the nature of the immunological paradox of pregnancy based on any of the existing paradigms. It is particularly important to move away from the view that trophoblast is like a conventional allograft that must resist or evade rejection. Instead, one should consider the maternal immune response to provide a balanced environment which encourages trophoblast invasion but, at the same time, curbs excessive and unsocial behaviour which could endanger the mother. In this way, a state of peaceful coexistence between two allogeneic tissues is achieved (Moffett & Loke 2004).

REFERENCES

Akira, S. & Hemmi, H. (2003). Recognition of pathogen-associated molecular patterns by TLR family. *Immunol. Lett.*, **85**, 85–95.

Bieche, I., Laurent, A., Laurendeau, I. *et al.* (2003). Placenta-specific INSL4 expression is mediated by a human endogenous retrovirus element. *Biol. Reprod.*, **68**, 1422–9.

Billingham, R. E., Brent, L. & Medawar, P. B. (1953). 'Actively acquired tolerance' of foreign cells. *Nature*, **172**, 603–6.

Blond, J. L., Lavillette, D., Cheynet, V. *et al.* (2000). An envelope glycoprotein of the human endogenous retrovirus HERV-W is expressed in the human placenta and fuses cells expressing the type D mammalian retrovirus receptor. *J. Virol.*, **74**, 3321–9.

Burnet, F. M. (1959). *The Clonal Selection Theory of Acquired Immunity*. Nashville, Tennessee: Vanderbilt University Press.

Crisa, L., McMaster, M. T., Ishii, J. K., Fisher, S. J. & Salomon, D. R. (1997). Identification of a thymic epithelial cell subset sharing expression of the class Ib HLA-G molecule with fetal trophoblasts. *J. Exp. Med.*, **186**, 289–98.

Crocker, P. R. & Varki, A. (2001). Siglecs, sialic acids and innate immunity. *Trends Immunol.*, **22**, 337–42.

Davies, B., Hiby, S. E., Gardner, L., Loke, Y. W. & King, A. (2001). HLA-G expression by tumors. *Am. J. Reprod. Immunol.*, **45**, 103–7.

Devergne, O., Coulomb-L'Hermine, A., Capel, F., Moussa, M. & Capron, F. (2001). Expression of Epstein-Barr virus-induced gene 3, an interleukin-12 p40-related molecule, throughout human pregnancy. *Am. J. Pathol.* **159**, 1763–76.

Fox, D. (1999). Why we don't lay eggs. *New Scientist*, **162**, 27–31.

Frendo, J. L., Olivier, D., Cheynet, V. *et al.* (2003). Direct involvement of HERV-W Env glycoprotein in human trophoblast cell fusion and differentiation. *Mol. Cell. Biol.*, **23**, 3566–74.

Frumento, G., Franchello, S., Palmisano, G. L. *et al.* (2000). Melanoma and melanoma cell lines do not express HLA-G, and the expression cannot be induced by gamma-IFN treatment. *Tissue Antigens*, **56**, 30–7.

Guidotti, L. G. & Chisari, F. V. (2001). Noncytolytic control of viral infections by the innate and adaptive immune response. *Annu. Rev. Immunol.*, **19**, 65–91.

Harris, J. R. (1998). Placental endogenous retrovirus ERV: structural, functional and evolutionary significance. *BioEssays*, **20**, 307–16.

Hiby, S. E., King, A., Sharkey, A. M. & Loke, Y. W. (1997). Human uterine NK cells have a similar repertoire of Killer Inhibitory and Activatory receptors to those found in blood, as demonstrated by RT-PCR and sequencing. *Mol. Immunol.*, **34**, 419–30.

(1999). Molecular studies of trophoblast HLA-G: polymorphism, isoforms, imprinting and expression in pre-implantation embryo. *Tissue Antigens*, **53**, 1–13.

Karre, K., Ljunggren, H. G., Piontek, G. & Kiessling, R. (1986). Selective rejection of H-2-deficient lymphoma variants suggests alternative immune defence strategy. *Nature*, **319**, 675–8.

Kaufmann, P. & Burton, G. (1994). Anatomy and genesis of the placenta. In E. Knobil & J. D. Neill, eds., *Physiology of Reproduction*, 2nd edn. New York: Raven Press, pp. 441–83.

King, A. & Loke, Y. W. (1991). On the nature and function of human uterine granular lymphocytes. *Immunol. Today*, **12**, 432–5.

King, A., Boocock, C., Sharkey, A., Gardner, L. & Loke, Y. W. (1996). Evidence for the expression of HLA-C class I mRNA and protein by human first trimester trophoblast. *J. Immunol.*, **156**, 2068–76.

King, A., Allan, D. S. J., Joseph, S. *et al.* (2000a). HLA-E is expressed on trophoblast and interacts with CD94/NKG2 receptors on decidual NK cells. *Eur. J. Immunol.*, **30**, 1623–31.

King, A., Burrows, T. D., Hiby, S. E. *et al.* (2000b). Surface expression of HLA-C antigen by human extravillous trophoblast. *Placenta*, **21**, 376–87.

Koopman, L. A., Kopcow, H. D., Rybalov, B. *et al.* (2003). Human decidual natural killer cells are a unique NK cell subset with immunomodulatory potential. *J. Exp. Med.*, **198**, 1201–12.

Lee, N., Malacko, A. R., Ishitani, A. *et al.* (1995). The membrane-bound and soluble forms of HLA-G bind identical sets of endogenous peptides but differ with respect to TAP association. *Immunity*, **3**, 591–600.

Lee, N., Goodlett, D. R., Ishitani, A., Marquardt, H. & Geraghty, D. E. (1998a). HLA-E surface expression depends on binding of TAP-dependent peptides derived from certain HLA class I signal sequences. *J. Immunol.*, **160**, 4951–60.

Lee, N., Llano, M., Carretero, M. *et al.* (1998b). HLA-E is a major ligand for the natural killer inhibitory receptor CD94/NKG2A. *Proc. Natl. Acad. Sci. U.S.A.*, **95**, 199–204.

Loke, Y. W. & King, A. (1995). *Human Implantation: Cell Biology and Immunology*. Cambridge: Cambridge University Press.

(2000). Decidual NK cell interaction with trophoblast: cytolysis or cytokine production? *Biochem. Soc. Trans.*, **28**, 196–8.

(2001). HLA class I molecules in implantation. In *Fetal and Maternal Medicine Review 12*. Cambridge: Cambridge University Press, pp. 299–314.

Loke, Y. W., King, A. & Burrows, T. *et al.* (1997). Evaluation of trophoblast HLA-G antigen with a specific monoclonal antibody. *Tissue Antigens*, **50**, 135–46.

Loke, Y. W., Hiby, S. & King, A. (1999). Human leukocyte antigen-G and reproduction. *J. Reprod. Immunol.*, **43**, 235–42.

Mallet, V., Blaschitz, A., Crisa, L. *et al.* (1999). HLA-G in the human thymus: a subpopulation of medullary epithelial but not CD83+ dendritic cells express HLA-G membrane-bound and soluble protein. *Int. Immunol.*, **11**, 889–98.

Matzinger, P. (1994). Tolerance, danger and the extended family. *Annu. Rev. Immunol.*, **12**, 991–1045.

Medawar, P. B. (1953). Some immunological and endocrinological problems raised by the evolution of viviparity in vertebrates. In *Society for Experimental Biology*. New York: Academic Press, pp. 320–38.

Medzhitov, R. & Janeway, C. A. (2002). Decoding the patterns of self and nonself by the innate immune system. *Science*, **296**, 298–300.

Mi, S., Lee, X., Li, X. *et al.* (2000). Syncytin is a captive retroviral envelope protein involved in human placental morphogenesis. *Nature*, **403**, 715–17.

Moffett, A. & Loke, Y. W. (2004). The immunological paradox of pregnancy: a reappraisal. *Placenta*, **25**, 1–8.

Moffett-King, A. (2002). Natural killer cells and pregnancy. *Nat. Rev. Immunol.*, **2**, 656–63.

Muir, A., Lever, A.M.L. & Moffett, A. (2004). Expression and functions of human endogenous retroviruses in the placenta: an update. *Placenta*, **25** (Suppl. A), S16–25.

Ober, C., Aldrich, C., Rosinsky, B. *et al.* (1998). HLA-G1 protein expression is not essential for fetal survival. *Placenta*, **19**, 127–32.

Oldenburg, P.-A., Zhelezynak, A., Fang, Y.-F. *et al.* (2000). Role of CD47 as a marker of self on red blood cells. *Science*, **288**, 2051–4.

Robertson, W.B. (1987). Pathology of the pregnant uterus. In H. Fox, ed., *Obstetrical and Gynaecological Pathology*. London: Churchill Livingstone, pp. 1149–76.

Schulte, A.M., Malerczyk, C., Cabal-Manzano, R. *et al.* (2000). Influence of the human endogenous retrovirus-like element HERV-E.PTN on the expression of growth factor pleiotrophin: a critical role of retroviral Sp1-binding site. *Oncogene*, **19**, 3988–98.

Slukvin, I.I., Lunn, D.P., Watkins, D.I. & Golos, T.G. (2000). Placental expression of the non-classical MHC class I molecule Mamu-AG at implantation in the rhesus monkey. *Proc. Natl. Acad. Sci. U.S.A.*, **97**, 9104–9.

Stoye, J.P. & Coffin, J.M. (2000). A provirus put to work. *Nature*, **403**, 715–17.

Sverdlov, E.D. (2000). Retroviruses and primate evolution. *BioEssays*, **22**, 161–71.

Vilches, C. & Parham, P. (2002). KIR: diverse, rapidly evolving receptors of innate and adaptive immunity. *Annu. Rev. Immunol.*, **20**, 217–51.

DISCUSSION

McLaren Perhaps we could concentrate on the uterine environment, which I think is where your balance is happening. As I understand it, if trophoblast, at least in the mouse, is engrafted anywhere else in the mouse, it provokes a normal T cell-mediated response, presumably against these class I HLA-C, -E and -G. Trophoblast can be immunogenic elsewhere, but in the uterus it isn't.

Trowsdale There is another paradigm that is probably worth considering. There's a recent paper from Alex Betz suggesting that in the mouse suppressor T cells play a role in pregnancy (Aluvihare *et al.* 2004).

McLaren That isn't totally new, is it? I remember suppressor T cells from some way back.

Trowsdale But they weren't respectable for a long time. Now they are fashionable.

Loke I'm glad you raised this question. Since implantation involves the close mixing of cells, the extent of this mixing is very important. This means we have to consider different types of placentation, because the strategies employed by different species will be very different. This is the case in the mouse. Mouse trophoblast is said to express paternally inherited H2 antigens, like a graft. This is not like human trophoblast, which has an unusual combination. If mouse trophoblast is like a graft, then I suppose that all species will require different strategies, such as suppressor cells, that humans do not need.

Cross   In the mouse, soon after implantation many immune and inflammatory cells come close to the implantation site, and they then normally vacate the region. All the NK cells are then stuffed in a little pocket of the uterus called the metrial triangle, several millimetres away from the nascent trophoblast giant cells. They are kept separate from each other. You can't capture a single histological section with those two cell types present together.

Loke   Are mouse giant cells class I negative or positive?

Cross   I don't know.

Moffett   This touches on a question I raised earlier. The trophoblast stem cells, both in human and mouse, are going to be incredibly valuable for answering this important question: does mouse trophoblast have H2? It seems surprising that we haven't yet established this. In all of these mouse experiments we have to ask the question about what the T cells are seeing.

Lever   Just to add to what John Trowsdale said about suppressor cells, in chronic hepatitis B infection there is good evidence that it is the presence of T suppressor or regulatory cells in the liver that inhibits the clearance of the virus. So they aren't active just in mouse.

Redman   John Trowsdale described a model involving T regulatory cells. There is an earlier model from Andy Mellor where he showed that indoleamine 2,3-dioxygenase, which is produced by trophoblast, could be immunosuppressive (Munn *et al.* 1998). He was able to induce H2-specific abortion by inhibiting the enzyme. It had no effect on H2-compatible mouse pregnancies, but it led to loss of fetus in the H2 incompatible mice.

S Fisher   He has made the knockout, and it does not phenocopy the chemical inhibitor. There is no problem in pregnancy.

Redman   What a shame.

Loke   We have discussed at length how relevant this sort of work is. Also, in relation to the T helper (Th)2/Th1 shift, in order to generate Th1 or Th2 response, you have to have some kind of antigenic stimulation to bring all this about. We have always asked, what is the antigenic source for maternal sensitisation since human trophoblast does not express the normal array of MHC antigens?

Redman   That's true. Certainly, the Th1/Th2 balance is antigen specific. But most people are now talking about type 1 and type 2 immune responses, which don't necessarily involve the T cells, but describe the way in which the cytokines are being produced by other immune cells.

Loke   What cells are involved, then?

Redman   The evidence that we have is that the shift involves more particularly the NK cells. They are producing type 1 or type 2 patterns of cytokines, which vary with normal or an abnormal pregnancy.

Moffett   About three years ago I was asked to write a paper on maternal T cells in pregnancy. I thought that because this subject is in such a mess, it would do me good to sit down and try to sort it out. I still haven't written the paper! But I think the reasons it is such a mess are worth clarifying. One is the big mouse–human difference, which we have already discussed. T cells are not activated against the trophoblast or fetus in humans. There must be many ways that they are prevented from being activated. The dendritic cells (DCs) in the decidua are rather unique. The other confusing thing is that people always muddle up the local response to the trophoblast in the uterus, and the systemic response of maternal T cells during pregnancy. Maternal T cell responses to many antigens – autoantigens, infectious antigens, trophoblast antigens – are altered. This is why women with systemic lupus erythematosis (SLE) or rheumatoid arthritis (RA) have different manifestations of clinical disease in pregnancy. But no one has convincingly shown that this deviation of T cell responses actually has any effect on the outcome of pregnancy. It is probably an epiphenomenon to do with all the steroids, hormones and so on that are produced during pregnancy. It isn't fundamentally important.

Braude The confusion that exists between mouse and human is actually having a detrimental effect on a lot of women. People are picking up snippets from the immunological literature, and there are patients going through IVF where they are receiving intravenous immunoglobulin weekly at £1500 a time. They are also receiving steroids as they go through their IVF cycle, along with heparin and aspirin. This is all based on anecdotal reports or very scant data. All the agents are being used for unlicensed applications so we can't turn round and say it is not harmful.

S. Fisher They also sometimes receive leukocyte injections.

Braude These have been stopped in the USA and UK. It was a treatment that was being suggested for recurrent miscarriage. The idea was that circulating anti-paternal cytotoxic (or 'blocking') antibodies were shown to be absent in people who frequently miscarried. Therefore it was proposed that if these women were injected with their partner's cells they would develop these 'blocking' antibodies and be protected from rejecting their fetus. What they failed to do was to measure levels in people who were not miscarrying. Professor Regan and I showed some years ago that normally pregnant women don't have them either (Regan *et al.* 1991). The hypothesis was flawed and many women were treated based on data where the control was missing.

Moffett This discussion has already drifted into the systemic response, which neither Charlie Loke nor I mentioned. If we want to look at the immune response, we have to look in the uterus, because this is where maternal immune cells actually contact trophoblast in vivo. The circulating syncytiotrophoblast that Chris Redman is talking about is class I negative and probably pretty immunologically inert. We have got into a muddle, and we need to be clear what we are talking about.

Loke   The phenotypic differences between the NK cells in the blood and those in the uterus are striking, even within the same woman. Functionally and phenotypically the populations are very different so we can't talk about them in the same way.

S. Fisher   Several years ago we published that trophoblast cells make bucketloads of IL10. By relatively simple observations we were able to show that IL10 is incredibly immunosuppressive. The mouse knockout showed that if you take away IL10 you get inflammatory bowel disease and other autoimmune conditions. You mentioned the relative anergy of NK cells. When NK cells are exposed to this very specific cytokine milieu in the uterus, it makes them quite unready to react against the trophoblast cells.

Moffett   You are making the assumption that they are there to react against the trophoblast cells. Why would you get in a whole lot of NK cells and then have to go to great lengths to turn them off again by making IL10 or class I? They must be there for some positive reason.

S. Fisher   If we look at this the way Anne Croy does, they help placental development. They are partnering the trophoblast, serving a decidua-like function.

Loke   Are you saying that NK cells are stimulated by the presence of trophoblast?

S. Fisher   Yes, the trophoblast brings them in. I think they are cooperating.

Loke   It is interesting to note that there are so many activating receptors on NK cells, rather than inhibitory receptors. Therefore, it is not a question of evasion or resistance. Natural killer cells have a positive role to play. They are not there just to resist trophoblast invasion.

Cross   In the mouse, Anne Croy has shown that in NK cell-deficient mice the spiral arteries don't undergo their modification so they remain constricted with lots of smooth muscle (Croy *et al.* 2000). Vasodilation occurs in a place far away from where there are any trophoblast cells. Is there any evidence that this might be true in humans or other species as well?

Moffett   Yes. The NK cells in humans make three angiogenic growth factors: Ang2, placental growth factor and vascular endothelial growth factor (VEGF). We think that in the non-pregnant uterus they have an important effect on the growth and modification of placental spiral arteries. Before any other morphological signs of menstruation can begin, these NK cells are already dying. The lack of these angiogenic growth factors may be the trigger for menstruation. If we look across species (Marilyn Renfree sent us some specimens from a wallaby), there is no decidua in this species: there is just a layer of epithelium. Intriguingly, the blood flow here is increased by angiogenesis. It is a completely different way of increasing the blood flow to the uterus than in humans. Around the uterine arteries in the marsupial there were little lymphocytes that looked extraordinarily like NK cells. The original role of NK cells is probably to regulate blood flow in the uterus. In humans, as the trophoblast got more and more invasive, these cells have probably taken on the additional role of influencing trophoblast development and behaviour.

Cross   Following the theme of dialogue between NK cells and trophoblast, we also need to consider decidual stroma cells as part of that dialogue. We have done a screen comparing gene expression in decidual stromal cells from a normal implantation site compared to one in which there is a failed conceptus generated in different ways. We found that there are some genes expressed in decidual stromal cells whose up-regulation is dependent on there being normal trophoblast present. At least one of these turns out to be a cytokine that can affect NK cell function. Therefore, there is a three-way cell conversation.

Burton   It could be four way. We have found that the NK cells also produce epidermal growth factor (EGF) when they are sitting underneath the glandular epithelium, so they may be supporting this epithelium.

Loke   It could even be a five-way dialogue. We haven't mentioned macrophages. These cells are likely to have a significant influence on the decidual environment.

Moffett   If we look at the evolution of KIR in primates, there are species-specific differences. Perhaps these correlate with the depth of invasion and bigger brain size. As we move up through the primates, more invasion is needed for a bigger brain, so perhaps this interaction between NK cells and the trophoblast becomes more important. In orang-utans, only half have HLA-C and it is all group 1. Rhesus macaques don't have any HLA-C, and they don't have interstitial invasion. Chimpanzees and gorillas have both group 1 and 2, but they have completely different KIRs to ours. These are species-specific genes. The requirement to have deeper invasion and a longer intrauterine period could be associated with this coevolution.

Trowsdale   It is interesting that HLA-C is a relatively new invention in some primates. The appropriate KIRs that go along with HLA-C are quite specific. It was thought until not long ago that KIRs were only in humans, because mice don't have KIRs. Now it has become much more complicated, like most things in biology. Mice do have a couple of KIRs but they are not expressed on NK cells in the same way. One is on the X chromosome. A range of other mammals have a mixture of KIRs and lectin-like molecules. The key development is that of HLA-C and appropriate KIRs in primates, including humans.

Braude   Ashley Moffett, you talked of NK cells as possibly regulating depth of invasion. Someone mentioned yesterday about these strange placentas that go straight through the myometrium. You will be aware that patients who have had a Caesarian section have a much higher preponderance of having morbidly adherent placentas – so-called placenta accretas. Is there a difference at those sites in terms of why they actually do this? Do they have a different type of invasion?

Moffett   In all the situations you described the decidua is absent or deficient. The two unique things about the decidua are the stromal cells and the NK cells. The functions of decidua are likely to be dependent on these two cell types.

Keverne   The KIR cells have activating and inhibitory pathways. Are they distinct signalling pathways, and can they both be switched on in the same cell?

Trowsdale   They can be switched on in the same cell. There appears to be a balance between activating KIRs and inhibitory KIRs on the same cell.

Keverne   So HLA-E and HLA-G could be triggering the KIR in order to do the positive thing that you were talking about in terms of releasing growth factors.

Trowsdale   Relevant to this is the notion of the NK cell not just being a killer cell. It doesn't necessarily kill, and it could well be just producing the appropriate growth factors and cytokines.

Keverne   Can you culture them from a stem cell population?

Trowsdale   With appropriate cytokines you can get T cells to be NK-like. There may be subsets of NK cells, with a regulatory role for example, in addition to the CD56^{brights} and CD56^{dims}. It will probably become more complex, but the crucial thing is that they are not necessarily just killing targets in a class I regulated way.

Keverne   These cells in the placenta may therefore be the regulatory ones rather than the killers.

Trowsdale   Possibly.

Starkey   What is the nature of the positive response? People wave their arms and call out cytokines, but does anyone have any favourite molecules that they think they make in response to seeing trophoblast MHC?

S. Fisher   When you talk about the fact that these NK cells make VEGF, trophoblast cells have all three VEGF receptors. There would be a good collaboration there. That is just one set of molecules.

REFERENCES

Aluvihare, V.R., Kallikourdis, M. & Betz, A.G. (2004). Regulatory T cells mediate maternal tolerance to the foetus. *Nat. Immun.*, **5**, 266–71.

Croy, B.A., Ashkar, A.A., Minhas, K. & Greenwood, J.D. (2000). Can murine uterine natural killer cells give insights into the pathogenesis of preeclampsia? *J. Soc. Gynecol. Invest.*, **7**, 12–20.

Munn, D.H., Zhou, M., Attwood, J.T. *et al.* (1998). Prevention of allogeneic fetal rejection by tryptophan catabolism. *Science*, **281**, 1191–3.

Regan, L., Braude, P.R. & Hill, D.P. (1991). A prospective study of the incidence, time of appearance and significance of anti-paternal lymphocytotoxic antibodies in human pregnancy. *Hum. Reprod.*, **6**, 294–8.

Final general discussion

McLaren	We've said very little so far about transport across the placenta, and whether trophoblast is involved in transport. Earlier there was mention of one hormone that got into the fetus and another that didn't. Does the placenta select in this way, and if so how?
Sibley	The evidence for selective transfer isn't really there. A lot of hormones do get into both sides, and directionality of transport is not clear. Many of the data are based on looking at circulating concentrations. It depends on where and when you are sampling. The best model for looking at this is in the perfused human placenta, where both sides are perfused. If you use this model then there does tend to be a preponderance of the hormone coming out on the maternal side. There will still be some on the fetal side, though. Whether this is really selective, or whether it is because on the fetal side you have it coming out of the trophoblast and having to cross the basement membrane and then the matrix, I don't know. You can certainly see it coming out of both sides in this in vitro preparation.
McLaren	S. K. Dey, this links up with something that you were interested in, which was the transport outwards of waste products.
Dey	That would suggest that there is a selective transport system, getting the waste products out from the fetal side to the maternal side.
Sibley	This doesn't need to be selective. For driving any sort of solutes across the placenta, the most important factor is concentration and electrical gradients. You are making more waste products, whatever they are, in the fetus, so there will tend to be a higher concentration gradient into the mother. Part of this discussion is how we characterise a selective process: for me this is where a transporter protein with high affinity for a particular solute is involved, with some sort of directionality. You can get fluxes in different directions merely through driving forces, not selectivity.

Biology and Pathology of Trophoblast, eds. Ashley Moffett, Charlie Loke and Anne McLaren.
Published by Cambridge University Press © Cambridge University Press 2005.

Dey   What about the ABC transporters, which transport drugs one way?

Sibley   Of the ABC transporters the one that is best characterised in the human placenta is P glycoprotein (PgP). This is exquisitely localised to the microvillous plasma membrane. A xenobiotic in the maternal circulation would tend to hit the maternal side of the placenta. It might get into the plasma membrane towards the syncytiotrophoblast, but PgP is localised to pump it straight back out again.

Loke   Surely the classic example of selective protein transport must be that of immunoglobulins. Of the five classes, only IgG gets across.

Sibley   I agree. This hasn't received as much attention as it has deserved.

Trowsdale The neonatal Fc receptor only transports subclasses of IgG. It also has another function in turnover of steady-state levels of IgG. It is not restricted solely to transport into the fetus.

Loke   This has great clinical implications. This is the reason why we get Rhesus erythroblastosis, because Rhesus antibodies are IgG. ABO erythroblastosis is less common because natural ABO antibodies are IgM and cannot cross the placenta.

Evain-Brion In human placental perfusion systems, most of the specific pregnancy hormones are secreted into the maternal compartment. If you find something in the fetal compartment it is just because the hormone is very highly secreted. This is the case for human chorionic gonadotrophin (HCG) and human placental lactogen (HPL). But there are no placental growth hormones in the fetal circulation. In the perfusion system, leptin is essentially secreted into the maternal circulation and there is very little secretion in the fetal circulation. What is circulating in the fetal circulation is coming essentially from fetal adipocytes.

Sibley   Is there a specific pathway that puts the leptin out through the maternal side, or is it because the leptin or whatever is being lost in the matrix within the villous chorionic villi?

Fowden   There is some evidence in the human that the umbilical vein has a higher leptin concentration than the umbilical artery. This suggests that there is a small output into the fetal circulation from the placenta.

Sibley   We agree that there will be more in the maternal circulation, but I am not sure that this describes a selective mechanism or a dilutional effect within the compartments of the placenta.

Loke   A trivial explanation could be anatomical. If substances are produced by the syncytiotrophoblast lining the intervillous space, then I would have thought that it is easier for these products to get into the maternal circulation rather than backwards into the fetus.

McLaren   Ashley Moffett, you mentioned that there were data that it would be good to have from trophoblast stem (TS) cells. Trophoblast stem cells in the mouse are available in two labs represented in this room. I don't know whether we have human TS cells yet, but we probably will. What were you actually thinking of?

Moffett   From the immunologists' point of view, the question that needs addressing is the H2 expression. This is difficult to do in mouse placenta. You could differentiate these along the lineages and look at H2 expression.

Kunath   I'm not sure that getting human TS cells will be possible.

McLaren   At least one could get the original trophoblastic cells, because the human embryonic stem (ES) cells differentiate into trophoblast. One could look at HLA types there.

McLaren   Colin Sibley, earlier you wanted to raise the question of fetal growth retardation and to what extent this could be dissociated from placental insufficiency.

Sibley   Yes. This was provoked by our discussion on blood flow. I'd like to broaden this to cover not just growth retardation but also the villous trophoblast. Blood flow is defective and undoubtedly contributes to growth restriction. This is most likely due to failure of extravillous trophoblast invasion. In addition, this can't explain all the features seen in growth restriction. For example, amino acid concentrations are low in the growth-restricted fetus and their transfer is not blood-flow limited. They are limited by transporter protein processes. We have shown with others that there are transporter protein defects in the villous trophoblast. This is one line of thought. I'm reminded of data showing that there is a strong association between pregnancy-associated plasma protein A (PAPP-A) in the first trimester and a range of pregnancy complications seen later on at term. Pregnancy-associated plasma protein A is a villous trophoblast marker, so there is that strong correlation. At the same time it was interesting to hear Chris' long-standing theory with regard to deportation of villous trophoblast particles. The flip side of the villous trophoblast damage is that there also appears to be a repair mechanism. Graham and I have alluded over the past few days to what happens if we grow villous trophoblast in explant cultures, which is that the outer layer of syncytiotrophoblast is shed, probably by apoptosis, but then within 4 days the cytotrophoblasts underneath are reactivated and form a new syncytiotrophoblast layer, which is there by about day 6 or 7. This suggests that there is a whole damage repair mechanism going on which we don't understand. Relating this to the in vivo situation in any normal pregnancy you can see areas of the placenta that are denuded, where there are bits of the placenta that don't have any syncytiotrophoblast on them. This brings us back to the immunologists. There is a lot of maternal plasma that is exposed to basement membrane of the placenta. There is a lot going on with the villous trophoblast which might all be connected. Transporter defects might be associated with failure of repair and damage, for example. This is what is seen in pre-eclampsia, and whether you get pre-eclampsia or growth restriction might be to do with exactly what sorts of damage you are seeing to the villous trophoblast as well as all the blood-flow issues.

McLaren   I found Chris' microparticles on the monocytes quite intriguing. They were most common in the third trimester, but they were also there in the second trimester in large amounts. I wondered whether one could FACS sort them and use the DNA as a non-invasive method of prenatal diagnosis.

Redman   They don't contain DNA. They are anuclear fragments. They are derived from the villous membrane. The DNA, if it has gone anywhere, is present in the plasma as soluble DNA. Some investigators are even investigating if measuring soluble DNA of fetal origin could be a predictive test for pre-eclampsia. The trouble is, you have to find a gene that is unique to the fetus, and unless the fetus is male it doesn't work. But Colin has raised a very important question that hasn't been addressed in this meeting: the whole process of how new syncytium is formed, and how this happens. Although there are some suggestions of what the mechanisms are, the total cycle of cell–cell fusion and reforming of the surface of the placenta awaits investigation.

Sibley   That was the major reason for me bringing it up. I think it is a fascinating cell biological question: how is the syncytiotrophoblast reformed? We watch it all the time in explants but we never study it.

Cross   In response to that, I think there is ample evidence as to how it occurs at a molecular level, primarily in mice although we do have some information in humans too. A transcription factor called GCM1 is expressed in syncytiotrophoblast precursors. When you force stem cells to express it they stop dividing. If you have two cells next to each other then they are in a position to fuse. We think that GCM is not required in both of the participating cells: it may be expressed in one, which then interacts with a non-GCM-expressing partner. Or that cell can fuse with the intact syncytium. We have actually seen GCM-positive cells fusing with an overlying syncytium. It can occur either way. With respect to GCM regulation, why does it come on in these fused cells? We don't know the initiation of it but one of the little arrows on my diagram came in from the allantoic mesoderm or the placental stromal cells. The maintenance of GCM expression is dependent on contact with these stromal cells. You can initiate it but it is not maintained unless there are stromal cells present. We would love to know the nature of the molecular signal that does this. GCM is a transcription factor and it has been shown that the promoter for syncytin contains GCM binding sites. In vitro it has been shown that GCM binds to the regulatory regions and if you cotransfect cells with a GCM expression vector and a syncytin promoter, you activate the origin.

Moffett   Is syncytin found in mouse?

Cross   No. There are certainly endogenous retroviruses, but to our satisfaction we haven't found a true syncytin homologue. Clearly, syncytiotrophoblast fusion occurs. We focused on the problem of thinking about initiation of the process. We have data that forcing expression of GCM in two cells wouldn't do it. We are trying to determine the molecular features of the partner cell that GCM fuses with and then we'll worry about what the cell adhesion molecules are. There is quite a bit of information that has emerged over the last few years, in both mammalian and *Drosophila* skeletal muscle, of transcription factors and adhesion molecules that mediate fusion in skeletal myogenesis. What we like about this model is that it is suggesting that cell–cell fusion is an asymmetric process. There is a founder cell (in the trophoblast system we would say this is the GCM-expressing cell) and then a fusion-competent cell (which would be the GCM non-expressing cell), which get together. We have cloned mouse homologues of the fly genes, and for all of these we find expression.

Sibley   Should we look for GCM expression in our regeneration human model?

Cross   Yes, that would be good. John Kingdom in Toronto is doing exactly that. He is using hyperoxia to kill the syncytiotrophoblast and then watching it reform.

McLaren   Charlie Loke, you mentioned endogenous retroviral proteins: was it in this context of syncytial cell fusion?

Loke   It has been proposed that syncytin is responsible for the formation of giant cells and syncytiotrophoblast. There are some people who feel that the whole evolution of viviparity is dependent on endogenous retroviral sequences in our genome, otherwise we wouldn't be able to develop the placental form of reproduction.

Lever   Jay Cross has summed up the data on HERV-W, which is the human endogenous retrovirus implicated in cell fusion whose envelope protein has been renamed syncytin. The GCM-related regulation and the fact that hypoxia leads to down-regulation of syncytin in vitro all points to this. In vitro experiments show that expressing syncytin in cells induces fusion. These all fit together indicating that this protein is one of the major proteins involved in the cell–cell interaction that leads to fusion. Human endogenous retrovirus-W is the only endogenous retrovirus that is exclusively expressed in placenta. Lots of the others are expressed in other tissues but not at the same high level. They may have other effects. For example, some of the envelope proteins have been shown to suppress natural killer (NK) cell activity.

Loke   Many years ago we became interested in endogenous retroviruses when we made an antibody towards the syncytiotrophoblast surface. This antibody doesn't react against any other cell type except syncytiotrophoblast. It also doesn't react against any kind of infected cells except one that is infected by an endogenous retrovirus. It seems, therefore, that endogenous retrovirus infection produces a cell surface component that is antigenically similar to that present on a normal syncytiotrophoblast.

S. Fisher I wanted to ask a question directed to people who do re-formation of the syncytium in culture. We certainly see trophoblast cells fuse and form a syncytium, but we never see regeneration of this incredibly complex branched microvillous surface that covers the normal placenta. It is the only place in your body where you have branched microvilli. We have never got this to go in culture. Have others?

Loke A long time ago we used to do these studies. We found that all multinucleated cells produced in vitro are in fact class I positive. We came to the conclusion that when cells fuse into multinucleated cells, they are representative of the extravillous giant cell differentiation pathway, rather then the villous syncytial pathway. They are class I positive, and they are HCG negative.

S. Fisher We have the same data with isolated cells, but I was talking about the explant model.

Sibley We take a term piece of villus and put it in an explant culture in the 'chip pan' model. This is a filter with fluid above and below. After 24 h we see the syncytiotrophoblast coming off. After about 5 days, although this is variable, you can see areas of new syncytiotrophoblast that can't be distinguished from the old one. The sorts of things that we measure, such as the transporter function, work normally. There is a range of morphologies, but at least part is indistinguishable from 'normal' syncytiotrophoblast.

Burton In the first trimester the picture is similar. It is a bit mucky in the explant in that the syncytium forms over degenerating masses. You wouldn't say it was necessarily a complete layer. In the miscarriages we see in vivo where the degenerate syncytium is sloughing off, the new syncytium underneath is virtually identical to the normal.

Sharkey Have you done electron microscopy?

Burton Yes. We can follow it round the villous surface from a degenerating mass to the area we know is new. Sometimes it becomes difficult to distinguish old and new. Occasionally we see the odd desmosome on the surface with a few remnants of syncytiotrophoblast. This tells us that what we are actually looking at is regenerated syncytium rather than the original. I wouldn't be surprised if there is a lot of syncytial turnover during that first trimester period.

McLaren On this speculative note we must regretfully come to the end of our discussion. But before we finish, I would like to say that I've enjoyed this meeting very much. I would like to thank Simon Goldhill and the research centre at King's College Cambridge, who have been very generous in supporting this meeting, and the Novartis Foundation and staff for their support and help during these two days, and I'd also like to thank all of you for your participation.

Index

Page numbers in *italic* refer to figures. Page numbers in **bold** denote entries in tables.

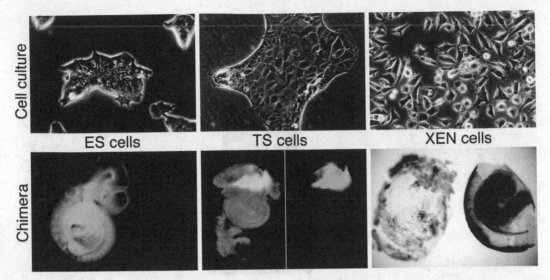

Plate 1 Embryonic stem (ES), TS and XEN cell cultures and chimeras. Representative cultures of three blastocyst-derived cell lines are shown (top panels): ES, TS and XEN cells. The bottom panels show mid-gestation chimeric embryos obtained with labelled cells. The EGFP–ES cell chimera has contributions throughout the embryo proper and the mesoderm of the definitive yolk sac (photo courtesy of Kristina Vintersten). The EGFP–TS cell chimera has contributions to the placenta, but not to the embryo proper. The LacZ–XEN cell chimera has labelled cells in the parietal yolk sac, but not in the visceral yolk sac or embryo proper.

The plates in this section are available for download in colour from
www.cambridge.org/9781107403154

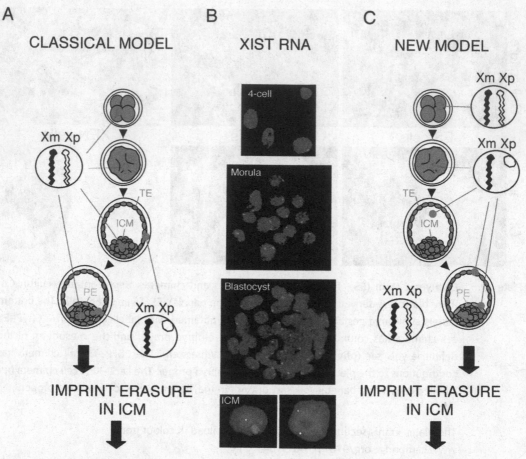

A **CLASSICAL MODEL**

Xm Xp

TE

ICM

PE

Xm Xp

IMPRINT ERASURE IN ICM

RANDOM X INACTIVATION POST-IMPLANTATION

B **XIST RNA**

4-cell

Morula

Blastocyst

ICM

C **NEW MODEL**

Xm Xp

Xm Xp

TE

ICM

Xm Xp

PE

IMPRINT ERASURE IN ICM

RANDOM X INACTIVATION POST-IMPLANTATION

Plate 2   Revision of the classical model for initiation of X inactivation during embryogenesis in the mouse. (A) In the classical model both X chromosomes are active (indicated as elongated chromosomes) up to the morula stage. Inactivation of Xp (indicated as compacted chromosome) was thought to occur coincident with differentiation of TE, and subsequently PE. In pluripotent ICM cells of the blastocyst, imprint erasure resets the programme and allows for random X inactivation to occur post-implantation, coincident with differentiation of epiblast cells. (B) RNA FISH analysis illustrates Xp *Xist* RNA domains (light grey dots) in XX embryos from four-cell through to blastocyst stage. In isolated ICM cells from late blastocysts approximately 50% of cells retain *Xist* domains. Low level *Xist* and *Tsix* expression (indicated by brighter dots representing overlapping red and green pinpoint signals) is seen in other cells. (C) In the revised model Xp inactivation is initiated together with Xp *Xist* expression at the two- to four-cell stage, and is maintained in all cells up until late blastocyst stage. At this time, cells allocated to the pluripotent epiblast lineage reactivate Xp, setting the ground state for subsequent random X inactivation in the embryo proper.

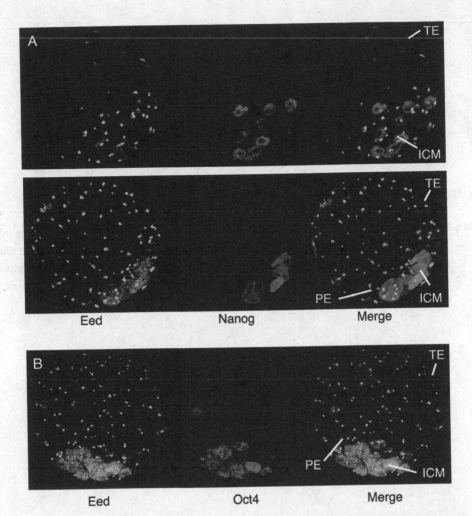

Plate 3   Development of the ICM. (A) Immunofluorescence analysis for the Polycomb-group protein Eed and the homeodomain protein Nanog in mid- (top) and late- (bottom) blastocyst stage XX embryos. Up to mid-blastocyst stage Eed is concentrated on the inactive Xp in both Nanog-positive (presumptive pluripotent epiblast) and Nanog-negative (presumptive PE) cells in the ICM region. The two cell types are arranged in a mosaic pattern within the ICM region. In late-stage blastocysts extinction of *Xist* RNA and delocalisation of Eed from Xi occurs in Nanog-positive cells. In addition the ICM reorganises into the prototypical structure of a single layer of PE overlying the pluripotent epiblast cells. Nanog-positive nuclei have higher overall levels of Eed protein than surrounding cells. (B) Staining of late-stage XX blastocyst for Eed and Oct4 protein. Oct4 is expressed both in pluripotent epiblast cells (high nuclear Eed level) and overlying PE cells (low nuclear Eed level).

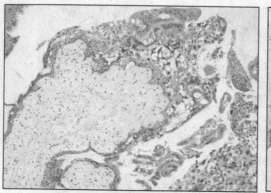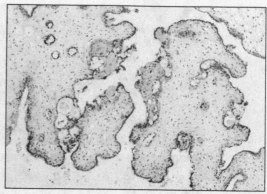

Plate 4   Photomicrographs of CHM (left) and PHM (right), demonstrating the differences in appearance. Complete hydatidiform moles exhibit a prominent 'budding' architecture with, often extensive, abnormal trophoblastic proliferation whilst PHM demonstrate villi with irregular outlines, having numerous pseudoinclusions and mild focal abnormal trophoblast proliferation (H&E, original magnifications ×100).

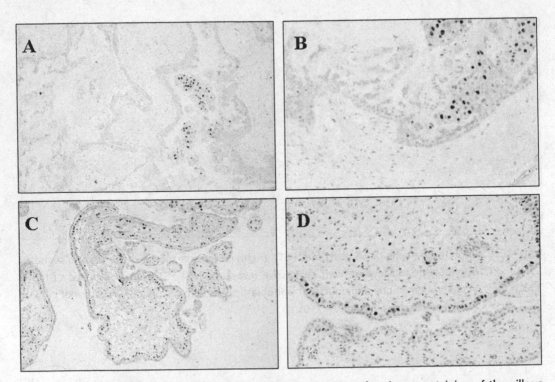

Plate 5   Photomicrographs demonstrating absence of p57 nuclear immunostaining of the villous cytotrophoblast and stroma in CHM (A and B) compared with extensive positive nuclear staining in a case of PHM (C and D). Non-villous trophoblast stains positively, acting as a control, in both cases. Original magnifications ×40 (A and C) and ×250 (B and D).

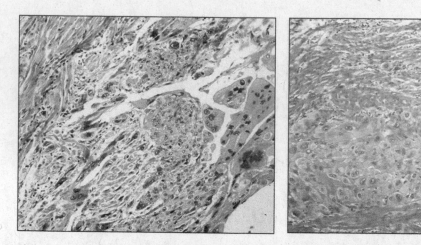

Plate 6   Photomicrographs of CC (left) and PSTT (right). Choriocarcinoma demonstrates biphasic trophoblastic proliferation with destructive invasion whilst PSTTs are composed of more bland predominantly mononuclear trophoblastic cells with an infiltrative pattern of growth (H&E, original magnifications ×250).

Printed in the United States
By Bookmasters